Quality Management
In Clinical Laboratories

Promoting Patient Safety
Through Risk Reduction And
Continuous Improvement

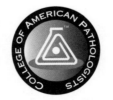

Advancing Excellence

College of American Pathologists
325 Waukegan Road
Northfield, Illinois 60093
800-323-4040

Paul Valenstein, MD
Editor

Caryn L. Tursky
CAP Editor & Designer

Library of Congress Control Number: 2005930424

ISBN: 0-930304-88-8

CAP Sponsoring Committees

Quality Practices Committee

Paul N. Valenstein, MD, Chair
Leonas G. Bekeris, MD
Richard C. Friedberg, MD, PhD
Christopher Mark Lehman, MD
Stephen S. Raab, MD
Stephen Gerard Ruby, MD, MBA
Afshin Salarieh, MD
Ana K Stankovic, MD, PhD
Milenko J. Tanasijevic, MD, MBA
Joseph A. Tworek, MD
Elizabeth A. Wagar, MD
David S. Wilkinson, MD, PhD
Christine Bashleben, MT(ASCP), CAP staff

Patient Safety and Performance Measures Committee

Richard C. Friedberg, MD, PhD, Chair
Lee H. Hilborne, MD
Harvey W. Kaufman, MD
Gregory Novak, MD
Francis Robert Rodwig Jr, MD, MPH
Deborah Ann Sesok-Pizzini, MD, MBA
Ronald L. Sirota, MD
Paul N. Valenstein, MD
Phillip A. Bongiorno, CAP staff

Contributing Authors

Bruce Jones, MD

Henry Ford Health System
Detroit, Michigan

Stephen Raab, MD

University of Pittsburgh Medical Center
Shadyside Hospital
Pittsburgh, Pennsylvania

Deborah Sesok-Pizzini, MD, MBA

University of Pennsylvania
Children's Hospital of Philadelphia
Philadelphia, Pennsylvania

Ron Sirota, MD

Advocate Lutheran General Hospital
Park Ridge, Illinois

Paul Valenstein, MD

St. Joseph Mercy Hospital
Ann Arbor, Michigan

Contents

Preface

To give this manual a uniform style and minimize duplication of content, I wrote the text. Even when others wrote the first draft of a section, I rewrote the draft and integrated it with the rest of the manuscript. I therefore take full responsibility for any statements that are incorrect, passages that are not clear, and for all decisions about presentation and organization of the material.

Very few of the ideas in this manual are my own. Credit for the creative content of this book goes to individuals who published the primary studies and review articles referenced in this manual and to the authors who wrote drafts of several sections. These individuals are acknowledged in the endnotes. Authorities within and outside the College of American Pathologists reviewed sections of the manuscript and corrected many errors I would otherwise have made. Some of these people are listed in the front matter as members of the CAP Quality Practices Committee or CAP Patient Safety and Performance Measures Committee. Some serve on other CAP committees or are part of the bright and knowledgeable staff employed by the College. Although it is not customary for individuals who work within an industry to thank their regulators, the staff of several US federal agencies have also made contributions to the management of laboratory quality. Their work, often done anonymously, has been borrowed freely.

I have made considerable effort to assure the accuracy of statements made in this manual about CAP policy and positions. However, my research into quality management and patient safety reminds me that the potential for error is always with us. Therefore I must remind readers that this manual is ultimately the work of its authors, and the opinions expressed herein may not accurately describe the views of the College of American Pathologists.

Paul Valenstein, MD, FCAP

Introduction

This manual was written for managers of clinical laboratories. The term "manager" includes laboratory directors, who have specific legal responsibilities when directing clinical laboratories in the United States, and pathologists and other supervisors who work under the general direction of a laboratory director or work for an organization that administers a clinical laboratory.

This is a practical "how-to" manual. It is designed to help readers:

❖ manage quality and patient safety in clinical laboratories;

❖ comply with quality and patient safety regulations and accreditation requirements; and

❖ develop and administer a quality management plan.

This manual addresses patient safety as an essential and inseparable component of laboratory quality. Patient safety is threatened wherever laboratory quality is wanting, and effective management of laboratory quality necessarily includes a consideration of patient safety. The patient safety movement has brought to light some of the human factors and cross-discipline issues that cause patient care to go awry and which were not adequately addressed by traditional, narrowly-focused quality control programs. Patient safety issues are discussed throughout this manual.

There are several aspects of laboratory quality that are not covered in this manual. First and foremost, we do not recapitulate each of the hundreds of quality and patient safety regulations issued by the federal government or all of the standards promulgated by major clinical laboratory accrediting organizations such as the College of American Pathologists. These regulations and standards undergo regular revision, and we refer readers to sources where current versions may be obtained. We discuss here only the most important standards and areas that have proven to be particularly problematic for laboratories. Regulations and accreditation standards for jurisdictions outside of the United States are not discussed in detail.

The manual does not deal directly with questions of patient and physician access to laboratory services, such as the number of phlebotomy sites a laboratory should deploy in a community or the appropriate hours of operation or test menu for a hospital-based or physician office laboratory. It can be argued that access to laboratory services represents a component of quality, but the literature relating access to patient outcomes is scant, and we have little intelligent guidance to offer readers in these areas.

We are aware of public interest in quality "report cards," quality awards, and "pay-for-performance" programs for hospitals, individual physicians, physician groups, and health care plans. Recent attention has been focused on creating report cards, awards, and quality incentives for clinical laboratories, although no program for laboratories has been widely adopted. We do not address the topic of quality report cards, awards, or incentives in this manual. Our focus is on management of laboratory services for the benefit of patients and the satisfaction of regulatory and accreditation requirements.

The management of quality in anatomic pathology is addressed in detail by a companion publication, *Quality Management in Anatomic Pathology: Promoting Patient Safety Through Systems Improvement and Error Reduction,* available from the College of American Pathologists.[1] The present publication speaks to general principals of quality management that are applicable to both anatomic and clinical pathology. In fact, the first case study presented in chapter 2 concerns an incident from the anatomic pathology section of a laboratory. Readers primarily interested in anatomic pathology quality management will find more detail in the companion publication.

Finally, we hasten to remind readers that there is more to the art and science of laboratory management than ensuring quality and patient safety. This manual does not concern itself with how to operate a laboratory that is safe for employees or the environment. This manual covers very few human resources or staffing issues. It does not deal with business strategy and tactics, budgeting, specimen logistics, marketing, sales, professional relations, facilities management, supply chain and inventory management, most of the field of clinical informatics, assuring the integrity of laboratory financial reporting, or regulatory compliance related to billing, inducement, and medical necessity. These important management topics impact quality and patient safety indirectly, but are left to other authors and other venues.

Case Studies

Five case studies have been developed to stimulate thinking and discussion about laboratory quality and patient safety. Each study is based on knowledge of an actual case, but the facts have been disguised and any resemblance to actual people or events is unintentional.

Readers are encouraged to identify quality and patient safety issues in each case study, and to think about how a manager should respond to the problems presented in each case, or work to prevent their occurrence in the first place. The remainder of this manual sets out a framework that managers may apply to these issues. But first, we turn our attention to the specifics of five cases.

Patient Misidentification

Case History

The worst day of Dr. Sandy Owens' professional life began on a Wednesday at 1:05 in the afternoon. Earlier in the morning, Dr. Owens had examined slides from a mastectomy specimen removed from Gretchen Gustoffen, a 42-year-old woman with a previous biopsy diagnosis of invasive ductal carcinoma. The initial sections from the mastectomy specimen revealed only mild fibrocystic disease, and Dr. Owens resigned herself to re-examining the gross breast specimen later in the day to find the carcinoma that had evidently been missed when the initial set of tissue blocks was selected for processing. As part of her follow-up, Sandy asked her transcriptionist to pull the slides from the original biopsy on Ms. Gustoffen, which she had interpreted three weeks previously. The slides were on her desk when she returned from lunch.

As Dr. Owens examined the original biopsy slides under the microscope, she could feel the muscles tightening in her upper back. There was no cancer to be found in any of the slides. She checked the numbers on the slide labels against the number on the biopsy report. She examined the slides a second time. She peeled back the slide labels and examined the histotechnologist's penciled accession numbers on the frosted surface, to be certain that the labels had been affixed to the proper slides. Finally, she brought the slides to a colleague for a disinterested re-examination. His interpretation was the same as hers: No cancer. Anywhere.

It took only 48 hours for the pathology department to complete its initial investigation. The mastectomy specimen was re-examined by two pathologists, and dozens of tissue blocks were selected for further study. No carcinoma was found in any of the tissue slides. All of the breast biopsy cases that had been interpreted on the same day as Ms. Gustoffen's initial biopsy were re-examined. One case—a breast biopsy from a Ms. Lydia Fields—had been reported by Dr. Owens as showing fibrocystic changes but in actuality contained invasive ductal carcinoma. Evidently, Ms. Gustoffen's and Ms. Fields' diagnoses had been reversed. But how?

A multidisciplinary committee was formed to investigate the incident in more detail. The committee included the chair of the department of pathology, the head of the hospital quality committee, the manager of histotechnology, the lead transcriptionist, and the manager of the ambulatory surgery suite where Ms. Gustoffen's and Ms. Fields' original biopsies had been performed. Because the incident qualified as a sentinel event under Joint Commission on Accreditation of Healthcare Organizations standards for hospital accreditation, the investigation of the incident included a root cause analysis.

The committee listed all of the steps in the process that begins with removal of a biopsy specimen in the ambulatory surgery suite and ends with issuance of a pathology report. Each step was examined to determine where the mix-up occurred and why it occurred. Some of the material that would have been helpful in the investigation had not been retained. For example, the specimen containers from both biopsies had been discarded because all of the tissue within the containers had been processed. It was also impossible to determine whether Ms. Gustoffen's slides and Ms. Fields' slides had been positioned next to one another in the same slide tray when given to Dr. Owens to examine.

From the information that was available, it appeared that the most likely explanation for the mix-up was that Dr. Owen had picked up Ms. Fields slides in error and had thought she was examining slides from Ms. Gustoffen's biopsy. However, the committee could not exclude the possibility that the correct slides had been examined and interpreted, that a transcriptionist had juxtaposed the diagnoses when typing them into the laboratory information system, and that Dr. Owens did not notice the reversed diagnoses when she electronically verified her reports in the computer. The potential for a specimen labeling error in the ambulatory surgery suite was considered but dismissed, because the two biopsy specimens were of significantly different size, and the gross description for each biopsy corresponded with the size of the specimen that each surgeon indicated he had removed. The potential for a mix-up in histology processing was also considered unlikely, as each biopsy involved multiple tissue blocks and the gross description of each biopsy specimen corresponded with the number of blocks that had been prepared.

Ms. Fields was notified about her carcinoma and eventually underwent a lumpectomy, which disclosed residual ductal carcinoma with negative margins. Ms. Gustoffen was notified about the diagnostic error by the surgeon who performed the mastectomy. Initially, Ms. Gustoffen was pleased to learn that she did not have carcinoma. Later, she became angry that she had undergone an unnecessary mastectomy.

Investigation of the incident at the hospital and imposition of corrective measures was complicated by the fact that the event was receiving a great deal of media attention, which involved the hospital's media relations staff. The committee looking into the problem felt pressured by the media relations department to speedily announce sanctions and changes to work practices. At the same time, the hospital's risk management staff was reluctant to have the incident discussed widely within the institution and was concerned that hasty imposition of corrective measures might be interpreted as some sort of admission by the hospital that standard practices were not being followed. The investigative committee tried to balance these competing priorities as best it could. During the investigation, Dr. Owens continued to practice but was told not to discuss the incident with anyone other than members of the investigatory committee and legal counsel. Although she felt profoundly disturbed by the course of events, Dr. Owens did not seek professional psychiatric help.

After two weeks, several new measures were adopted by the hospital and its pathology department to decrease the likelihood that a similar incident would recur. Slides from each biopsy case were to be placed in their own slide tray. Biopsy cases from the same anatomical site (breast, colon, etc) were to be staggered with intervening cases from other body sites. Patient names and accession numbers were both to be dictated by pathologists before any diagnosis was dictated. Transcriptionists were instructed to check the name and accession number in each dictation against the printed gross pathology report before transcribing dictations into the laboratory information system. When reports were electronically verified, department pathologists committed to compare the name and accession number on the computer screen to the name and accession number on the gross pathology report, which was to be returned by the transcriptionist to the pathologist's office prior to electronic verification. None of these interventions had been reported in the literature to decrease error rates. So far as the committee could tell, none had ever been systematically studied. Since this type of error had never occurred before at the hospital, it was generally agreed that there was no point in conducting a local experiment to determine whether these changes were likely to be effective. The Joint Commission on Accreditation of Healthcare Organizations (which accredited the hospital) and the College of American Pathologists (which accredited the laboratory) were both contacted and apprised of the local investigative committee's work.

The committee investigating the incident contacted the vendor of the hospital's laboratory information system to determine whether the vendor would be willing to include a check digit in surgical pathology accession numbers to minimize data entry errors, and whether the computer applications that transcriptionists and pathologists used to enter and verify reports could be modified so that double entry of accession numbers was required to call up or verify a case. The vendor was not interested in making these changes. There were two other hospitals in the city in which Dr. Owens practiced. Both of these hospitals used labeling, transcription, and verification procedures similar to the procedures used at Dr. Owens' hospital when the mix-up occurred. Neither of the other hospitals made any changes to their workflow processes as a result of the incident.

The committee looked into Dr. Owens' past performance. No lawsuits had been filed against her, and she had an exemplary 12-year practice history at the institution. During the day in which Ms. Gustoffen's and Ms. Fields' biopsies were interpreted, Dr. Owens had a larger-than-usual number of biopsies to interpret, but days with equal volumes had been recorded several other times during the year. Dr. Owens received two phone calls from clinicians with questions about chemistry testing, attended a one-hour meeting of the hospital library committee, and spent a half-hour reviewing quality control results in the chemistry section of her laboratory on the day in which Ms. Gustoffen's biopsy was interpreted. Based on this information, the committee decided not to recommend any action against Dr. Owens or to restrict her clinical activity, and the pathology department did not make any changes to pathologist staffing or work schedule. The committee that investigated the incident reviewed the workload of surgical pathology transcriptionists, but did not believe the workload to be abnormally taxing on the day in question and indicated that the transcriptionist pool was adequate for the workload overall. Accordingly, no changes were made in transcriptionist staffing.

Questions for Discussion

Do identification errors occur often in clinical laboratories? How often do they impact care? How should rare but serious incidents such as this be investigated? Is a local laboratory equipped to carry on an investigation of rare incidents, or should efforts be concentrated at a higher level, involving multiple institutions, whereby more incidents of the same type are likely to occur? Were the corrective measures adopted by this hospital appropriate? Were they timely? Were they sufficient? Should they be adopted by the other two hospitals in the city? Nationally? Should Dr. Owens have personally informed Ms. Gustoffen about the medical error, or relied as she did on the operating surgeon to communicate with his patient? What are the responsibilities of laboratory computer vendors for designing systems to prevent clerical errors? How can other protective systems be designed to correct human slips before they cause harm to patients?

Reagent Failure

Case History

At 10:00 AM, Terry Weimer, the laboratory director of Colbert Community Hospital, received a phone call from his laboratory manager about problems with troponin-I testing.

Colbert Community Hospital is an independent, 150-bed, not-for-profit hospital that serves the community of Colbert and the surrounding, mostly rural region. During the daytime hours, three technologists normally work in the laboratory, along with the manager. In the evening, one to two technologists work in the laboratory, and during the night shift the laboratory is staffed by a single technologist. Dr. Weimer is part of a group of 12 pathologists that oversees several hospital laboratories, including the laboratory in Colbert Community Hospital. He spent 12 hours per week overseeing the Colbert laboratory, either on-site or through telephone conversations. The laboratory manager also spent 20 hours per week on site in the laboratory and managed the laboratory of another hospital during the remainder of her work week.

According to the laboratory manager, one of the day shift technologists noticed that the laboratory had not reported a troponin-I result of 0 ng/mL in two days. Shortly after the technologist noticed this problem, an internist called with the same concern: he had not seen a troponin-I result with a value of 0 ng/mL in several days.

Troponin-I is a marker of acute myocardial injury. In the Colbert laboratory, troponin-I testing is performed on an automated analyzer, using reagents supplied by the analyzer's manufacturer. Values less than 0.3 ng/mL are considered normal, and most healthy patients have no detectable troponin-I in their blood. Values between 0.3 and 2.0 ng/mL are considered "borderline," and values above 2.0 ng/mL are considered indicative of a myocardial infarction. The Colbert analyzer was calibrated two weeks previously. Calibrator solutions were supplied by the analyzer manufacturer, and the manufacturer indicated calibration was stable for 30 days, so long as quality control testing was performed every 8 hours and the results were found to be acceptable. Control specimens were purchased from a different manufacturer. Three levels of controls were tested every 8 hours: a low, intermediate, and high value (L1 to L3).

When the laboratory manager reviewed the quality control records for the past three weeks, she noted two issues. The target range for the high value (L3) control was stated by the control manufacturer to be between 22.3 and 48.9 ng/mL (depending on the assay system used).

However, for several months the L3 control had been running above this range, with results in the mid-50s. This problem had been called in to the manufacturer of the test system and had been noted by at least three neighboring hospitals using the same lot of test reagents and same L3 controls. The assay manufacturer, Bishop Diagnostics, had been unable to detect a problem with its assay and had issued a letter suggesting that the laboratory switch to control solutions produced by Bishop. Technologists had been told, for the time being, to ignore the high results obtained with the L3 control until the cause of the elevation could be determined. The high results were within 2 standard deviations of the laboratory's own mean for the L3 control, even though they had remained above the control manufacturer's upper target value of 48.9 ng/mL through at least one calibration of the instrument.

Of more concern was the fact that, for the past two days, testing of the L1 control solution did not produce values in the target range (0.8 to 2.7 ng/mL) on the midnight shift. While L1 testing had been averaging 2.5 ng/mL up until two days ago, the L1 test results on the midnight shift from the previous two days had been 3.1 and 3.4 ng/mL. In addition to being out of the control manufacturer's target range, these values were more than 3 standard deviations above the mean of the laboratory's previous L1 testing results. The technologist who was working the midnight shift the past two days apparently noted this problem, but ran patient specimens anyway and released results. The problem had not occurred during the day and afternoon shift, although the results of L1 control testing on days and afternoons did appear to be drifting upward, and one test of the L1 control on the afternoon shift was above the target range and more than 3 standard deviations above the historic L1 mean. Upon retesting, the L1 control produced a result of 2.7 ng/mL.

Colbert's proficiency testing results for the past two years disclosed no problems with troponin-I testing. The medical technologist on the night shift had received training in quality control principles as part of his education at an accredited medical technology program. The Colbert laboratory did not provide education in quality control principles as part of its new laboratory employee training program.

The laboratory director asked the laboratory manager to retest samples from all patients who had troponin-I assays performed during the midnight shift over the past two days. Eight patients had been tested, all from the Emergency Department, and all originally had "borderline" values (0.3 to 2.0 ng/mL). There were no "positive" results (greater than 2.0 ng/mL) and no "normal" results (less than 0.3 ng/mL). After retesting the eight specimens on the day shift, six of the specimens produced retest results less than 0.3 ng/mL (normal), and the other two remained in the borderline range.

The manufacturer of the troponin-I reagents, Bishop Diagnostics, was a publicly traded United States company. Several years prior to the incident, Bishop Diagnostics entered into a consent decree with the US Food and Drug Administration (FDA) for failing to follow the FDA's Good Manufacturing Practices (GMP) / Quality System (QS) Regulation. Bishop agreed to pay a fine of several million dollars and discontinue the manufacture of a number of reagents. One of the areas of noncompliance identified during FDA inspections was process validation. The company was not able to provide the FDA with satisfactory evidence that its manufacturing processes could consistently produce a product that met its predetermined specifications. The consent decree entered into by Bishop and the FDA did not restrict Bishop's production of troponin-I test systems, and the particular reagent system used by Colbert Community Hospital had been approved by the FDA for sale in the United States.

The laboratory director and laboratory manger knew of Bishop's problems with the FDA when the instrument used to test troponin-I was purchased. The decision to purchase the instrument was made by a purchasing committee for a group of hospitals on the basis of price and performance.

The laboratory director contacted the director of the Emergency Department (ED) to determine how patients might have been affected by a report of artificially elevated troponin-I values. Chart review disclosed that the eight patients with borderline values had all been held in the ED for observation. Some additional testing had been performed, but no patient was admitted or had been subjected to invasive studies. All eight patients were discharged from the ED without a diagnosis of myocardial infarction, although one was diagnosed with "probable angina." The ED director determined that the patients had not been harmed as a result of falsely elevated troponin-I values, and that there was no need to notify the patients about this problem. Bills for the ED visits, which included charges for "observation," were not adjusted.

The laboratory director and manager emphasized to all technologists in the laboratory the importance of not releasing patient test results when quality control test results violated control rules, unless they were specifically told to do so by the laboratory manager or laboratory director. Bishop Diagnostics was contacted about the problem but did not have a suggested solution. In the interim, the laboratory director and laboratory manager decided together that serum from a patient with no detectable troponin-I would be added as a fourth control to be run on every shift. Patient test results were to be rejected if testing of this sample produced a result above 0.2 ng/mL. Laboratory reports were corrected for the six patients who had "borderline" results that were normal on retesting. A note was appended to the result indicating that the value may have been falsely elevated due to analytic problems. The test instrument was recalibrated, and the problem did not recur.

Four months after this incident, the manufacturer of the test system issued a written communication indicating that certain lots of troponin-I reagent were demonstrating an upward shift in patient and control values. This shift occurred with values between 0 and 2.0 ng/mL. The manufacturer believed the problem occurred because of premature degradation of one of the assay reagents, which was supposed to be stable on the instrument for 24 hours. The manufacturer recommended that the implicated lot of reagents be discarded, quality control testing be increased to every 4 hours, that a very low-value control (or negative patient specimen) with an expected value of less than 0.3 ng/mL be added, and that the instrument be recalibrated whenever this control produced a value greater than 0.5 ng/mL or a value more than 2 standard deviations above the laboratory's mean for the new control. This practice was adopted by the Colbert laboratory.

Questions for Discussion

How significantly was quality and patient safety compromised by this problem? What was the cost of this problem? Who incurred these costs? What factors may have caused this problem? What role did decisions made by the laboratory director, laboratory manager, technologist on the night shift, reagent manufacturer, purchasing department, and others play in causing this problem? What protective systems prevented this problem from becoming worse than it was? After investigation of the problem, was appropriate action taken? Should patients have been notified? Were adequate steps taken to prevent this problem from recurring? How often do problems of this type occur in clinical laboratories?

Laboratory Mismanagement

Case History

Vincent Marconi leaned back in his chair and contemplated the task before him. He had 45 days to bring one of the most closely scrutinized hospital-based laboratories in the United States back into regulatory compliance before the laboratory lost its license to serve Medicare and Medicaid patients, effectively putting the lab (and perhaps the entire hospital) out of business. The previous laboratory administrator, Joe Connors, had been discharged. The president and chief executive officer of the hospital had resigned, along with the laboratory medical director. Vincent considered the events over the past two years that had led the First Union Hospital laboratory to its present state of affairs.

First Union Hospital of Newark, New Jersey, is a licensed, 221-bed, not-for-profit hospital that serves the 54,000 residents of Newark's Central Ward. Patients are predominately African-American, with a median income slightly above the US poverty level, but the hospital also staffs the student health services for nearby Rutgers University and Essex County College. In 2002, First Union lost $1,412,000 from operations, which was in stark contrast to the hospital's major competitor, New Jersey University Medical Center. University Medical Center is a 618-bed state-operated institution located on a 69-acre campus in the heart of Newark. University Medical Center is Newark's largest employer and enjoyed an operating surplus in 2002 of $4,400,000.

The First Union Hospital laboratory included chemistry, hematology, microbiology, transfusion medicine, and anatomic pathology sections. Sixty percent of First Union's laboratory specimens came from inpatients, 30% from hospital-sponsored clinics, and the remaining 10% from outreach activity.

In 2002, when troubles began, the laboratory director of the First Union Hospital was a pathologist named Thomas Shenan. Dr. Shenan was board-certified in both clinical and anatomic pathology, but mostly practiced surgical pathology because of the heavy anatomic pathology case load in the department. Dr. Shenan was joined by two other pathologists, all employed by First Union Hospital, and the three pathologists together performed 16,008 surgical pathology interpretations in 2002, along with 620 nongynecologic cytology interpretations and 105 bone marrow evaluations. For two years, the pathologist had asked the hospital's chief operating officer for funding to hire a fourth pathologist, but the financial condition of the hospital had precluded new recruitment.

Dr. Shenan delegated most of First Union's laboratory director duties to the laboratory administrative director, Joe Connors, who also served as the supervisor of clinical chemistry. Like Dr. Shenan, Joe was frustrated by the hospital's financial situation, which prevented the laboratory from hiring as many medical technologists as Joe believed were required to do the job. Dr. Shenan and Joe Connors together presided over scheduled monthly laboratory quality meetings, but it became clear after events unraveled at First Union that the quality meetings often were canceled. During all of 2002 and 2003, only seven meetings had been held.

In May 2002, the First Union laboratory acquired a used robotic immunochemistry instrument, the RoboLab, which was manufactured in Germany. The RoboLab was the first major analyzer to be acquired by the First Union laboratory in the past two years, and

Mr. Connors had personally invested many hours convincing First Union's Chief Financial Officer that acquisition of the instrument made financial sense. Mr. Connors had calculated that the RoboLab would allow First Union to bring HIV and hepatitis B and C testing in-house. These three tests were being sent to a reference laboratory at considerable expense.

Although the RoboLab was manufactured in Germany, the reagents used by First Union to test for HIV and hepatitis B and C were produced by a United States company and had been approved by the FDA for sale in the US as a "moderately complex test." Approximately 1100 United States laboratories performed HIV and hepatitis B/C testing using the RoboLab with the same test reagents used by First Union. Control reagents were provided by a separate manufacturer. When the RoboLab was delivered, a technician from the company provided a lead technologist in the chemistry section with one week of on-site training on the instrument. Subsequently, First Union laboratory staff attempted to validate tests for HIV, hepatitis B, and hepatitis C, following the methods recommended by the reagent and instrument manufacturers.

Hepatitis B testing was easily validated, but HIV and hepatitis C testing proved to be more difficult and were never fully validated. Most of the time, the testing of control solutions fell within the manufacturer's recommended range, but on several occasions during the validation period, testing of control solutions did not produce acceptable results. In addition, the machine jammed periodically, and on three occasions a technician had to be summoned from the manufacturer to repair the instrument. Some technologists believed that the machine was carrying over specimens from one sample to another, and the instrument periodically failed self tests (internal diagnostics).

The hospital began clinical testing using the RoboLab in June of 2002. As recommended by the reagent manufacturer, calibrator solutions were run in triplicate to establish a "cut-off" value that would be used to separate "positive" from "negative" assays. When one of the three calibrators did not produce a result within the manufacturer's recommended range, or when the spread among the three calibrator values exceeded the manufacturer's limits, technologists were instructed by Mr. Connors to ignore the aberrant calibrator results and to substitute the average of the two acceptable results. This "editing" of calibrator values occurred on several separate instances. During this period, First Union staff repeatedly called the manufacturer of the RoboLab about instrument issues, and eventually the manufacturer provided First Union with a second instrument to use along with the original RoboLab.

One month after HIV and hepatitis testing of patient samples had commenced, the lead technologist in the special chemistry section filed a complaint with the state of New Jersey and also with Joe Connors, alleging that testing was not being performed properly and that patients were being put at risk. The state of New Jersey did not act on the allegations because state inspectors believed the allegations were "too vague" to be actionable. Joe Connors did not take any action. A second employee complained to Joe Connors' superior that laboratory management was not attending to quality issues in special chemistry. Joe Connors was contacted by the hospital administrator to look into the allegation, but instead he informed technologists in the special chemistry section that if they did not stop complaining to hospital administrators, their jobs would be at risk. At the time, First Union Hospital had not designated a compliance officer to confidentially receive employee complaints.

During the period when clinical HIV and hepatitis C testing was in progress, the state of New Jersey received a separate complaint about the First Union laboratory related to inadequate turnaround time of test results. An inspection team from the New Jersey

Department of Community Health conducted a two-day unannounced inspection and cited the laboratory for failure of the laboratory director to exercise his responsibilities and for failure to perform proper quality assurance in several areas. However, HIV and hepatitis C testing practices were not cited by the state inspectors.

Also during the period when HIV and hepatitis C testing was in progress, the College of American Pathologists (CAP) conducted a routine accreditation inspection of the laboratory. The inspection team, which consisted of two pathologists and five medical technologists, found several deficiencies relating to laboratory management and quality assurance, including failure to implement a quality plan. However, HIV and hepatitis C testing practices were not cited by the CAP inspectors as being deficient. First Union laboratory was given 30 days to correct the deficiencies that were identified by CAP inspectors and to document compliance with CAP standards. Although the process of document exchange between First Union and the CAP lasted more than 30 days, the CAP eventually reaccredited the laboratory under its "deemed authority" from the Centers for Medicare and Medicaid Services (CMS). The CAP inspection team was unaware of complaints that had been received by the state of New Jersey or the inspection by the New Jersey Department of Public Health.

In late 2003, another technologist in the laboratory, Tawana Davis, sent a written complaint to the state of New Jersey indicating that quality control results for HIV and hepatitis C testing were being improperly altered. Ms. Davis also alleged that she had become infected with HIV while attempting to repair the RoboLab. The state of New Jersey conducted a complaint survey of the First Union laboratory and during the inspection identified several instances in which manufacturer's recommended procedures were not being followed and proper quality control practices were not being applied.

In early 2004, a local newspaper became aware of the story and featured it prominently in a series of articles. A follow-up inspection of the laboratory and other parts of the hospital was conducted by the Centers for Medicare and Medicaid Services regional office, the state of New Jersey, and the Joint Commission on Accreditation of Healthcare Organizations (JCAHO). Congressional hearings into laboratory quality were scheduled. The College of American Pathologists conducted a special investigation of the First Union laboratory and cited the laboratory for a number of deficiencies. In the flurry of public attention that followed, resignations of the laboratory's administrative director, medical director, and the hospital's president and chief executive officer were announced. HIV and hepatitis testing were discontinued by First Union and sent to a reference laboratory. A consulting firm was engaged to manage the laboratory and address citations issued by the state of New Jersey, CMS, CAP, and JCAHO. Vincent Marconi, who worked for the consulting firm, agreed to become the new administrative director of the First Union laboratory.

During the period when HIV and hepatitis C testing was performed on-site, First Union proficiency testing results for HIV and hepatitis C disclosed no deficiencies. All results, which were reported to the proficiency testing vendor as "positive" or "negative," were graded as "satisfactory." Review of proficiency testing records from more than 1000 laboratories that used the RoboLab to perform HIV and hepatitis testing disclosed a deficiency rate that was no higher than the rate observed with other analytic platforms.

In time, Vincent Marconi and the staff at the First Union laboratory and hospital were able to satisfy the state of New Jersey, CAP, JCAHO, and CMS that the laboratory and hospital were in conformance with applicable standards for administrative oversight and quality control. However, funding problems and staff morale at First Union remained problematic. Six months later, First Union hospital workers participated in a one-day strike to protest compensation, staffing levels, and working conditions. The new medical director of the laboratory told Mr. Marconi that she was not interested in actively managing the laboratory, due to her heavy anatomic pathology workload, and that she expected Mr. Marconi to keep the laboratory in conformance with regulations and standards.

Approximately 2000 patients who had been tested for HIV or hepatitis C by First Union were offered the opportunity to be retested at no charge. Of the 380 patients who availed themselves of this opportunity, three were found to have discrepant results. Two patients who had previously tested negatively for HIV were found to have HIV antibodies upon retesting, and one patient who had previously tested negative for hepatitis C was found to have hepatitis C antibodies on retesting. No previously positive patients retested as negative. Because more than a year had elapsed between the time of original testing and retesting, it was not clear for the three patients with discrepant results whether the original results were incorrect or the patients had seroconverted between their initial test and their retest.

Questions for Discussion

What were the consequences of this quality failure for First Union patients and employees, and for First Union as an institution? What roles did education, training, management, instrument manufacturers, and local economics play in causing the problems at First Union? What legal responsibilities for laboratory quality are vested in a laboratory director and a laboratory's owner? Can the laboratory director's duties and responsibilities be delegated? What options are open to a medical director if he or she is having difficulty bringing a test system or a laboratory section up to standards? What options are open to an administrative director? How should a laboratory respond to complaints about quality received from employees? Can external inspection from a state department of health, the CAP, JCAHO, or CMS reliably detect the type of problem that arose in First Union? Can external proficiency testing? What other safeguards can be employed to identify episodic problems in laboratories?

Communication Failure

Case History

"At least it wasn't a subpoena," thought Paul Newcombe as he reread the letter. Apparently the hospital in which Dr. Newcombe practiced was being sued by the estate of a man who had died two years ago. The hospital's counsel wished to speak with Dr. Newcombe at his "earliest convenience," explained the letter, because the plaintiff's lawyer had indicated he would depose Dr. Newcombe—the laboratory director—in relation to the complaint.

On the telephone with the hospital's counsel, Paul learned more about the case. The patient who died was a 58-year-old man who had suffered a myocardial infarction two months before his death. He was treated at Dr. Newcombe's hospital, and during the hospitalization, a pacemaker was inserted to correct rhythm abnormalities that developed as a consequence of myocardial damage. The patient was discharged with good cardiac function, but about five weeks after discharge, he complained of fever and malaise. He was readmitted to the hospital for a four-day work-up and was then discharged. At some point during his hospitalization, a blood culture that eventually grew *Staphylococcus aureus* was obtained. The patient was never treated for *S. aureus* infection during the hospitalization or in the days thereafter. He was admitted to another hospital with *S. aureus* sepsis one week after discharge and expired. The patient's estate was suing the cardiologist at Dr. Newcombe's hospital for failing to treat the patient's staphylococcal infection, and was suing Dr. Newcombe's hospital for not having "adequate policies and procedures in place to notify doctors of laboratory results that became available after discharge." Paul Newcombe was not named in the suit. Paul scheduled a time to talk face-to-face with the hospital attorney, who promised he would send Paul a copy of the complaint. Paul also wrote down the patient's name and medical record number, and indicated he would look for records relevant to the complaint.

Dr. Newcombe asked the manager of the microbiology laboratory to pull the laboratory's procedure related to notification of critical results and to print a copy of the electronic work card from the patient's positive blood culture. Meanwhile, he walked down to the medical records department to take a look at the patient's medical chart. He learned from the chart that the patient had chronic renal failure. The patient's nephrologist was listed as the attending physician for the four-day hospitalization that was the focus of the lawsuit. Most of the patient's care in the hospital had been managed by a consulting cardiologist, Dr. Giordoni. The blood culture that grew staphylococci was ordered by a third-year medical resident. After he obtained a printout of the work card from microbiology, Dr. Newcombe began to put together the sequence of events.

The patient's blood culture had been ordered and drawn on the day of his admission. Four days later, the automated blood culture instrument used in the laboratory detected growth, and the blood culture bottle was Gram stained, revealing Gram-positive cocci in clusters. The laboratory's "critical value" notification policy specified that positive blood cultures detected within 48 hours of collection were to be called to a physician responsible for the care of the patient; after 48 hours, positive blood cultures could be reported through the laboratory computer systems without telephone notification. Although the laboratory policy did not require technologists to call blood cultures that first turned positive after four days of incubation, the technologist working up the culture evidently decided to call a physician about the result anyway. A note was made in the work card that the technologist had communicated the Gram stain's results by telephone to a "Dr. Roux" at 3:00 in the afternoon. Paul did not recognize the name Dr. Roux, so he called the credentialing office and learned that Dr. Roux was a house physician employed by the hospital. His name was not mentioned in the patient's chart. According to the medical record, the patient had been discharged from the hospital at 9:00 AM—before the result was called. It was not clear to Dr. Newcombe whether Dr. Roux ever communicated the results of the blood culture Gram stain to the attending nephrologist or the consulting cardiologist.

Dr. Newcombe knew that a number of years back the laboratory had developed a procedure to alert clinicians to laboratory results that became available after a patient was discharged. He called the manager of the laboratory's information system to ask about the procedure. "Almost all attending physicians receive a discharge laboratory report one day after discharge, which lists all laboratory results that are available at the time the report is printed," the manager of the computer system told Dr. Newcombe. "In addition, physicians receive a copy of any new laboratory results that become available after this report is printed. All of these reports are filed in the physician's mailbox. Of course, some physicians have informed us that they do not want to receive these reports, and we have excluded them from the discharge report list." Dr. Newcombe was relieved to hear that the attending nephrologist was not one of these physicians. The laboratory did not have a procedure to send postdischarge laboratory reports to consulting physicians or ordering physicians.

When contacted by Dr. Newcombe, Dr. Roux could not recall the phone call he had received from a microbiology technologist two years previously, informing him that a recently discharged patient was growing Gram-positive cocci in clusters four days after his blood culture had been obtained. Dr. Roux indicated that even if he had received the call, he probably would not have done anything about it because blood cultures with Gram-positive cocci in clusters that took four days to grow were most likely contaminants, and that the attending physician would need to make a decision about whether to treat the patient based on the final culture results. The attending physician could not recall whether he received a laboratory report after discharge indicating that the blood culture was growing *Staphylococcus aureus*. However, he said that follow-up care was to be provided by Dr. Giordoni, the consulting cardiologist, because the patient's problem was believed to be cardiac and not renal. Dr. Giordoni, who was named as a defendant in the suit, had scheduled a follow-up appointment with the patient for one week after discharge. He was adamant that he had never received any blood culture report from the laboratory. He indicated that with a pacemaker in place, the patient was a candidate for a staphylococcal infection, and he would certainly have treated the patient had he known about the patient's blood culture results.

Questions for Discussion

Might this patient's clinical course have been different if his cardiologist knew about the results of the patient's blood culture? Is a blood culture showing Gram-positive cocci in clusters after four days of incubation a "critical result"? What is a critical result? To whom should this result be communicated? The ordering physician (a resident in this case)? The admitting physician (a nephrologist in this case)? The consulting physician (a cardiologist in this case)? What responsibility does the laboratory have to communicate preliminary and final results after a patient has been discharged? What should a laboratory do when a physician asks not to be notified about preliminary test results or about final results that become available after discharge? What should the laboratory do when a caregiver cannot be contacted or refuses to accept a critical result over the telephone?

Fraud

Case History

AccuPap Diagnostics was a for-profit, free-standing, cytology laboratory in Nashville, Tennessee, that served the offices of 55 local gynecologists and general practitioners, and also processed "overflow" gynecologic cytology cases from six area hospitals.

AccuPap was a joint venture owned by a pathologist and two nonphysician business partners. The AccuPap laboratory had been in business for six years, maintained a CLIA certificate, and had been accredited on two successive occasions by the College of American Pathologists.

In March of 2004, the CAP received a written complaint from a woman who indicated she was an employee of AccuPap Diagnostics. The woman alleged that AccuPap was reusing single-use cytology processing filters to save money. The employee further alleged that management was aware that the reuse of filters deviated from the filter manufacturer's instructions, and that management did not change AccuPap's practice when she had brought it to management's attention. She indicated that when performing Pap smear interpretations on persons known to the owners of AccuPap Diagnostics, the owners instructed specimen prep technicians not to reuse cell filters.

Ten days after receipt of the complaint, the CAP received a letter from the legal counsel of AccuPap. The letter indicated that allegations made by the AccuPap Diagnostics employee were untrue, that the employee was being terminated, that AccuPap considered itself to have been libeled, and that AccuPap was prepared to take legal action against the discharged employee if she did not cease and desist from making further untrue allegations.

Three days later, the CAP sent an inspector to Nashville to perform a nonroutine (unscheduled) survey of the laboratory. Following the nonroutine inspection, a special inspection team was assembled, which included a nationally known cytopathologist. The team inspected the AccuPap facility two weeks thereafter. The team was not able to directly document that cytology cell filters had been reused, but a review of AccuPap records disclosed that the number of cell filters the laboratory had ordered during the past year was less than one-half the number of Pap smear interpretations that had been reported during the same period. Although AccuPap steadfastly denied reusing filters, it could not satisfactorily explain this discrepancy. The CAP inspectors concluded that it was highly likely the laboratory was reusing Pap smear filters, which were explicitly labeled as single-use devices by the manufacturer.

In addition to the likely reuse of cell filters, the CAP inspectors found that some cytotechnologists were exceeding the maximum daily screening limits specified in the Clinical Laboratory Improvement Amendments of 1988 (CLIA). The CAP withdrew its accreditation of the laboratory two weeks after the inspection and notified the Tennessee Department of Public Health.

The state launched its own investigation of the laboratory and also concluded that cell filters had been improperly reused. In addition, the state cited the laboratory for failing to conduct required control testing on equipment and reagents, and for failing to notify local health departments of sexually transmitted diseases, as required by law. The Tennessee Department of Public Health, in conjunction with the regional office of the US Centers for Medicare and Medicaid Services, suspended AccuPap Diagnostics' CLIA laboratory license because it considered the laboratory "an immediate jeopardy to the health of its patients and that of the general public."

AccuPap Diagnostics was closed in June of 2004. Its owners indicated that they planned to sell the laboratory, but no buyer could be identified, and the equipment from the laboratory was eventually put up for auction. More than 100,000 women had been tested by AccuPap during the period in which cell filters had been reused. Approximately 5000 were reported to have had cytopathologic abnormalities. These abnormalities ranged from atypical squamous cells of undetermined significance (ASCUS) to high-grade squamous intraepithelial lesions

(HSIL). Because of the potential for carryover of cells from one specimen to another when filters were being reused, it was possible that some of these reported abnormalities represented false-positives.

Questions for Discussion

Is it ever appropriate to compromise quality in the interest of improving financial performance? What if compromises do not cause practices to fall out of conformance with regulations or accreditation standards? What if compromises are required to preserve the financial viability of a charitable institution? In this case, management clearly crossed the line and committed fraud. Can fraud be prevented? What controls are applied in other industries to discourage fraudulent behavior? Is fraud a major cause of quality problems in clinical laboratories? Have you ever committed fraud? Have you ever backdated a quality control record? Have you ever "signed off" on quality control records you did not actually examine? Have you ever been less than forthcoming with a laboratory inspector?

Approaches to Managing Quality and Patient Safety

There are dozens of philosophies about how to promote quality and safety. Some have been in existence for years and are actively applied in many enterprises; others are best described as "fads" that exist mainly in the minds of consultants and leave little lasting impact. Some approaches are too theoretical to be useful in daily management, dwelling excessively on defining quality and safety in multiple ethereal dimensions, and devoting little attention to the less glamorous task of making it happen in the real world.

This chapter describes major approaches to managing quality and patient safety that we believe useful to clinical laboratory managers. There is no statutory requirement that laboratory directors in the United States apply any of these methods to managing the quality of their operations, but it is difficult to imagine a director overseeing quality without some sort of consistent management philosophy.

In this chapter, we review the history and key contributions provided by each school of thinking and appraise the strengths and limitations of each approach to quality management. Several of these approaches evolved from a common historical ancestry and provide overlapping recommendations.[2]

Statistical Process Control

Statistical process control (SPC), which is sometimes called statistical quality control, refers to the use of statistical methods to monitor and ultimately control the quality of a process. Statistical process control allows organizations to assess the quality of a product or service efficiently, by making relatively few measurements, and signals operators when a process is not performing adequately. Statistical process control may also be used to determine whether quality improvement activities are having their intended effect.

Statistical process control is used in hundreds of industries throughout the world. In clinical laboratories, SPC is used to assess the performance of automated analyzers, but many laboratory managers do not realize that the principles of SPC may be applied to managing the quality and safety of preanalytic and postanalytic processes. In this section, in addition to describing SPC, we illustrate the application of SPC to preanalytic and postanalytic issues.

History

For all practical purposes, statistical process control began with Walter Shewhart (1891-1967). Shewhart received a bachelor's and master's degree from the University of Illinois, and a doctorate in physics from the University of California at Berkeley in 1917. After working for a year in academia, Shewhart joined the Western Electric Company, which served as the manufacturing arm of Bell Telephone and was responsible for building the equipment required for the nation's first telephone system.

Western Electric's largest manufacturing operation was the massive Hawthorne Works in Cicero, Illinois. At its peak, 40,000 employees labored at the Hawthorne facility, and some

5000 were involved in quality inspections. In an operation as large as Hawthorne, the economic stimulus to improve manufacturing quality and reduce the cost of inspection was immense. Shewhart spent six years making theoretical and empirical inquiries into the causes of quality failure at Western Electric and developed methods to economically improve monitoring of the production process. One of these methods was the control chart, which Shewhart proposed to his supervisors in an historic memorandum on May 16, 1924.

Shewhart recognized the impossibility of producing suitable product with perfect consistency. Some variation was inevitable. Yet the burden of inspecting every product at every step in the manufacturing process was too costly. When could variation in production safely be left to chance, with the knowledge that the variation was unlikely to impact quality, and when did variation signal that something was amiss which required corrective action? Shewhart defined two types of variation: *chance-cause* (also called *common-cause*) variation, which resulted from the inescapable vagaries of operating within the physical world; and *assignable-cause* (also called *special-cause*) variation, which resulted from specific circumstances that could be identified and corrected.

Processes that displayed only chance-cause variation were said to be in a state of *statistical control*. That is, variation in these processes followed predictable statistical laws. Parts produced by processes in statistical control did not require universal inspection because the probability that an individual part would meet performance standards was very high. In contrast, processes not in statistical control suffered from assignable-cause variation and more often produced parts that were defective.[3] In Shewhart's own words, "While every process displays variation, some processes display controlled variation, while others display uncontrolled variation."

To Shewhart, the goal of the production manager was to eliminate assignable-cause variation and bring production processes into statistical control, where remaining variation was small and could be left to chance.[4] Shewhart's *control chart* allowed the production manager— with relatively little investment of time in inspection—to distinguish between processes in statistical control (which demonstrated only common-cause variation) and processes that were impacted by assignable-cause variation (which required investigation and remediation).

In 1931, Shewhart summarized his findings and coined the term "statistical quality control" in his classic monograph, *Economic Control of Quality of Manufactured Product*.[5] Two years later, his methods were adopted by the American Society for Testing Materials (ASTM). H.F. Dodge and H.G. Romig at Bell Telephone Laboratories extended Shewhart's methods by developing more efficient schemes for acceptance sampling. Their combined work was instrumental in improving the quality of US wartime production, and after the war was taught to Japanese industry as part of US-led efforts to improve the Japanese postwar economy.

In 1939, Shewhart wrote *Statistical Method from the Viewpoint of Quality Control*, in which he first articulated his elegantly simple model for quality improvement in the real world setting: *Plan-Do-Study-Act (PDSA)*. The PDSA model (also called Plan-Do-Check-Act) was later popularized by W. Edwards Deming and is sometimes incorrectly attributed to Deming. In 1950, Levey and Jennings[6] introduced the Shewhart control chart into the clinical laboratory, and in recognition of their contribution, laboratory control charts are often called "Levey-Jennings" charts.

Key Points

Steps in Statistical Process Control. Statistical process control progresses sequentially through a series of steps depicted in Figure 1.[7] Although the ultimate goal of SPC is to improve quality, immediate attention is focused on reducing variation rather than improving performance. Through the systematic reduction in variation, performance ultimately improves. The use of graphical SPC tools illustrated in Figure 1 is optional, but the basic steps of SPC should not be taken out of sequence.

1. Define the process to be controlled. This often involves use of a *flow chart* (sometimes called a *process map*).

2. Specify operational definitions of satisfactory performance. An operational definition allows staff to determine whether the process conforms to standards in a practical way, using available tools. In clinical laboratory medicine, an operational definition of satisfactory performance might consist of instructions about how to measure turnaround time of specimens coming from the Emergency Department, along with an objective standard for what constitutes acceptable turnaround time.

3. Make preliminary measurements at various stages in the production process, and focus on the most problematic steps. For example, in one laboratory concerned about lost specimens, most specimen loss might occur when "split" specimens that need to be processed in several areas are not properly divided. Often, as few as 20% of the steps are responsible for 80% of the defects. The steps deserving of greatest attention may be illustrated with a *Pareto chart,* which is a histogram that shows the relative importance of different groups of data.[8] Sometimes, customer complaints or a log of incidents is used to determine which steps to focus attention upon.

4. Measure key production steps systematically and plot on a *run chart.* A run chart displays performance over time, but does not have control limits and does not specify a "target" performance. Each point on a run chart can represent the mean performance of every specimen in a "run" or the mean performance of a randomly selected sample. The run chart is used to determine whether a process is in statistical control or whether it suffers from assignable-cause (special-cause) variation. There is no single mathematical procedure that can be used to determine whether a process is in statistical control, but for most applications within the laboratory, "eyeball" examination of a run chart is sufficient to determine whether assignable-cause variation exists. Any clearly discernable pattern to variation over time indicates that the process is being influenced by special causes. If the variation has no pattern and individual values gravitate randomly around their mean, then the process is likely to be in statistical control.

5. Identify causes of variation. Very few processes within the clinical laboratory are likely to be in statistical control, except results obtained by automated equipment. Therefore, most processes are being influenced by specific identifiable causes of variation. Sources of assignable-cause variation are manifold; they might range from periodic staffing shortages to the introduction of poorly trained employees to breakdowns in information systems. A *cause-and-effect diagram* (often called a *fishbone diagram* or *Ishikawa diagram*) lists all of the inputs that affect a process and that may be responsible for assignable-cause variation.

Figure 1. Statistical Process Control in Practice

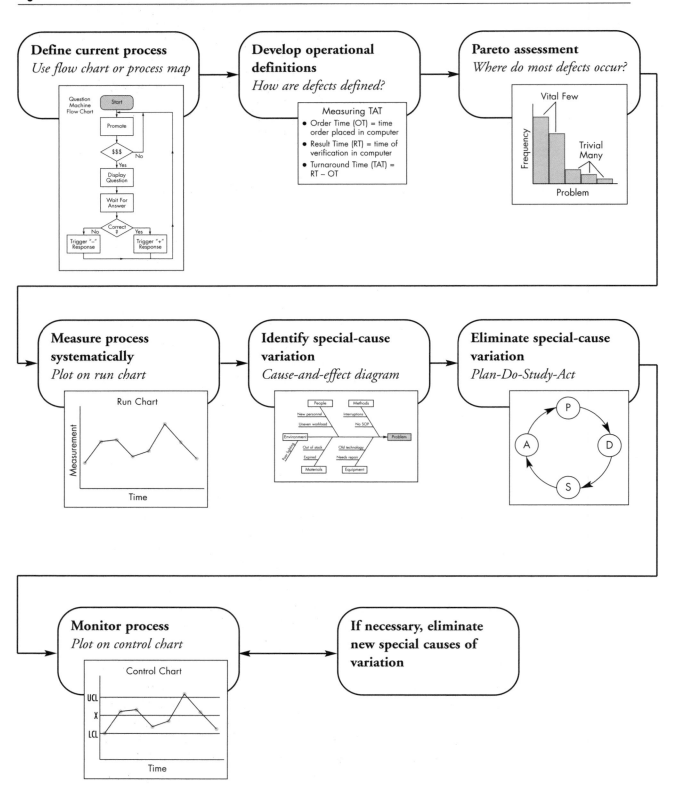

Brainstorming with a cause-and-effect diagram is often a useful exercise in identifying factors that may be producing assignable-cause variation.

6. Eliminate assignable-cause variation. Use the Plan-Do-Study-Act methodology to determine whether an experimental change to a suspected cause actually reduces variation. For example, if it is hypothesized that variation in the size of the transcriptionist pool causes variation in the turnaround time of surgical pathology reports, carry out an experiment to determine whether cross-training and stabilization of the transcriptionist pool actually reduces variation. If it does, implement the change on a permanent basis. The elimination of assignable-cause variation in a process can take years of effort and involve rigorously standardizing work methods, training staff, and convincing physicians, physician offices, and patient care units to standardize their own processes.

7. Once special-cause variation has been eliminated, plot performance on a *control chart*. The use of control charts is discussed below. A surprisingly small number of samples are required to follow a process with a control chart, once the process is in statistical control. Control charts alert operators when assignable-cause variation reasserts its ugly head and is in need of remediation. Control charts can also be used to test whether changes designed to improve performance are having their intended effect.

8. When an operation exceeds control limits, identify and eliminate the cause of variation.

Using control charts in practice. There are several kinds of control charts, but most processes in the clinical laboratory can be followed with one of two basic chart types. Processes that can be measured with continuous variables, such as a serum sodium assay or Emergency Department test turnaround time, are followed using an *X-bar control chart*. Processes that are binomial (eg, yes/no or defective/not defective), such as whether or not a critical result was called, are followed using a control chart called a *p-chart*. Exhibit 1 provides an example of how to create and use an X-bar control chart for a preanalytic variable. Exhibit 2 provides an example of how to create and use a p-chart for a postanalytic attribute.

Exhibit 1. Using the X-bar Chart: A Control Chart for Continuous Variables

In this example, an X-bar control chart will be constructed to track turnaround time of stat electrolyte results from the Emergency Department (ED). Laboratory and ED staff have already met for a number of months and established a process for efficiently transporting specimens to the lab. They have agreed to measure the turnaround time from specimen drop-off in the laboratory to verification of results in the laboratory computer. The process seems to be in reasonable statistical control—performance from one day to the next does not vary much. Therefore, the control chart represents an economical way to track performance over time and make sure the process does not require special attention.

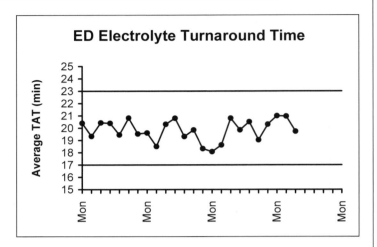

When ED staff bring specimens to the laboratory, they time-stamp the paper requisition that accompanies the specimen. Every day, a technologist selects at random four requisitions that include requests for a stat electrolyte panel. The technologist looks up the time each panel was verified in the laboratory computer. The interval from the time stamped on the requisition to the verification time is the turnaround time for that specimen. While it might seem easier to track turnaround time of all specimens using the log-in time automatically recorded in the lab computer instead of using the time stamp, staff know that specimens are not always logged in promptly.[9] One of the advantages of the control chart is that only four samples need to be tracked every day to monitor quality. This allows laboratory staff to concentrate on measuring what is really going on—when specimens are actually dropped off—rather than using a more convenient (but less accurate) source of information.

The laboratory technologist plots the average of the four daily turnaround times on the control chart, as illustrated. The technologist e also records the average of the four values on a form. If the average falls outside the control limits on the chart, the manager is notified. It is highly likely that something has happened to disturb the process, and further investigation is required. Otherwise, the technologist goes back to his or her remaining work.

How are upper and lower control limits established for an X-bar chart? Every four weeks, the manager looks at the table of turnaround times from the previous four weeks.

If m is the mean of the turnaround time values in the previous four weeks, SD is their standard deviation, and n is the number of measurements made per day (4 in this example), then:

$$Lower\ Control\ Limit = m - \frac{3SD}{\sqrt{n}}$$

$$Upper\ Control\ Limit = m + \frac{3SD}{\sqrt{n}}$$

If a lower control limit is below 0, it can be ignored. In this illustration, the average turnaround time (m) is 20 minutes, and the standard deviation of daily turnaround times over the past four weeks is 2 minutes, so:

$$Upper\ Control\ Limit = 20 + \frac{(3)(2)}{\sqrt{4}} = 23$$

There are more sophisticated approaches to creating control charts for variables, but this method is adequate to track most preanalytic and postanalytic processes that are described using continuous variables.

Exhibit 2. Using the p-Chart: A Control Chart for Attributes

In this example, a p-chart will be constructed to track the fraction of critical values called to outpatient physicians. The laboratory director knows that it is sometimes difficult to call outpatient critical values because caregivers cannot always be reached by phone when critical values are discovered. The director wishes to monitor how faithfully critical values are called, and to be alerted when the laboratory's rate changes. The variable being studied—whether or not a critical value was called—is an attribute. It can take only two values: called and not called. Therefore, a p-chart for attributes is used to track performance, rather than an X-bar chart for continuous variables.

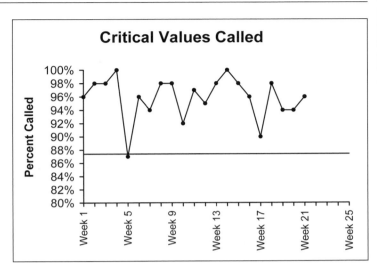

To use a p-chart, a sample size must be sufficiently large that most samples contain at least one defect. Since the laboratory calls most critical values—about 96%—a sample size of 50 critical values is used. With a sample of 50, it is likely that at least one call will not have been made. To keep the work of collecting information manageable, samples are collected weekly. Every week, 50 critical values in the chemistry and hematology area are identified using the laboratory computer. A lead technologist then checks to determine whether there is documentation in the computer that the critical value was called.

The lead technologist calculates the fraction of critical values called in the sample of 50 values. If there is documentation that 48 of the 50 critical values were called in the first week, then the fraction called is 48/50 or 96%. The technologist plots this value on the p-chart, as illustrated, and alerts the manager if values fall below the lower control limit. In this example, the performance in week 5 was below the lower control limit; the manager was alerted and talked with the technologist responsible for calling critical values on the afternoon shift. For the other weeks, no special action was taken because control limits were not violated.

How are control limits calculated for a p-chart? The manager calculates average performance using data from the previous 20 weeks.

If p is the average fraction of successful calls made during the 20 previous samples, and n is the size of each sample, then the control limits are:

$$Lower\ Control\ Limit = p - 3\sqrt{p(1-p)/n}$$

$$Upper\ Control\ Limit = p + 3\sqrt{p(1-p)/n}$$

If an upper control limit is over 100%, as in this example, it can be ignored. In this illustration, the average fraction of successful calls in the previous 20 weeks (p) was 96%, and the number of critical results sampled each week (n) was 50. Therefore:

$$Lower\ Control\ Limit = .96 - 3\sqrt{\frac{(.96)(.04)}{50}} = 87.7\%$$

There are more sophisticated approaches to creating control charts for attributes, but this method is adequate to track most preanalytic and postanalytic processes that are described using attributes.

Important Caveats. Experience with control charts in the clinical laboratory and other industries leads us to provide the following cautionary comments.

❖ Control charts should only be used to monitor processes that are normally in reasonable statistical control. If a process that is subject to substantial assignable-cause variation is plotted on a control chart, control limits will be exceeded frequently. Work will be repeatedly stopped, and operators may not have the time to identify all the causes of variation and bring the process into statistical control. When a laboratory has operated for years with a preanalytic or postanalytic process that is not in statistical control, management and staff should apply Plan-Do-Study-Act or some other approach to systematically eliminate assignable-cause variation, while continuing to operate the laboratory. Only after the preanalytic or postanalytic processes is brought into reasonable statistical control should control charts be used.

❖ Once a process has been brought into statistical control, production is normally stopped when the process jumps out of control. For example, when a control solution is tested and the result falls outside of control limits, clinical testing should stop. Some operators continue to test patient specimens while retesting the control solution, under the mistaken assumption that something is "wrong with the control." It is much more likely that something is wrong with the testing process itself, and that this problem is affecting patient results as well as control results.[10] When statistical process control is applied to preanalytic or postanalytic processes, it may not be practical to bring testing to a halt, but the reasons for the variance still require investigation.

❖ Control limits are often confused with performance targets. They are not the same thing. A control limit alerts an operator that a process is probably out of statistical control. A process that is out of statistical control may still be meeting performance targets, if the process has room for slippage before quality is affected. Conversely, a process that is in statistical control may not be meeting performance targets, if the process itself isn't up to the task. For example, most current analytic methods for measuring creatinine are simply not adequate for detecting small changes in renal function. Achieving statistical quality control in the laboratory is unlikely to remedy this situation; better methods for measuring creatinine or alternative markers for renal failure are needed.[11]

❖ When a process receives specimens from multiple sources (such as a laboratory receiving specimens from multiple nursing units), and there is a problem with specimen quality, it may be advantageous to create separate control charts for the quality of specimens from each patient care unit, rather than aggregate specimens from all care units into a single chart. Both approaches will work, but separate control charts for each patient care unit are more likely to detect a problem with a particular unit than a single control chart that includes all patient care units combined. The same point can be made about the use of control charts to follow turnaround time of multiple types of stat tests. Using separate control charts for each analyte will detect a problem with a particular assay more quickly than an aggregate control chart that includes multiple analytes.

❖ It is important that inspection be brought into statistical control, as well as the product. When making measurements that involve time, temperature, or weight, this is not normally a problem. Time, temperature, and weight can be measured accurately and reproducibly. However, inspection of cytology or surgical pathology diagnoses raises questions about the accuracy and consistency of the inspector, and whether the inspector is biased by knowledge of the initial diagnosis. For example, it is becoming increasingly common for institutions to require that a second pathologist re-examine slides associated with high-risk surgical pathology diagnoses. While this may be a healthy trend, comparatively little attention has been given to the accuracy and consistency of the pathologist re-examining the case or whether this pathologist is blinded to the original diagnosis.

❖ When defects in a final product become very rare (less than one defect per week), statistical process control can no longer be applied to the entire process. For example, the current incidence of hemolytic transfusion reactions is on the order of 1 in 20,000 transfusions. There is little point in plotting a hospital's hemolytic transfusion reactions on a p-chart; hemolytic reactions occur too infrequently, and control limits could never be established in any sort of meaningful time frame. Instead, statistical process control should be applied to each individual step in the process that is used to select and administer blood products. These include phlebotomy and labeling, accessioning and record keeping, blood typing and antibody screening, and the release and transfusion of blood products. Because the blood administration process involves multiple redundant checks, the frequency of errors in individual steps is much higher than the overall rate of hemolytic transfusion reactions. These individual steps are suitable for monitoring with statistical process control, even though the overall process is too reliable to plot on a control chart.

Appraisal of Statistical Process Control

Statistical process control takes time to work. It is for the quiet and long-suffering incrementalist and for the organization that is willing to maintain consistency of purpose over many years. Statistical process control is not for the impatient manager who wishes to make a big impression by hitting the home run, or for an organization that is prone to move from crisis to crisis in a reactive manner.

As a result of regulations described in the next chapter, SPC is used throughout the United States to control the quality of analytic processes in the clinical laboratory. Yet the application of SPC to preanalytic and postanalytic processes in the laboratory is still uncommon.

There are several reasons why SPC has failed to take hold in preanalytic and postanalytic domains. First, basic knowledge about statistical process control fundamentals is lacking in many operations. Few workers in a typical laboratory have much confidence in their knowledge of statistics. Secondly, SPC for automated analyzers is often embedded in the design of the analyzer or in commercially purchased software packages. Operators who have been trained to use these analyzers often do not understand the control measures being applied. Third, much of the variation in preanalytic laboratory processes is introduced by physicians and staff in patient care areas, and laboratory managers have been reluctant to insist that these "suppliers" control variation in their processes. Fourth, as we have mentioned, many managers lack the patience to take a long-term incremental approach to quality improvement, or find themselves managing in an environment that emphasizes short-term results. Finally, clinical laboratories are surprisingly complex operations, even in small hospitals. In small, complex facilities with limited budgets, it may not be possible to economically apply statistical process control to all preanalytic and postanalytic processes.

In our experience, many preanalytic and postanalytic problems are addressed reactively, in response to complaints or incidents, rather than proactively, using statistical methods to drive out the variation that produced the incidents in the first place. Making changes in response to incidents can sometimes help, but may also make things worse. Both Shewhart and Deming showed that making corrections in response to deviations can lead to over-compensation, and may increase variation and degrade quality beyond its normal levels. This paradox should sound a note of caution to those who base their entire quality management program on reactive responses to incidents, such as the root cause analyses described elsewhere in this chapter. Statistical process control has a better track record.

Total Quality Management

Total quality management (TQM) is a practical philosophy of excellence. It arose with the postwar renaissance of Japanese industry and was shaped principally by two American advisers, W. Edwards Deming and Joseph Juran, and the president of the Japanese Union of Scientists and Engineers, Kaoru Ishikawa.[12]

Total quality management concerns itself with how best to organize a business to apply statistical process control to quality and productivity. Total quality management cannot be separated from statistical process control any more than a tree can be separated from its roots. However, TQM is more than statistics: fundamentally, it is about how to equip an organization and its employees to pursue a statistical approach to quality instead of using traditional management approaches, which TQM's founders considered ineffective.

History

W. Edwards Deming (1900-1993) studied statistics under Sir Ronald Fisher and statistical process control with Walter Shewhart. He took a doctorate in mathematical physics from Yale and demonstrated that many of Shewhart's methods for improving manufacturing could be applied with equal effect to the clerical processes used in the 1940 US census. After the Second World War, Deming worked for the Supreme Command of the Allied Powers in Tokyo, assisting with their preparation for a census of Japan to be conducted in 1951.

As Deming worked in Japan, a number of Japanese engineers began to wonder whether the methods of Shewhart might be used to make Japanese industry more productive. In March of 1950, Deming was invited to be an advisor to the Japanese Union of Scientists and Engineers (JUSE) and began teaching senior managers and engineers the principles of statistical process control. He became convinced that the Japanese, who had not historically produced internationally competitive products, could successfully "invade the markets of the world" within five years if they committed themselves to the principles of total quality management. Deming's conviction was largely realized. In 1960, Deming was honored by the Japanese Emperor with the Second Order of the Sacred Treasure for his teachings to Japanese industry.

Deming was a bald man with a large forehead and thick dark-framed glasses who aptly fit the stereotypic caricature of an "egghead." His written sentences are short and choppy, and his tone, impatient. His writing has a restless urgency that propels the reader onward. Deming's lifetime of consultative experience with dozens of manufacturing and service industries gives his work a credibility unmatched by today's quality consultants.

Joseph M, Juran (1904-) was born in poverty in Romania and emigrated at age five to the United States. He obtained a BS in engineering from the University of Minnesota and went to work for Bell Telephone at the massive Hawthorne Works in Illinois, rising slowly through the ranks and eventually being appointed as one of two engineers for the emerging Inspection Statistical Department.

Juran introduced the Pareto diagram into quality management, encouraging managers to first concentrate on the *vital few* (the 20% of causes that lead to 80% of problems) and leave other causes—the *trivial many*—for later.[8] In comparison to Deming, Juran took a less statistical and more strategic approach to the management of quality. He defined a role for upper-level management that involved quality planning, but did not require as much familiarity with statistical principles.

Kaoru Ishikawa served as president of JUSE and developed a core training program in quality management that included seven quality tools he believed all employees should be taught. Many of these tools are illustrated in Figure 1. Ishikawa is also credited with the development of quality circles and the cause-and-effect diagram.[13]

Key Points

Quality Exists Only in Relation to the Customer

Total quality management defines quality as something that satisfies the consumer's needs. Any activity or process that does not help address a customer's needs is unnecessary. However, the TQM movement recognizes that customers cannot always articulate their needs, and that producers may be in a better position than customers to develop effective solutions. The TQM approach therefore encourages a rich and iterative exchange between customer and supplier, in which the two work together to develop better and better solutions to addressing the customer's needs.

Internal Customers and Suppliers

> ### Exhibit 3. Identifying Customer and Supplier Relationships
>
> **Your Department**
> Where in the total organizational structure does your department fit? What products and services does it provide? What processes are used to provide these products and services? What would be the effect if your department stopped producing its products and services?
>
> **You**
> Where do you fit into your department? What is your job? What do you create or produce? How do you do this? How do you know if you produce good or poor results (ie, are there standards or criteria for good performance)? How are the standards established?
>
> **Your Customers**
> Who are your immediate customers (the individuals who receive directly the products or services that you produce)? How do your customers use what you produce? What would happen if you did not do your job right? How do you find out if you are not meeting the needs or requirements of your customers (eg, from the customer, your boss, reports)? How far beyond your immediate customer can you trace the effects of what you do? How is your work initiated (eg, assignment from boss, request of customer, self initiated)?
>
> **Your Suppliers**
> Who supplies you with material, information, and services that you need to do your job? What would happen if your suppliers did not do their jobs? Do they have performance standards? How do their errors affect you? How do they find out if they are not meeting your needs or requirements? Are you working with them? Are you fulfilling your obligations to them?

Total quality management conceptualizes business as a value stream in which each operation receives input from suppliers, adds value, and passes the resulting product along to the customer. A particular department's "suppliers" and "customers" may be found within a single organization—not every department deals with external suppliers or external customers. Deming used several questions, which appear in Exhibit 3, to help individuals and departments identify their suppliers and customers, and the type of value they provide.[14] These questions might fruitfully be posed to any clinical laboratory employee or section manager. They can help focus a department's quality management activities on immediate customers within an organization, particularly when the ultimate consumer is too distant to identify.

Central Importance of Statistical Process Control

Although the technical solutions to improving quality vary with each industry and process, the primary method for improving quality in the TQM framework is statistical process control. Deming identified 14 points that he believed essential to creating an atmosphere in which statistical process control could flourish (Exhibit 4). Many of these points require abandonment of management practices still used today, such as always purchasing supplies from the lowest bidder, holding individuals accountable for system problems, or managing to numerical goals and quotas. Deming provided specific examples of continuous quality improvement efforts that failed to take hold because managers ignored statistical control principles or some of his 14 points. In his own words:

> A program of improvement sets off with enthusiasm, exhortations, revival meetings, posters, pledges, [but no statistical process control]. Quality becomes a religion. Quality...shows at first dramatic improvement, better and better by the month. Everyone expects the path of improvement to continue... Instead, success grinds to a halt. At best, the curve levels off. It may even [deteriorate]... Despondence sets in. Management naturally becomes worried. They plead, beg, beseech, implore, pray, intrigue, supplicate heads of the organizations involved in production and assembly with taunts, harassment, threats, based on the awful truth that if there be not substantial improvement, and soon, we shall be out of business.
>
> What has happened? The rapid and encouraging improvement seen at first came from removal of special causes, detected by horse sense. All this was fairly simple. But as obvious sources of improvement dried up, the curve of improvement leveled off and became stable at an unacceptable level.
>
> It is interesting to note that when an attempt at improvement commences with the program of action in the 14 points...the curve of improvement follows for the first few months or even as long as two years about the same curve as the one shown. The difference is that with a sound program, the curve for improvement of quality and productivity does not level off. Improvement continues so long as the management leads the program.[15]

Exhibit 4. Deming's 14 Points for Management of Quality

1. Create constancy of purpose for improvement of product and service.

2. Adopt the new philosophy.

3. Cease dependence on mass inspection; build quality into production processes.

4. End the practice of awarding business on price tag alone. Instead, reduce total cost.

5. Constantly and forever improve the system of production and service.

6. Institute training on the job.

7. Institute leadership and supervision.

8. Drive out fear; create trust.

9. Break down barriers within the organization.

10. Eliminate slogans, exhortations, and targets for the work force, asking for zero defects and new levels of productivity. Instead, focus on the system.

11. Eliminate numerical goals and quotas. Eliminate management by objectives. Substitute leadership.

12. Remove barriers that hinder the hourly worker and manager and rob them of pride in their work.

13. Institute a vigorous program of education and self-improvement.

14. Engage everyone from top management down to accomplish the transformation.

Quality Planning

Total quality management requires the active involvement of an organization's leadership. However, as TQM developed it became clear that leaders could not effectively involve themselves with improving individual production processes or applying statistical techniques. Instead, Juran emphasized leadership's role in quality oversight, which he called "quality planning." Planning for quality included setting the proper ethical tone—the enterprise truthfully represents its products to consumers, takes affirmative steps to make its products conform to contractual specifications, and accepts responsibility for quality failures. Planning also requires that leadership take responsibility for the design of products so that they meet customers' needs, and for seeing that control functions are in place to ensure quality and correct deficiencies.

Appraisal of Total Quality Management

Total quality management has a proven track record in hundreds of manufacturing companies and dozens of service organizations. Total quality management assumes different forms in different industries (see, for example, the next section on the Toyota Production System), but it is difficult to take issue with any approach to quality that has demonstrated such widespread effectiveness over the course of several generations.[16]

While TQM has many successes, TQM has only limited penetration in the health care industry. Health care has a paternalistic tradition, and the definition of quality is not easily ceded to the customer by professionals who believe they "know better."

On a more practical level, fully implementing TQM requires that management make fundamental changes in many time-honored practices, particularly in customer and supplier relations and in human resource practices. When the laboratory is part of a larger organization such as a hospital, these changes must usually be made throughout the organization, rather than only within the laboratory.

Toyota Production System (Lean Production)[17]

The Toyota Production System (TPS) does not represent a distinct philosophical approach to managing quality. Instead, TPS provides a particularly salient example of total quality management applied within an individual company. The Toyota Production System has been studied in detail by a number of authors,[18-20] and the application of TQM at Toyota over the course of more than half a century has resulted in the development of production methods and an organizational culture that have relevance for the clinical laboratory industry today. The term *lean production* was applied to Toyota's methods by three enterprising business authors who published several well-written and widely read analyses of Toyota's production methods in the 1990s.[19] Today the term lean production refers to any production process based on the methods applied at Toyota.

The Toyota Production System has some unique characteristics, but many TPS elements can be found in other organizations within and outside of Japan. For example, just-in-time inventory management is well developed at the Dell computer corporation, and continuous flow practices are being applied in many industries, including histopathology laboratories.[21]

History

Four individuals played pivotal roles in developing the Toyota Production System: Sakichi Toyoda, who founded the Toyoda Group in 1902; Kiichiro Toyoda (son of Sakichi Toyoda), who headed the automobile manufacturing operation between 1936 and 1950; Eiji Toyoda (nephew of Sakichi Toyoda), who became managing director in 1950 and chairman in 1981; and Taiichi Ohno, founder of the *Kanban* system of just-in-time production and inventory management.[22]

Sakichi Toyoda invented a power loom in 1926 that automatically shut down when a thread snapped, preventing production of poor quality material. He later sold his automatic loom patents to a company in England to finance an automobile manufacturing operation, which he launched with his son Kiichiro. At the time, Ford Motor Company was the largest manufacturer of automobiles in Japan, and Kiichiro traveled to Ford's River Rouge plant outside of Detroit and spent a year studying the American automotive industry. He returned with a determination to adapt the system to smaller production quantities, which required a predictable supply of inventory and rapid change over of dies and other heavy equipment. The system was referred to as *just-in-time* within the Toyoda Group.

Eiji Toyoda, a nephew of Sakichi Toyoda, also traveled to the United States to study the American automotive industry. He learned about Ford's employee suggestion system and used it as the basis for the Toyota commitment to continuous improvement (*Kaizen*).

Taiichi Ohno joined the Toyoda Automatic Loom Works after graduating from Nogoya Technical High School in 1932 and expanded upon the just-in-time concepts developed by Kiichito Toyoda to reduce waste. Ohno recognized the central importance of managing inventory and worked out important production timing problems so that the task performed by each worker in an assembly line required the same amount of time. This enabled work to progress using a rhythmic coordinated series of handoffs. Although Ohno is credited with developing much of the Toyota Production System, he himself indicated that most of the credit belonged to Henry Ford and to the supply systems developed by US supermarkets to stock store shelves in the 1950s.

Key Points

Scholars who have studied the Toyota Production System do not agree upon all of TPS' essential features, but the following elements are regularly emphasized.

Rigid Specification of Work Methods

Each job is defined and documented in great detail, down to the direction in which a worker will turn before performing an assembly operation.

Simple and Direct Internal Handoffs

Transfer of work from one station to another is accomplished using well-defined processes that often employ *visual controls*—simple signals that new work has arrived. A visual control might consist of placing a component to be installed in a specified location where it can be easily seen. Workflow of the entire line is often displayed on a lighted board that all employees in a plant can easily see. The development of simple methods for transferring work allows each station in the assembly process to "pull" work from the preceding station.

Defined Connections With Customers and Suppliers

External handoffs from suppliers to Toyota are simple and rigidly defined, as are handoffs from Toyota to retailers or consumers. In this manner, customers pull product from the manufacturing operation, and the manufacturing operation pulls material from external suppliers.

Kanban (Just-in-Time)

The net result of defining the activity of each work station, ensuring that the activities performed at each work station take the same amount of time, and the act of pulling product through the organization allows the production process to achieve smooth, near-continuous flow, which in turn minimizes the requirement for on-site inventory. Supplies arrive "just in time," markedly reducing storage requirements and capital tied up in inventory.

Jidoka

Jidoka refers to building quality into the production process to minimize the potential for human error. For example, a parts basket might be designed with an electronic sensor that records when a part needed for engine assembly is removed from the basket. This sensor is connected to the engine assembly line so as to prevent engines from being transferred on to the next workstation if a worker forgets to remove a required part from the basket. In another example, a worker can stop the entire automobile production line when trouble appears at one station, to ensure that the orderly sequence of assembly is not disrupted.

Kaizen

Kaizen refers to a commitment to continuous incremental improvement. Improvements are made by teams called *quality control circles* (almost never by individuals acting alone). QC circles generally include a teacher who helps the team apply scientific methods and statistical quality control. QC circles form and disband spontaneously, often with only low-level management oversight; change is made at the lowest possible level in the organization.

Appraisal of the Toyota Production System

The Toyota Production System (lean manufacturing) has produced a track record of quality and economy that cannot be ignored. The concepts applied in TPS are not intellectually demanding but turn out to be difficult to apply in practice. Strict standardization of work methods and handoffs, simplification of work pathways, devolving quality management to low-level QC circles, instituting pull relationships with customers and suppliers, and developing "self-healing" production processes that automatically prevent defective work from advancing down the production line are in some ways at odds with the American ethos, which places a high value on individual autonomy and accountability. Further, the *batch-and-queue* approach to mass-fabrication has a long and storied history in the United States and is difficult to replace with the *continuous flow* approach to production used in the Toyota Production System. To illustrate the difficulties of applying lean production in the laboratory environment, readers might ask themselves whether histotechnologists will agree to process surgical specimens individually as they come into the department, rather than wait for batches to accumulate before grossing, processing, embedding, sectioning, staining, and cover slipping. How eagerly will pathologists agree to interpret individual cases as they come out of the histology laboratory, without waiting for a few "trays" of slides to accumulate?

We believe the simplification and rigid standardization of work processes and handoffs has much to offer the clinical laboratory. But other elements of TPS may be difficult to adopt in a laboratory so long as caregivers and suppliers remain committed to performing work in batches.

It is interesting to note that within the Toyota corporation itself, many of the key methods for producing quality product have never been written down. Nor can Toyota's key methods be articulated by most of Toyota's workers.[20] Toyota's success appears to rely on an implicit, almost cultural commitment to systematic quality improvement that is widely shared, but not centrally orchestrated. This observation should give pause to managers who believe quality is best assured by creating company-wide quality management documents or a laboratory-wide quality management program.

COSO

Manuals and textbooks about laboratory quality typically do not reference literature from the accounting profession. However, the revelation of several well-publicized quality failures within clinical laboratories due to negligence and fraud have caused us to look beyond the medical literature for more robust approaches to quality management. The auditing industry has studied the causes of fraud and negligence and developed several approaches to help managers and governance assure the reliability of financial reporting. Some of this thinking is applicable to the management of quality in the clinical laboratory.

History

The Committee of Sponsoring Organizations of the Treadway Commission (COSO) was formed in 1985 as an alliance of five professional organizations: Financial Executives International, the American Accounting Association, the American Institute of Certified Public Accountants, the Institute of Internal Auditors, and the Institute of Management Accountants (formerly the National Association of Accountants). COSO convened a commission headed by James C. Treadway, Jr., to report on fraudulent financial reporting. The Commission issued its landmark report in October 1987.[23] The report studied "causal factors that can lead to fraudulent financial reporting" and identified ways to reduce their incidence.

The Treadway Commission based its report on extensive research and interviews with experts in all stages of the financial reporting process, including individuals within management, audit committees, external and internal auditors, regulators and educators, and other outside advisors. The Commission then provided each of these groups with recommendations based on the report's findings. At the time of its completion, the project was considered the most comprehensive study of its kind and is still referenced in the business community today.[24]

Subsequent to the publication of the Treadway Commission report, COSO conducted a seminal study of internal controls—the processes that managers use to exert control over an enterprise. The report, *Internal Control-Integrated Framework,* was first published in 1992.[25] This multi-volume report offered users a definition of internal controls and a guide to assessing and improving a company's internal control systems.

Key Points

Although intended primarily for the accounting and business community, *Internal Control-Integrated Framework* provides a useful framework for quality management. It identifies five essential components of internal control that form the basis of all good quality management programs: (1) a control environment, (2) risk assessment, (3) control activities, (4) information and communication, and (5) monitoring.

The *control environment* is the "tone" of an organization—the integrity, ethical values, and operating style of managers and staff. Organizations with a good control environment set realistic goals that do not create undue pressure on management or staff. In the management of quality and patient safety, a good control environment encourages adherence to procedure, while at the same time empowering all employees to speak openly about quality or safety concerns.

Risk assessment involves the identification and analysis of risks that might cause an organization not to meet its objectives. Risk assessment also forms a basis for determining how risks should be managed. Risks that can compromise clinical laboratory quality and patient safety are manifold; they include improperly identified specimens, improper transmission of orders, defective analytic reagents or equipment, fatigued or ill-trained operators, and misrouted or ambiguous reports, among many others. Major risks to clinical laboratory quality are discussed in chapter 5.

Control activities are the policies, procedures, and inventions that address and mitigate risks. Control activities occur throughout the organization, at all levels and in all functions. In the clinical laboratory, they include a range of activities as diverse as preventative maintenance of machinery, quality testing of new reagent lots, external laboratory proficiency testing, competency testing for staff, credentialing and privileging of pathologists, segregation of duties, and correlation of current and historical findings.

Information and communication involves the identification, acquisition, and dissemination of information in a form and time frame that enable people to carry out their control responsibilities. In the context of laboratory quality, this means that information about quality problems are shared widely within the organization and are seen by individuals in a position to correct the problems.

Monitoring involves the periodic assessment of how well the organization's control systems perform over time. In the clinical laboratory, monitoring may take the form of monthly or quarterly tabulations of particular problems (such as is carried out in the CAP Q-Tracks program) or a special one-time audit undertaken to explore quality in an area that had not been previously studied (such as a CAP Q-Probes study). Some monitoring is internal and some monitoring external (such as external inspections and proficiency testing).

Appraisal of the COSO Framework

The COSO framework places a healthy emphasis on organizational tone and ethics, encouraging reporting of quality deviations detected at any level in an organization. The framework emphasizes the explicit identification of risks, which helps focus quality management efforts on areas with the greatest need. The accounting profession also recognizes that individuals placed under too much pressure or provided with too much temptation may not follow proscribed procedures or behave honestly. An emphasis on *segregation of duties* (with individuals checking one another's work) and other control mechanisms helps reduce temptation to act in a manner that may compromise quality or patient safety. In a clinical laboratory, bench technologists perform a check on the integrity of management, much as managers check the integrity of their organizational subordinates.

An obvious limitation of the COSO framework is that it was designed to provide an organization with financial controls and as such offers only generic guidance to laboratory managers interested in controlling quality. The College of American Pathologists, JCAHO, the Clinical and Laboratory Standards Institute (CLSI [formerly NCCLS]), and the International Organization for Standardization (ISO) provide more laboratory-specific guidance. More fundamentally, the COSO system is designed to manage an organization to the objectives of administrators and governance, rather than its customer. Some of the other schools of quality management take a different approach, placing the customer's objectives first. Finally, COSO has little to say about how to design workflow to reinforce quality and minimize errors; too often, reliance is placed on a separate monitoring function to detect problems rather than redesign of work processes to prevent problems from occurring in the first place. In accounting, errors discovered after the fact can usually be corrected; in medicine, this may not be possible, and prevention is preferable.

Consensus Standards

One approach to managing quality in the clinical laboratory is to ensure that operations conform to written consensus standards developed by standards-creating organizations. Written standards are typically developed by large groups of knowledgeable individuals who have carefully considered areas where quality may be compromised.

In this section, we describe the efforts of two large standards organizations—ISO and CLSI (formerly NCCLS)—to formulate written quality standards for the clinical laboratory. ISO and CLSI, along with CAP, JCAHO, and CLIA regulations, have gone the furthest in identifying risks to the practice of high-quality laboratory medicine and in suggesting controls that can be applied by laboratory management. ISO's and CLSI's contributions are discussed in this section. The College of American Pathologists, JCAHO, and CLIA are discussed in the next chapter because they relate to regulatory compliance in the United States.

History

ISO

The International Organization for Standardization (ISO) is the world's largest developer of standards.[26] Founded in 1947 as an outgrowth of the National Standardizing Association, which focused on mechanical engineering and disbanded during World War II, ISO is a nongovernmental network of the national standards institutes of 146 countries. National standards organizations from most major developed nations are members of ISO. The United States is represented by the American National Standards Institute (ANSI).

ISO standards are developed by technical committees comprising experts on loan from the industrial, scientific, and business sectors. Several United States laboratorians serve on ISO technical committees. Approved ISO standards are assigned unique numbers; when citing the standard, the number is sometimes followed by the year in which the standard was approved.

The major ISO standards relevant to quality management in clinical laboratories are the ISO 9000 series and ISO 15189.

The ISO 9000 series is a family of generic standards concerned with quality management, which ISO defines as what an organization does to (1) meet customer quality needs, (2) meet applicable regulatory requirements, and (3) continually improve performance. ISO 9000 specifies attributes that must be demonstrated by every organization's quality management systems, defines a number of quality-related terms, and provides information about auditing organizations (the process of checking that an organization's quality management systems conform to the ISO standard).

The ISO 9000 series was first published in 1987. The current version of ISO 9000 was released in 2000 (ISO 9001:2000). The three major documents in the ISO 9000 family are: ISO 9000:2000, Quality management systems – Fundamentals and vocabulary; ISO 9001:2000, Quality management systems – Requirements; and ISO 9004:2000, Quality management systems – Guidelines for performance improvements. The ISO 9001 quality system "requirements" document can be applied to any organization, large or small, public or private, whatever its product—including "products" that are actually a service. ISO 9001 is applicable to private business enterprises, public organizations, and government departments. ISO 9001 concerns the way an organization goes about its work, but not with the result of this work (at least, not directly). While ISO 9001 lays down what requirements a quality system must meet, it does not dictate how standards should be met in a particular organization, which leaves flexibility for implementation in different business sectors and different national cultures. In 2003, more than half a million organizations were registered as having quality systems compliant with ISO 9001:2000 (sometimes referred to as ISO 9001-certified). The United States ranks sixth among nations in the number of ISO: 9001-certified organizations.

In 2003, ISO published a quality standard specific to medical laboratories, ISO 15189:2003. Based on the ISO 9000 series, ISO 15189 specifies particular requirements for medical laboratories to demonstrate quality and competence.[27] The standard covers all aspects of laboratory operation, including patient preparation and identification, the collection and examination of clinical samples, and the maintenance of employee competence. Some nations require ISO 15189 accreditation of a laboratory in a manner more or less analogous to CAP accreditation in the United States, although third parties (rather than ISO itself) will accredit laboratories as being compliant with the ISO 15189 standard. The CAP plans to offer an ISO certification option to laboratories that wish to document that they meet ISO 15189:2003 standards. ISO certification is not required in the United States.

Clinical and Laboratory Standards Institute

The Clinical and Laboratory Standards Institute (CLSI, formerly NCCLS) was formed in 1967 as the National Committee on Clinical Laboratory Standards; the organization changed its name to CLSI in 2005. CLSI is a global (but primarily US-based), nonprofit, standards-developing organization for the health care community. Standards are developed through an involved consensus process that includes representatives from industry, academia, and the provider community. CLSI became accredited by the National Bureau of Standards (currently the National Institute for Standards and Technology [NIST]) in the 1970s. Initially involved with housing the National Reference System for the Clinical Laboratory (a set of reference methods designed to improve comparability of test results), the organization moved on to develop its own laboratory standards and guidelines in the 1980s. CLSI standards have met with varying acceptance in the laboratory community. Some standards are little known. Others, such as CLSI standards in clinical microbiology, have become *de facto* interpretive standards for antimicrobial susceptibility testing in the United States.[28]

Because the CLSI consensus processes takes time, the organization often publishes draft or proposed versions of standards or guidelines, sometimes years before their final adoption. CLSI documents are designated by a one- or two-letter prefix that indicates the type of standard (eg, HS = healthcare services, M = microbiology), the number of the standard, a suffix letter that indicates the document's status (A = approved, P = proposed), and a suffix number that indicates the edition (if more than one edition exists). Thus, HS01-A2 falls within the health services section (HS), is the first standard/guideline within the section (01), has been approved (A), and has been released as a second edition (2).

In addition to developing its own standards, CLSI serves as the secretariat for (administers) the ISO Technical Committee on Clinical Laboratory Testing and in vitro Diagnostic Test Systems (ISO/TC 212) for ANSI. CLSI has fostered a global approach to its standards and has aligned itself with the ISO series of documents.

CLSI has published three guidelines of particular relevance to quality management in the laboratory:

- ❖ HS01-A2. *A Quality Management System Model for Health Care*
- ❖ GP26-A3. *Application of a Quality Management System Model for Laboratory Services*
- ❖ GP22-A2. *Continuous Quality Improvement: Integrating Five Key Quality System Components*

Key Points

Quality Management Systems

ISO and CLSI provide a distinctive approach to quality management, emphasizing the adoption of systems. Whereas CLIA '88 and the CAP emphasize specific quality activities to be performed (such as monitoring refrigerator temperatures or incoming reagents), and whereas statistical process control requires the application of certain quality methods (such as using control charts), ISO and CLSI emphasize the operation of certain systems within an organization. The systems required of laboratories by ISO and CLSI are shown in Exhibit 5.[29] CLSI systems are referred to as quality system essentials (QSE).

Policies, Processes, and Procedures

CLSI distinguishes between policies, processes, and procedures. *Policy* specifies intent and direction for the organization. An example of a policy might be a laboratory's commitment to issue a corrected report within one hour of an error being identified. A *process* describes the sequence of specific activities that will transform a policy into action. A process might be a flow chart describing the sequence of activities, from the discovery of a laboratory error to the issuing of a corrected report. Processes are often depicted diagrammatically or with a table that enumerates the sequence of activities and the individual responsible for each activity. A *procedure* documents instructions for how a specific activity should be carried out by an individual. A procedure might list the steps required to issue a corrected report in the laboratory information system.

Exhibit 5. Quality Systems	
CLSI Quality System Essentials	**ISO 9001:2000 Quality Systems**
Organization	General Management Commitment Quality Policy Planning Responsibility, Authority, and Communication Management Review Provision of Resources
Personnel	Human Resources
Equipment	Control of Measuring and Monitoring Devices
Purchasing and Inventory	Purchasing
Process Control	Planning and Product Realization Customer-Related Processes Design and Development Production and Service Provision
Documents and Records	Documentation Requirements
Information Management	Analysis of Data
Occurrence Management	Control of Nonconforming Product
Assessments	General Monitoring and Measurement
Process Improvement	Improvement
Customer Service and Satisfaction	Customer Focus
Facilities and Safety	Infrastructure Work Environment

Path of Workflow and Patient Safety

CLSI emphasizes the importance of documenting and optimizing the laboratory "path of workflow." This path of workflow begins outside the laboratory's boundaries, with a caregiver's request for a laboratory examination, and ends outside the laboratory's boundaries, when the laboratory result influences a provider's decision making. In CLSI's view, many patient safety problems arise because the actual path of workflow in a laboratory is poorly understood and does not correspond to the idealized workflow path imagined by management.

Risk Assessment

Both ISO and CLSI identify specific risks to which clinical laboratories are vulnerable. Many of these risks are discussed in chapter 5.

Appraisal of the ISO and CLSI Framework

ISO and CLSI recognize that quality failures may occur on many levels. A laboratory may have well-developed procedures and adequately trained staff, but might have an inadequate path for workflow, with poorly defined handoffs that result in lost specimens and unnecessary delay. Each ISO and CLSI quality system is designed to address a type of vulnerability. The ISO and CLSI conception of quality is therefore sophisticated and robust.

On the other hand, both ISO and CLSI have been criticized as lacking specificity. It is not clear from reading ISO or CLSI standards exactly what the laboratory manager should do. Two clinical laboratories could follow CLSI guidelines and find themselves with very different quality programs that have little overlap. Outside of the United States, ISO accrediting organizations have been criticized for lack of consistency in applying ISO standards, a shortcoming that in part reflects the generic nature of ISO standards. ISO and CLSI standards have also been criticized for placing too much emphasis on structure and process, with too little attention applied to the outcome of care. Finally, some authorities have questioned whether promoting adherence to "paper standards" is the best route to ensuring quality. The quality-promoting interventions used in the Toyota Production System, while in many ways compatible with ISO standards, were created by a distinctive culture, without any reference to a set of paper standards.

Failure Mode and Effects Analysis / Root Cause Analysis[30]

History

Failure mode and effects analysis (FMEA) was developed as an engineering tool to reduce the potential for failures in complex systems. Although every inventor tries to anticipate what could go wrong with a new design, an organized process for evaluating prospectively the potential for system failure was first formalized in 1949 with the introduction of military procedure MIL-P-1629, which describes the FMEA process.[31] Failure mode and effects analysis was used for aerospace and rocket development, and was adopted in the 1970s by the Society of Automotive Engineers (SAE standard J1739) for the prospective analysis of potential automotive safety failures.

Fundamentally, FMEA evaluates each individual step in a process, or component in a design, for its potential to fail and cause harm. Today, a number of health care organizations have adapted FMEA to identify potential failures in clinical processes. Most notable of these is the Veterans Administration effort, which introduced a form of FMEA in 2001 called the Healthcare Failure Mode and Effects Analysis (HFMEA™).[32]

Root cause analysis differs from failure mode and effects analysis in that it is applied retrospectively, after a significant adverse event has already occurred. The goal of a root cause analysis is to find out what happened, why it happened, and what can be done to prevent it from happening again. Unlike FMEA, root cause analysis was not formalized as a quality improvement technique by the military, and proponents of root cause analysis recommend different approaches to determine the root causes of problems.

Key Points

Classic FMEA

A failure mode and effects analysis involves assembling a multidisciplinary team to prospectively evaluate a process or design. Individuals who participate in the FMEA should have subject matter expertise and daily experience with the process under evaluation. The FMEA team is responsible for identifying the major steps in the process that are subject to failure. Flow-charting the process helps identify individual steps and their relationship to outcomes. Each type of failure that could conceivably occur in the process or system is termed a *failure mode*. Once the different failure modes are identified they are listed on a work sheet that is used for scoring. Each failure mode is scored in terms of: (1) *severity*, the magnitude of the problem that will result if failure occurs; (2) *occurrence*, the likelihood that the failure will occur; and (3) *detectability*, the likelihood that a failure will be detected in time to prevent adverse consequences.

Scores for each component range from 1 to 5. Classically, each failure mode is then assigned a *risk priority number*, or RPN, which is the product of the severity, likelihood, and detection ratings. The higher the RPN, the more critical the step to patient safety. Steps with high RPN scores are redesigned by reworking the process to decrease the consequences of failure or the likelihood of failure, or by instituting safety checks to promote the timely detection of failure before care is impacted.

Modern FMEA

Today, FMEA places less emphasis on improving the detection of failure and more emphasis on preventing failures from occurring. Instead of an RPN, a *criticality score* or *hazard score* is calculated for each failure mode. The criticality/hazard score is the product of the failure mode's severity and its likelihood of occurring. Attention is focused on correcting failure modes with the highest criticality/hazard score.

Cumulative Effect of Vulnerabilities

The probabilistic underpinnings of FMEA make clear how processes that are composed of multiple sequential steps will fail frequently, even when each step in the process is highly reliable. For example, a process composed of 25 sequential steps, each with a 99.9% success rate, still has more than a 2% chance of failure if each step in the process requires the successful execution of the preceding step. The cumulative effect of individual vulnerabilities argues for redesigning processes so they are simpler and can withstand the failure of one or two individual steps.

Root Cause Analysis

Like FMEA, a root cause analysis is conducted by an interdisciplinary team, involving experts from frontline services. The team conducting the root cause analysis is expected to dig deeply into the circumstances surrounding an event to identify factors that caused a problem. Identifying root causes may be difficult. For example, "human error" is not considered a root cause. Instead, root cause analysis posits that every instance of human error has at least one preceding (underlying) cause. This may be the omission of a step in a written medical procedure, fatigue due to inadequate rest, or engagement in at-risk behavior (performing a task by memory instead of using a checklist). In addition to root causes, contributing factors that allowed the root cause to produce an adverse event may be identified.

To be credible, a root cause analysis is supposed to include participation by the leadership of an organization as well as those most closely involved in the processes. The root cause analysis should be impartial and impersonal, focusing on problems with systems rather than with individuals. A credible root cause analysis should include consideration of the relevant literature as well as the facts surrounding a particular case.

Appraisal of Root Cause and Failure Mode and Effects Analysis

Failure mode and effects analysis and root cause analysis help organizations think about vulnerabilities using a disciplined approach. However, both present some practical problems in health care. For example, the Joint Commission on Accreditation of Healthcare Organizations (JCAHO) requires accredited hospitals to perform at least one proactive risk assessment annually, using FMEA or another forward-looking method.[33] Although FMEA may be a powerful tool for proactive analysis of potential failures, there are so many activities that go on in a typical hospital that the performance of a single failure mode and effects analysis per year will leave many patient safety vulnerabilities unexamined. Further, rating the consequences of a system failure may be difficult in medicine because some failures increase organizational cost while others compromise patient health. Combining cost and health data into a single scale may be problematic.[34] Finally, individuals participating on a FMEA team often are asked to reassign their responsibilities to other workers during the failure mode and effects analysis; this may not be practical in many health care settings. To reduce the time spent in failure mode and effects analysis, it has been recommended that an FMEA "super-user" be present to facilitate the process.

The Joint Commission on Accreditation of Healthcare Organizations also requires JCAHO-accredited hospitals to perform a credible root cause analysis within 45 days of any *sentinel event*—an event that caused death or serious patient injury. The value of root cause analysis in health care has been questioned by some authors. Routine use of root cause analysis as a patient safety strategy may be wasteful in situations where analysis is unlikely to reveal remediable "errors" or to suggest better systems of care that will prevent errors. Hofer and Hayward[35] point out that the ability to establish causality through *post hoc* review is the linchpin behind the recommendation for widespread root cause analysis of sentinel events. When causality cannot be established, as is often the case in complex care scenarios, it is impossible to know whether any changes adopted as a result of the root cause review will be effective. In our own practices, we have had mixed experience with root cause analysis. Some root cause analyses have been useful in elucidating causes and suggesting particular remedies; others have not been particularly helpful.

Monitoring

Monitoring the performance of operations is part of every sensible approach to quality management. Monitoring helps determine whether processes that once functioned adequately have drifted out of control and are in need of corrective action. Monitoring also helps determine whether recently implemented process improvements had their desired impact.

But can monitoring, in and of itself, *improve* performance? In other words, will the simple act of monitoring a process improve its quality without any other intervention? There is some evidence that individuals perform better when they know their performance is being measured, although the literature needs to be interpreted cautiously.

History

In 1898, an experimental psychologist and bicycling enthusiast named Norman Triplett reported that the performance of bicycle racers varied with different types of competition.[36] Fastest speeds were obtained when cyclists were pitted against one another. The next best times were recorded when the riders were being paced by a tandem cycle, and worst performances occurred when a cyclist raced only against the clock. Triplett believed that the physical presence of competitors was responsible for these differences. He conducted a second experiment with 40 school-age children who were asked to turn a fishing reel as fast as possible for a short period of time. Children who worked in pairs had superior performance to those who worked alone, even though every subject had an identical reel to turn.

The phenomenon described by Triplett—improved performance in social settings—was later termed *social facilitation*. Triplett studied performance in the presence of coactors who were engaged in the same task as a subject. But in 1900, Meumann demonstrated that performance could also be improved when subjects were tested in the presence of a passive audience.[37] Subjects in an exercise workout room demonstrated greater exercise tolerance when exposed to spectators than when exercising alone.

Social facilitation has been studied by psychologists under a wide range of conditions, including a variety of competitive and noncompetitive tasks, with subjects variously aware of one another's presence. Social facilitation has even been demonstrated in several animal species (for example, chickens eat more grain when in the vicinity of other chickens).

A landmark study that illustrates social facilitation in the work setting was conducted in the 1920s and early 1930s at the Western Electric Hawthorne Works plant in Cicero, Illinois.[38] One of the conclusions from the Hawthorne Works experiments is called the *Hawthorne effect* and describes improved performance produced by the psychological stimulus of being singled-out in the work setting and made to feel important.

The first phase of the Hawthorne Works studies, known as the Illumination Experiments, was conducted between 1924 and 1927 under the direction of Vannevar Bush. The purpose of the study was to find the level of illumination that made the work of female coil winders most efficient. Workers were divided into test and control groups. Lighting for the test group was increased systematically from 24 to 70 foot-candles. Production of the test group increased as expected, but production of the control group increased approximately the same amount.

Harvard University School of Business professors Elton Mayo and Fritz Roethlisberger were recruited to explain these curious findings. They conducted a second phase of tests, called the Relay Assembly Test Room Experiments, between 1927 and 1932. Mayo selected six women for the test whose prior relay assembly production rates were known. These women were assigned to a special test room and worked under different test conditions. Their production rate was monitored automatically; as each woman completed assembly of a relay, she dropped the relay down a chute, activating an electric counter.

The experiments consisted of 23 changes in the working environment. Production of relays increased no matter how physical conditions were varied. In fact, when conditions were returned to their original state, productivity remained 25% above its original value. Mayo concluded that attention from investigators and interaction among group members, rather than the work conditions themselves, were responsible for the subject's increased productivity.[39]

Key Points

Types of Tasks

Social facilitation tends to be most pronounced with easy or well-rehearsed ("overlearned") tasks, such as drawing blood or performing order entry. The presence of an audience or coactors may interfere with effectiveness in performing complex or less-familiar tasks—a phenomenon familiar to anyone who has experienced stage fright. Therefore the use of monitoring as a tool to stimulate quality improvement is most effective when applied to well-defined, simple, and familiar processes.

Extinction

The Hawthorne effect typically diminishes over time, usually after 3 to 24 months. The psychological arousal that initially enhances performance moderates as operators become used to being observed or operating in a social group. When monitored performance improves steadily over the course of more than two years, the improvement is unlikely to be due to social facilitation. In the majority of CAP Q-Tracks studies, in which laboratories committed to continuously monitor an aspect of laboratory quality over time, continued program participation has been associated with improved performance over the course of more than four years.[40] In these cases, more than the Hawthorne effect is at work.

Communication

The beneficial effects of monitoring are most pronounced when the results of monitoring are widely communicated. Private feedback of monitoring results to individual operators will not provide the same degree of psychological stimulation as sharing the results from each operator with a larger group.

Benchmarks

Quality performance in laboratories is commonly compared to past local performance or to industry benchmarks. Benchmarks are useful for managers interested in determining whether a local quality or safety problem exists. However, there is no evidence that operator performance is enhanced by the incorporation of benchmarks into a monitoring program. In fact, some experimental psychology literature suggests that the benefits of social facilitation are diminished when an aggressive target is incorporated into a monitoring program.

Appraisal of Monitoring

Laboratories invariably engage in some quality monitoring simply to determine if performance meets industry norms or has deteriorated from previous levels. For example, in one of the authors' laboratories, ongoing monitoring of blood culture contamination revealed a spike in contamination rates when nurses in a patient care unit started drawing all of their blood cultures from indwelling catheters instead of using dedicated phlebotomy. Monitoring is very useful to determine whether changes made to production processes are having their intended effect. Concurrent monitoring can detect problems before results are released (such as when control samples are run along with patient specimens to test instrument performance, or concurrent second-pathologist review of surgical pathology diagnoses are performed to reduce diagnostic error rates). These types of monitoring are well-established practices of proven benefit.

In our view, however, the value of monitoring to motivate employees and drive organizational change is often overstated. The benefits of monitoring as a motivating force are modest and short lived, often extinguishing themselves when the novelty of being observed wears off. Use of monitoring as the primary strategy to improve quality is rarely enough. Genuine quality improvement usually requires that procedures or processes be changed.

Passive monitoring of quality without any active intervention has been likened to the study of statistics about accidents. The study of accident statistics will teach you about the frequency of accidents at home or on the road or in the workplace, but will not reduce the frequency of accidents.

Human Error Research[41]

Many quality and patient safety problems encountered in clinical laboratories are the result of human errors—operators failing to follow a step in an established procedure or making an error in judgment. The playwright Aeschylus reminded his audience in the fifth century BC that even "the wisest of the wise may err." For the rest of us, errors are commonplace, and the damage they produce has stimulated inquiry into the factors that cause humans to blunder and whether changes to our work environment might reduce our propensity to err.

History and Classification of Error

The medical community has not made significant strides in understanding errors, in part because the profession has internalized a duty to perform faultlessly and is loathe to discuss errors openly. Error prevention in medicine has been characterized as following a *perfectibility model,* in which the elimination of errors is pursued through education and motivation.[42] Given the lack of understanding about error mechanisms in health care, it is fortunate that cognitive psychologists and human factors researchers in other disciplines have developed an understanding of human errors and approaches that can be used to minimize the impact of errors on quality. In general, these investigators accept the premise that humans err frequently, and that systems which rely on vigilance or error-free performance will inevitably fail.

The modern cognitive classification of errors was developed in the 1980s and 1990s and is attributed to Reason[43] and Rasmussen.[44] Errors are divided into two major types: (1) *errors of automatic action* (commonly referred to as *slips* and *lapses*), and (2) *errors of judgment* (commonly referred to as *mistakes*).

Errors of Automatic Action

As early as 1932, Bartlett[45] recognized that most purposeful human activity consists of automatic learned sequences of actions, which are executed unconsciously without express effort on the part of the actor. For example, putting on a shirt, dialing a familiar phone number, or entering the names of patients and tests into a computer all are unconscious, automatic, learned actions. Bartlett called these automatic action sequences *schemata* and found that a typical adult commits thousands of schemata to memory. Schemata are activated by conscious intention, but once activated, the sequence of action proceeds rapidly with little conscious thought. To carry out an automatic action correctly, an operator must understand how to execute a set of instructions he or she has learned, but need not understand the reasons behind them. Through training and practice, the operator becomes sufficiently proficient to perform actions without the need to refer repeatedly to directions. Most actions performed during activities of daily living (and at work in the laboratory) are automatic actions. When humans perform actions automatically, we are said to be operating in *schematic control mode.* Schematic control mode activity requires less mental effort than conscious purposeful action and allows tasks to be performed more rapidly than if each step had to be thought through.

Errors of automatic action are classified as either slips or lapses. Slips are execution errors, where an automatic action in a schemata is either incorrectly performed or is incorrectly added. They are errors of commission. Lapses involve the omission of an automatic action in a sequence. Both types of error are potentiated by loss of attentional stimuli or distractions.

Slips may take several forms. Among the most common are the following:

❖ *Capture slips* occur when an actor does something unintended because the actor fell into a more familiar pattern. For example, an order entry clerk might transcribe a test order into a computer with a "routine" priority instead of "stat" priority, because most of the tests he or she transcribes are ordered on a routine basis, and the keystroke sequence for ordering routine tests is more familiar than the keystroke sequence for ordering a stat request.

❖ *Associative activation slips* occur when an actor makes a faulty mental association between two stimuli. A technologist may be used to turning off a centrifuge when the centrifuge beeps. The technologist may erroneously turn off the centrifuge when the fire alarm is being tested, even though the fire alarm and centrifuge beep make very different sounds.

❖ *Loss of activation slips* occur when an actor loses track of the stimulus that initiated an action, due to temporary memory loss. For example, a pathologist may fail to order estrogen receptor analysis on a breast cancer because he or she was momentarily distracted by a telephone call.

Errors of Judgment

When situations are novel or are otherwise unsuited to the schematic control mode, humans operate in *attentional control mode*. The attentional control mode requires conscious thought (reasoning and judgment) and considerably more mental effort than the schematic control mode. An operator may make judgments by applying a decision rule that has been committed to memory (eg, "when the warning light goes on, the instrument is to be turned off") or may evaluate acquired knowledge using any number of more complex cognitive processes. The attentional control mode is much slower and less reliable than the schematic control mode but is adaptable to more varied situations.

Mistakes, or errors of attentional control mode, also take several forms:

❖ *Rule-based mistakes* occur when the wrong rule is chosen due to the misunderstanding of the situation or misapplication of the rule. For example, a clinician in the Emergency Department may be confused by a poorly formatted toxicology report that does not clearly distinguish between the patient's result (no drug detected) and reference information, which includes interpretive breakpoints for a positive drug screen (such as a listing of minimal drug concentrations that would be detected as "positive"). The physician incorrectly begins treatment for a drug overdose because he or she has misunderstood the situation and applied a decision rule for treating a drug intoxication that does not exist.

Application of a defective or poorly formulated rule is another form of rule-based mistake. For example, in anatomic pathology, there are many published rules and criteria to distinguish between atypical ductal hyperplasia and ductal carcinoma in situ of the breast; however, most of the rules are difficult to apply in practice and therefore very often result in diagnoses which are not reproducible.[46]

❖ *Knowledge-based errors* result from a lack of knowledge or from defective or "buggy" knowledge, inaccessibility of learned knowledge during a given situation, or misapplication of knowledge. Availability bias (choosing a course of action because it is the one that comes most readily to mind) and overconfidence bias (fixation on a particular course of action with active pursuit of supporting evidence and dismissal of contradictory evidence) are two common types of knowledge-based errors.

Active and Latent Errors

In addition to thinking about errors from a cognitive perspective, errors may be classified according to their impact. System engineers recognize two types of errors: active and latent.[47]

Active errors are errors whose effects are immediately felt (eg, a worker drops a tube of blood and it breaks; the specimen must be redrawn). Active errors occur at the so-called "sharp-end" of a chain of events—at the last interface between a human operator and a problem. When they occur, they usually are obvious and appear to have caused the problem at hand. Because of their proximity to a problem, operators who make active errors are often blamed. Active errors are difficult to anticipate and are therefore very difficult to prevent or eradicate.

Latent errors are errors that are embedded in a system upstream from the problem they produce. Latent errors are caused by faulty decisions that result in defective practices and procedures. These defective practices usually do not exert their ill effects until an unpredictable or unanticipated trigger or set of circumstances precipitates or catalyzes their negative consequences. They are not as obvious as the active error at the end of a chain of events; however, they often potentiate or cause the active error to occur. For example, a courier who breaks several specimens in the trunk of his vehicle while driving over a deep pothole committed an active error—driving without care. The manager of the couriers, who failed to install padded specimen holders in vehicle trunks to protect specimens against bumps, committed a latent error many months earlier. Exposing latent errors requires careful system analysis. Both failure mode and effects analysis and root cause analysis are methods that can effectively expose latent errors.

Human Factors Engineering

Human factors engineering, or ergonomics, is the study of physical, psychological, and physiological variables that affect human performance in an operational system. Human factors engineers study variables that impact upon human performance, and seek to optimize the design of the human-machine interface, respecting known limitations in human performance such as reliance on memory. The goal is to design instruments and technology that are "user friendly" and less error prone. Human factors engineers focus on the placement of instrument switches, knobs, dials, and indicator lights in arrays that are easily understood and which are naturally mapped so as to prevent error. For example, they have discovered that the use of multimodal switches (ie, switches that perform more than one function when other switches are pushed simultaneously) are very confusing to most operators and predispose to error. Human factors engineers try to use discrete switches for each function wherever possible.

Attention to human factors in the design and selection of laboratory instruments and technology defends against error. Usability testing and comparison of instruments with regard to their ease of use and propensity for human error is a necessary part of quality management in the laboratory.

The System Approach to Error Reduction

While it is impossible to eliminate all error, error can be defended against. Defending against error requires a *system approach,* rather than a *person approach.*[48] While the person approach to error focuses primarily on human operators as a cause for error, the system approach looks at all the blunt-end latent variables in a system that can cause error and seeks to eradicate those flaws. It does not focus primarily on the sharp-end, where the last human operator sits, because it is fundamentally easier to modify systemic latent flaws than it is to eliminate human fallibility, which is inherent in human performance (eg, poor memory, reaction to fatigue or stress).

The system approach views the human operator as just one part of the system in which he or she operates. Other parts of the system include its goals, the overall culture of the organization, technology, equipment, the physical environment, policies, and the procedures and variables that affect team function. All of these system components profoundly affect system fallibility.

Key Points

Researchers who have studied human errors and accidents in industry have developed robust recommendations that are applicable to the management of quality in clinical laboratories. Some of the most salient recommendations follow:

- ❖ Human error can never be eliminated. Minimization of accidents requires a multifaceted approach that combines error reduction strategies with the design of systems to withstand or recover from individual errors.

- ❖ A number of internal and external factors increase propensity for both slips and mistakes. These precursors of error include physiologic factors (such as fatigue, alcohol or drug abuse, illness); psychological factors (such as personality types, boredom, frustration, fear, anger, over-stimulation, stress, an excessively "busy" work environment with frequent interruptions); and environmental factors (such as noise, temperature extremes, visual distractions, and ill-fitting equipment).[49] Factors known to promote errors should be minimized in the work environment. Most individuals perform best with a small amount of tension in the workplace, but not excessive levels of stress. Because individuals vary in their response to stress, the same work environment will not be optimal for all operators.

- ❖ Efforts at error reduction should have a system rather than a person focus. Because latent errors are more amenable to analysis, and because latent errors often cause or potentiate active error at the sharp end of a process, efforts at error reduction should focus on eradication of latent errors rather than active errors.

- ❖ Most of our actions are carried out unconsciously while in schematic control mode. For this reason, most human errors are slips or lapses (failure of schematic control mode), and not mistakes (failures due to lack of knowledge or misapplication of knowledge). It follows that reliance on education alone—the transmission of knowledge—will not be an effective strategy for reducing most errors. Practice of work-related tasks is a necessary and important error-reduction strategy.

❖ Tasks should be designed to minimize reliance on the weakest elements of human cognition: short-term memory and problem solving. The use of checklists (instead of memory) and rule-based decision making (instead of knowledge-based problem solving) should be encouraged.[50]

❖ When rule-based systems are used to guide actions, they should be kept simple, because humans cannot reliably apply large sets of rules. In some instances, instead of human operators, instruments can be programmed to apply rules. For example, modern antimicrobial susceptibility test systems used in the microbiology laboratory incorporate expert logic that screens test results for conformance to national susceptibility databases and national interpretive standards.[51] Technologists and pathologists need not determine which of several dozen susceptibility interpretation rules should be applied in a particular case.

❖ Errors can be reduced by incorporating *forcing functions* (constraints) into devices so as to make them inoperative unless certain preconditions are met. For example, many point-of-care glucose meters will not operate unless quality control testing has been successfully completed. This "lock-out" design feature helps protect against slips from operators who might otherwise forget to perform required control testing. Many patient identification numbers contain check digits that prevent entry of juxtaposed numerals into computer systems.

❖ Feedback should be designed into processes or instruments to alert operators that an error has occurred. For example, while it is currently impossible to physically require nurses to bleed air out of intravenous lines before inserting them into patients, modern intravenous pumps have bubble detectors that alert nurses to the presence of bubbles. Many of the visual controls used in the Toyota Production System are in fact visual feedback systems that alert workers to deviations in the production process caused by human error. It need hardly be said that a feedback system which lacks specificity (frequent false alarms) may do more harm than good, in that it trains operators to ignore warning signs of dangerous situations.[52]

❖ Instruments and work processes can be designed with "buffers" that absorb errors and make systems impervious to individual mishaps. The automatic spelling corrector that runs in the background as this manuscript is being typed into a computer is an example of a buffer that protects the work product (this manual) from the author's typographical errors.

❖ When errors cannot be prevented or reliably detected, redundancy can be applied to protect a work process from individual human blunders. In the clinical laboratory, for example, the practice of manually checking tests entered into a computer against test requisitions is associated with more accurate order fulfillment.[53]

❖ Instruments and technology should be selected with human factors in mind. Designs that respect the limitations of human performance are safer and less error prone.

Before selection of major instruments or technology, the workers who will use the instrumentation or technology should perform usability tests to determine which instruments may be best suited to the operators who will actually use them.

❖ The creation of a culture of safety is paramount for error reduction and error prevention. Organizational culture must be committed to error prevention and improvement of safety as an explicit and stated goal. Characteristics and practices of high reliability organizations should be adopted wherever possible in the laboratory (see "Culture of Quality and Safety" in chapter 5).

Appraisal of Human Errors Research

We believe the recommendations made by cognitive psychologists and human factors researchers to reduce the frequency and impact of human errors are extremely valuable. Clinical laboratory managers should not design work processes around the "perfectibility" of pathologists, clinical caretakers, technologists, or suppliers. The work environment should be simplified and structured to reduce the probability of error, and attention should be paid to designing work processes and equipment to withstand and buffer remaining errors so that patient care is not affected.

The selection of analytic equipment, and particularly laboratory information systems, should be made with an eye to their potential to detect and correct operator errors, which will inevitably occur in every laboratory. The incorporation of check digits into identification numbers (including specimen accession numbers), the use of bar codes and/or radio frequency identification devices, the incorporation of intelligent lock-out features in instrument interfaces, and the application of rule-based reminders during order and result entry will have more impact on quality and patient safety than glitzy "management reports" that alert managers to problems long after they have occurred.

Concluding Remarks

The approaches presented in this chapter represent the major schools of thinking that we believe applicable to the management of quality and patient safety in the clinical laboratory. Together, these approaches provide insight into reducing the frequency of almost any type of quality or safety problem that might be encountered by the laboratory manager.

Most other schools of quality management can be traced back to the methods outlined in this chapter. For example, the *six sigma* quality movement consists largely of the vigorous application of statistical process control, coupled with formal training requirements and recognition of participants in the quality management process (six sigma "green belts," "black belts," etc).

Laboratory managers may elect to use any of the approaches presented in this chapter, according to the particular needs of their organizations and their own management styles. In the next chapter, we discuss laboratory quality and patient safety practices that are required in the United States as the result of law, regulation, or deemed authority.

Regulation and Accreditation

In the United States, clinical laboratories must conform to a variety of laws and regulations. This chapter reviews the major legislative and regulatory requirements that relate to quality and patient safety.

Principal Regulations

Federal Regulations

The *Clinical Laboratory Improvement Amendments of 1988 (CLIA)* is the primary federal legislation related to clinical laboratory quality and patient safety. CLIA was enacted after a series of revelations in *The Wall Street Journal* about "pap mill" laboratories that were making minimal efforts to control the quality of their output. All clinical laboratories in the United States must comply with the provisions of CLIA, whether or not they serve patients enrolled in federal health insurance programs.[54] CLIA is primarily administered by the Centers for Medicare and Medicaid Services (CMS), an agency of the United States Department of Health and Human Services (HHS). The Food and Drug Administration (FDA), another agency of HHS, administers the sections of CLIA that pertain to classification of tests; the Centers for Disease Control and Prevention (CDC), a third agency of HHS, maintains an active interest in CLIA. The CDC and CMS web sites are currently the best source for obtaining copies of CLIA regulations (www.cdc.gov and www.cms.hhs.gov/clia/). Since CLIA regulations have undergone numerous modifications over the past several years, it is important that laboratories comply with the current set of regulations.

Another important federal regulation that relates to the quality of laboratory operations is the *Health Insurance Portability and Accountability Act of 1996* (*HIPAA*). HIPAA contains standards governing the privacy and security of health information. HIPAA is administered by CMS and the Office of Civil Rights, both agencies of HHS. Copies of HIPAA regulations may be obtained from www.hhs.gov/ocr/hipaa/.

A group of regulations administered by the FDA concerns medical devices and biologics. The FDA defines a *medical device* as any instrument, apparatus, or other article that is used to prevent, diagnose, mitigate, or treat a disease or to affect the structure or function of the body, with the exception of drugs.[55] Included in the definition of medical devices are diagnostic test systems (reagents and instruments) and computer software used to manage the collection or administration of blood products. *Biologics* include blood and blood products, vaccines, and certain other therapeutic agents derived from living organisms.

Regulations related to medical devices and biologics that are important to the clinical laboratory are the FDA's *Medical Device Amendment of 1976, Safe Medical Devices Act of 1990, and Good Manufacturing Practices (GMP) / Quality System (QS) Regulation of 1996*. These regulations stipulate that manufacturers must obtain premarket approval from the FDA before selling diagnostic test systems and other medical devices (the premarket approval process is often called the 510(k) process), that instruments and reagents be designed and manufactured in accordance with a set of principles that ensure delivery of a consistent and useful product, and that manufacturers report adverse events associated with medical devices and biologics to the FDA. Information about these regulations can be found at the FDA web site (www.fda.gov). The regulations pertaining to medical devices and biologics place some reporting requirements on hospital-based clinical laboratories when adverse patient events are encountered.[56] These regulations also require that laboratories perform certain user validation testing of computer software that pertains to blood procurement and transfusion operations.[57]

Most tests offered by clinical laboratories will have been approved by the FDA's 510(k) premarket approval process. In addition, clinical laboratories may develop tests that use purchased analyte-specific reagents which are not subject to 510(k) approval. Analyte-specific reagents are antibodies, specific receptor proteins, ligands, or nucleic acid sequences intended for diagnostic use, but which are not part of test systems that have received 510(k) approval. When a clinical laboratory employs purchased analyte-specific reagents in a diagnostic test (including histopathology), the use and labeling of results must conform to 1998 FDA regulations CFR 809.10(e), 809.30, and 864.4020.[58]

State Regulations

Most quality and patient safety requirements for clinical laboratories are federal. States issue requirements for notifiable infectious diseases that must be reported by laboratories to local public health departments. Two states, New York and Washington, have exempted themselves from CLIA by creating internal state programs that are functionally equivalent to CLIA. New York State and Washington State require that clinical laboratories participate in a state-sponsored proficiency testing (PT) program and a state-sponsored laboratory accreditation program. In these states, PT from other vendors may be purchased but may not be substituted for participation in state PT programs. The state of Maryland maintains a cytology proficiency testing program in which Maryland laboratories must enroll. Several states (Massachusetts, California, and others) require licensure of medical technologists; licensure of technologists is not required by federal regulations. Several states other than New York and Washington have registration and inspection requirements beyond those required by the federal government, even though laboratories in these states are also subject to CLIA standards.

Other Regulations

Some managed care organizations specify laboratory quality requirements that must be met by providers wishing to serve managed care organizations' beneficiaries. In our experience, the quality requirements of managed care organizations have generally focused on routine outpatient test turnaround time, the availability of "stat" testing, patient waiting time for phlebotomy in laboratory ambulatory service centers, and Pap smear turnaround time.

Outside of the United States, many countries require clinical laboratories to comply with ISO standards. Since ISO does not certify laboratories directly, compliance with ISO standards is certified by other organizations that are accredited to issue ISO certification. United States clinical laboratories interested in serving populations outside the United States or serving organizations that conduct international business (such as performing drug testing studies for multinational pharmaceutical companies) may wish to obtain ISO certification. The College of American Pathologists plans to offer ISO certification to qualified laboratories, but this service is not available at the time of this writing. ISO certification is optional for clinical laboratories testing patients within the United States.

Many clinical laboratories in the United States are part of hospitals accredited by the Joint Commission on Accreditation of Healthcare Organizations (JCAHO).[59] The JCAHO hospital accreditation program requires hospital-based laboratory staff to participate in hospital investigations of sentinel events and "near miss" events that involved the laboratory. Certain hemolytic transfusion reactions and wrong-site surgeries involving the laboratory are considered JCAHO sentinel events. Laboratories that are part of JCAHO-accredited hospitals must also adhere to the Joint Commission National Patient Safety Goals. The JCAHO hospital accreditation program is separate from the JCAHO laboratory accreditation program, which is discussed elsewhere in this chapter.[60]

Overview of Regulatory Requirements

Types of Testing

Every clinical laboratory test system sold by a manufacturer is classified into one of three groups: *waived, moderate complexity,* and *high complexity.* The FDA is responsible for classifying each laboratory test system, and the type of quality control activities that must be conducted varies for each class of tests. The classification assigned to every test kit can be obtained from an FDA-approved test insert, the *Federal Register,* or from the FDA web site (www.fda.gov/cdrh/CLIA/). If a test has not been classified by the FDA, it should be considered highly complex.

Most test systems are classified by the FDA on the basis of the complexity of the testing procedure, not the analyte being measured. For example, there are "waived" rapid tests to detect group A streptococcus antigen, which are simple to perform, and "moderately complex" rapid group A streptococcus antigen kits, which involve more steps. Both the waived and moderately complex tests measure the same antigens of *Streptococcus pyogenes.* Many caregivers are under the misimpression that all office-based or point-of-care tests are waived. This is not the case. Many tests suitable for office or point-of-care use are moderately complex tests. Some waived and nonwaived tests share the same CPT code.

Waived tests are not subject to CLIA quality standards because regulators consider these tests to be so easy to perform correctly that the chances of an error are negligible.[61] However, even laboratories performing only waived tests must apply to and be approved by CMS before they may conduct clinical testing. A waived test must be performed exactly as specified by the manufacturer for it to remain "waived." If performance of a waived test kit is modified from the manufacturer's directions in any way (change in procedure, change in interpretation of results, change in the type of specimen to which it is applied, change in specimen storage conditions, etc), the test becomes subject to CLIA standards and is no longer considered waived.

Nonwaived tests (moderately and highly complex tests) are subject to CLIA quality standards. Moderately and highly complex tests have similar validation and quality control requirements in CLIA, but some requirements for highly complex tests are slightly more stringent. Any moderately complex test that is modified by the user becomes a highly complex test. These validation and quality control requirements for highly complex tests also apply to any test developed by the laboratory that uses a purchased reagent not licensed by the FDA (so-called analyte-specific reagents, which include many immunoperoxidase stains and molecular probes).

Special use and labeling requirements apply to assays that use analyte-specific reagents for in-house testing. Analyte-specific reagents are classified by the FDA as Class I, II, or III according to whether they are used adjunctively with conventional histopathologic examination or whether independently reportable diagnostic information is generated, as with HER2/*neu*. Specific use and labeling requirements are addressed in the CAP Laboratory Accreditation Program checklist.

Types of Laboratories

In 2005, there were approximately 190,000 clinical laboratories in the United States registered under CLIA. Each clinical laboratory is classified according to the complexity of the most complex test the laboratory performs. Thus, a laboratory that performs only waived tests is a "waived laboratory." A laboratory that performs only waived and moderately complex tests is a "moderately complex laboratory." Any laboratory that performs even one highly complex test is a "highly complex laboratory." Laboratories that conduct only provider-performed microscopy are placed in their own special category.

Waived laboratories are not subject to most regulatory requirements related to quality and patient safety. However, waived laboratories must still meet the data privacy and security provisions of HIPAA and notify public health departments of reportable diseases, as required by state law.

Moderately and highly complex laboratories must satisfy the quality and patient safety provisions in CLIA, which are detailed in the next chapter. Approximately 15,500 laboratories met CLIA definitions for moderate or high complexity in 2005. CLIA requirements for moderately and highly complex laboratories are virtually identical, but highly complex laboratories have some additional personnel requirements beyond those of moderately complex laboratories. Moderately and highly complex laboratories must also meet HIPAA privacy and security requirements and report notifiable infectious diseases to state agencies.

Laboratory Director

All clinical laboratories in the United States must designate a laboratory director. Requirements placed upon directors of moderately and highly complex laboratories are significant, and we suspect that some laboratory directors do not fully understand their legal obligations. In Exhibit 6 we list the regulatory responsibilities of directors of moderately complex laboratories. For laboratories performing nonwaived tests, the director may delegate performance of some of his or her duties, but the director remains responsible for ensuring that all duties are properly performed.

The pathologist laboratory director is professionally responsible and legally accountable for laboratory results. Penalties that may be levied against a laboratory director for serious CLIA infractions include prohibition from owning, operating, or directing a laboratory for a two-year period. Laboratory directors who intentionally violate CLIA provisions are subject to imprisonment or fines, or both.

Exhibit 6. Responsibilities of the Laboratory Director Under CLIA

The laboratory director is responsible for the overall operation and administration of the laboratory, including the employment of personnel who are competent to perform test procedures, and record and report test results promptly, accurate, and proficiently and for assuring compliance with the applicable regulations.

The laboratory director must—

(1) Ensure that testing systems developed and used for each of the tests performed in the laboratory provide quality laboratory services for all aspects of test performance, which includes the preanalytic, analytic, and postanalytic phases of testing;

(2) Ensure that the physical plant and environmental conditions of the laboratory are appropriate for the testing performed and provide a safe environment in which employees are protected from physical, chemical, and biological hazards;

(3) Ensure that— (i) The test methodologies selected have the capability of providing the quality of results required for patient care; (ii) Verification procedures used are adequate to determine the accuracy, precision, and other pertinent performance characteristics of the method; and (iii) Laboratory personnel are performing the test methods as required for accurate and reliable results;

(4) Ensure that the laboratory is enrolled in an HHS approved proficiency testing program for the testing performed and that— (i) The proficiency testing samples are tested as required under subpart H of this part; (ii) The results are returned within the timeframes established by the proficiency testing program; (iii) All proficiency testing reports received are reviewed by the appropriate staff to evaluate the laboratory's performance and to identify any problems that require corrective action; and (iv) An approved corrective action plan is followed when any proficiency testing results are found to be unacceptable or unsatisfactory;

(5) Ensure that the quality control and quality assessment programs are established and maintained to assure the quality of laboratory services provided and to identify failures in quality as they occur;

(6) Ensure the establishment and maintenance of acceptable levels of analytical performance for each test system;

(7) Ensure that all necessary remedial actions are taken and documented whenever significant deviations from the laboratory's established performance specifications are identified, and that patient test results are reported only when the system is functioning properly;

(8) Ensure that reports of test results include pertinent information required for interpretation;

(9) Ensure that consultation is available to the laboratory's clients on matters relating to the quality of the test results reported and their interpretation concerning specific patient conditions;

(10) Employ a sufficient number of laboratory personnel with the appropriate education and either experience or training to provide appropriate consultation, properly supervise and accurately perform tests and report test results in accordance with the personnel responsibilities described in this subpart;

(11) Ensure that prior to testing patients' specimens, all personnel have the appropriate education and experience, receive the appropriate training for the type and complexity of the services offered, and have demonstrated that they can perform all testing operations reliably to provide and report accurate results;

(12) Ensure that policies and procedures are established for monitoring individuals who conduct preanalytical, analytical, and postanalytical phases of testing to assure that they are competent and maintain their competency to process specimens, perform test procedures and report test results promptly and proficiently, and whenever necessary, identify needs for remedial training or continuing education to improve skills;

(13) Ensure that an approved procedure manual is available to all personnel responsible for any aspect of the testing process; and

(14) Specify, in writing, the responsibilities and duties of each consultant and each person engaged in the performance of the preanalytic, analytic, and postanalytic phases of testing, that identifies which examinations and procedures each individual is authorized to perform, whether supervision is required for specimen processing, test performance or results reporting, and whether consultant or director review is required prior to reporting patient test results.

Laboratory directors who cannot fulfill their responsibilities, due to lack of resources, control, or cooperation, should vigorously attempt to obtain the support required to bring their laboratory into conformance with standards, citing their responsibilities under CLIA. The fiduciary duty of a laboratory director to patients and the public transcends the director's obligation to the laboratory's owner, much as the fiduciary duty of a certified public account to stockholders and the community transcends the accountant's obligation to management. If all attempts with a laboratory's owners to secure required support fail, a laboratory director should consider resigning from the directorship position.

Personnel Requirements

CLIA regulations set minimal education and experience requirements for directors of all laboratories performing nonwaived testing. Regulations also specify minimal education and experience requirements for clinical consultants, technical consultants, supervisors, and personnel performing tests. Qualifications vary somewhat depending on the type of laboratory (moderately complex versus highly complex, etc). Each laboratory performing nonwaived testing is expected to engage at least one individual qualified to serve in each role required by CLIA (clinical consultant, technical consultant, etc); the same individual may serve in two or more roles, if qualified. Pathologists who provide professional services in hospital-based laboratories must generally be credentialed by the hospital medical staff; requirements vary among hospitals. CLIA requires that laboratory staff performing testing must periodically demonstrate their competence to perform the work they have been assigned to complete.

Quality of Testing Processes

For laboratories performing nonwaived testing, regulations specify that certain activities be performed to ensure the quality of preanalytic, analytic, and postanalytic processes. Requirements for analytic processes include the validation of new tests and minimum ongoing quality control activities. Specific standards are discussed in the next chapter of this manual.

Facilities

Laboratories that perform nonwaived testing must have adequate facilities. Special facility requirements are provided in CLIA for transfusion services and molecular diagnostics.

Records

For laboratories performing nonwaived testing, records and clinical materials of different types must be maintained for specified periods of time. Details are provided in the next chapter (Exhibit 61). Neither statutory nor case law clearly defines the legal ownership of clinical materials. The processing of some histopathology specimens transforms them into durable goods (eg, slides and blocks) that may fairly be claimed to be the property of the institution. Nevertheless, the laboratory is expected to preserve these clinical materials in a safe location for the future benefit of the patient. When diagnostic material is sent to another institution for special studies and not returned, the consulting laboratory becomes a secondary custodian of the referred material it retains.[1]

Incident Management

Laboratories that perform nonwaived testing are required by CLIA to investigate and address complaints that are brought by laboratory users or by individuals working within the laboratory.

Quality Planning

CLIA requires that laboratory management produce and implement a quality plan that is approved by the laboratory director. (See chapter 7.)

Privacy and Security

Laboratories that store personally identifiable health information in electronic form must protect patients' privacy. In general, identifiable health information cannot be used or disclosed without patient permission for any purpose other than treatment, payment, and health care operations. Disclosure of test results to physicians who have ordered a test is, of course, permitted. Disclosure of information to other providers actively caring for a patient is generally permitted, provided the information is requested for the purposes of treatment. The ability of laboratories to disclose result information to patients is usually defined by state laws and varies from state to state.

Laboratories that store personally identifiable health information must also protect the security of this information. Certain administrative, physical, and technical safeguards are required to protect data from loss or degradation and to protect the data from unauthorized access.

Privacy and security rules apply to all laboratories, including waived laboratories. (See the discussion on "Information Management" in chapter 5 for more detail.)

External Inspections

Waived laboratories are normally exempt from external federal inspections.[62] All laboratories performing nonwaived testing are regularly inspected to test conformance with CLIA standards. These inspections may be announced or unannounced. Normally, laboratories are inspected every two years, but inspections may be initiated more frequently in response to complaints or problems, or to validate the accuracy of previous inspections. Inspection may be carried out by CMS or its agents (such as state public health departments), or by representatives of approved accreditation programs (such as the CAP Laboratory Accreditation Program). There are no routine laboratory inspection requirements for HIPAA or other federal regulations pertaining to quality and patient safety. Laboratories in JCAHO-accredited hospitals may be involved in hospital accreditation inspections conducted by JCAHO. The Joint Commission on Accreditation of Healthcare Organizations has introduced a *tracer methodology* into its inspection process, whereby individual patients and patient specimens are tracked as they progress from one area of a hospital to another. Laboratory staff may become involved in a JCAHO inspection that "traces" a specimen into the laboratory or a report emanating from the laboratory. In addition, blood banks that modify blood products, collect blood products, or ship blood products interstate are subject to inspection by the FDA.

Proficiency Testing

Federal regulations require that all laboratories performing nonwaived tests enroll in an external proficiency testing (PT) program for certain analytes and demonstrate satisfactory PT performance. The analytes for which PT is required are called *regulated analytes*. The CAP PT program is one of several approved PT programs that can be used to satisfy this requirement. The criteria for satisfactory PT performance are specified in CLIA regulations. When multiple test platforms are used to measure an analyte, only the most commonly used platform is subject to proficiency testing.

For nonwaived tests that measure something other than a regulated analyte, CLIA regulations do not require enrollment in PT, so long as the laboratory verifies the accuracy of the assay twice yearly. CAP accreditation standards are more rigorous with regards to PT than CLIA standards. The CAP requires laboratories to enroll in a CAP-approved PT program for all analytes in which an approved PT program is available, rather than only the "regulated" analytes named in CLIA regulations.

The purpose of proficiency testing is to determine whether a laboratory is proficient at using its primary test system to measure an analyte, compared with other laboratories using the same test system. Proficiency testing does not measure the accuracy of laboratory results.[63]

Laboratory Registration

All clinical laboratories in the United States must apply to the government. Waived laboratories obtain a certificate of waiver which exempts them from CLIA quality and safety standards and external inspections, so long as these laboratories use only waived tests and follow manufacturers' testing instructions.[62] Laboratories performing moderate and high complexity testing receive a registration certification.[64] CLIA applications may be made to the United States Department of Health and Human Services or to state departments of public health, which act as agents of the federal government. In the process of applying, a laboratory must provide the names of the laboratory director and the laboratory owner(s), the disciplines in which testing will be performed, and the number of tests that the laboratory anticipates will be performed. The laboratory also must indicate whether it will be inspected by a CMS agent or an approved authority, such as the CAP. A laboratory representative must attest that the laboratory will be operated in accordance with CLIA requirements. A fee must be paid to obtain a CLIA certificate of waiver or CLIA registration certificate.

With very few exceptions, laboratories with different physical locations must register separately with CLIA even if they have common ownership.[65] All laboratories that are registered are assigned a unique CLIA number. There are no separate registration requirement for clinical laboratories related to HIPAA, medical device, or biologics regulations. Several states require laboratories to be registered with the state as well as HHS.

Certification and Accreditation

Registered laboratories that perform moderate and high complexity testing and which are subject to CLIA must progress to either certification of compliance or certification of accreditation. Certification of compliance is awarded when a laboratory agrees to be inspected by CMS or its agent (generally a state department of public health) and the laboratory passes a CMS inspection.[66] Accreditation is granted by a nonprofit organization, such as the CAP, that has been approved ("deemed") by CMS to have requirements that are equal to or more stringent than key ("condition-level") CLIA requirements. When an organization such as the CAP accredits a laboratory, CMS issues a "certificate of accreditation," which substitutes for a certificate of compliance.

Although most hospital-based and commercial laboratories are accredited by the CAP, other organizations have been approved to accredit laboratories under CLIA. These organizations can be found at www.cms.hhs.gov/clia/accrdorg.asp. As of this writing, approved accrediting organizations in addition to the CAP are the American Association of Blood Banks, American Osteopathic Association, American Society of Histocompatibility and Immunogenetics, COLA, and the Joint Commission on Accreditation of Healthcare Organizations. JCAHO accreditation of a hospital as being compliant with CMS *Conditions of Participation* for hospitals does not satisfy CLIA requirements for hospital-based laboratories. Hospital-based laboratories that elect to be accredited by JCAHO, rather than by the CAP or some other organization, must enroll in JCAHO's separate laboratory accreditation program.

CAP standards for laboratory accreditation, including checklist questions, are available without charge to the public on the CAP web site (www.cap.org). JCAHO standards for laboratory accreditation are available to the public for a fee. JCAHO standards may be purchased through the JCAHO web site (www.jcaho.org). All inspecting agencies, including CMS, CAP, and JCAHO, charge laboratories fees to cover the costs of inspections.

Third-party Reporting

Laboratories must report certain notifiable diseases to local public health departments, as required by state law. All laboratories must report to HHS or its agents within 30 days any change in the laboratory's ownership, location, name, or director. Laboratories performing nonwaived testing must also report within 6 months when they perform any test within a specialty area that is not included on the laboratory's certificate of compliance. According to regulations, laboratories must report to HHS changes in test methodology for any test included in the certificate of compliance. In practice, this requirement is not enforced so long as laboratories report method changes that change their classification as moderately or highly complex laboratories, or change the specialty disciplines for which they must be certified. Laboratories accredited by the CAP must report all of the above changes to the CAP as well as HHS, and must also report any adverse publicity or other developments that might indicate laboratory practices are being compromised.

Hospital-based laboratories must notify the FDA of any adverse events related to medical devices, transfusion-related fatalities, and any deviations from blood bank procedures that could impact the safety or potency of blood products. Some reporting to device manufacturers and blood suppliers is also required.

Laboratories that are part of JCAHO-accredited hospitals may participate in hospital analyses of sentinel events that involve the laboratory. JCAHO strongly encourages hospitals to report certain sentinel events to JCAHO, including hemolytic transfusion reactions involving administration of blood products with major blood group incompatibilities.

States and the federal government periodically require additional reporting, usually in the form of surveys and questionnaires sent to laboratories. Surveys may be related to public health issues, bioterrorism, or other miscellaneous topics.

Regulatory Noncompliance

There are a number of routes through which laboratory operations may be discovered to be out of regulatory compliance. Most commonly, a laboratory director or some other individual who works in a clinical laboratory directly observes that a practice within the laboratory does not conform to regulatory requirements. On other occasions, an external inspector may observe a practice that does not comply with regulations. A laboratory worker may self-report a deviation to a private accrediting agency such as the CAP or to state regulators. Complaints from laboratory users, patients, or business associates may be sent to the laboratory or other agencies. Finally, a laboratory may demonstrate unsatisfactory performance on proficiency testing.

Regulatory noncompliance in clinical laboratories is commonplace. During routine CAP inspections of laboratories, more than two-thirds of facilities are found to have at least one deficiency with CAP accreditation standards, and more than half of inspected laboratories demonstrate three or more deficiencies during routine inspection.[67] Anecdotal experience tells us that many more deficiencies are discovered by laboratory management and staff during the course of normal operations but are corrected before external inspections are conducted, as a part of normal quality management activities.

Laboratory management has a legal obligation to bring a laboratory into regulatory compliance when deficiencies are discovered. Passing an external inspection or external proficiency test does not relieve management of its obligation to correct known deficiencies. For CLIA regulations, the laboratory director is held responsible for assuring regulatory compliance. For HIPAA and most other federal regulations, the laboratory's owners are held responsible for assuring compliance. As a practical matter, every individual affiliated with a clinical laboratory should strive to identify and correct regulatory deficiencies.

The College of American Pathologists may become aware of a compliance problem with an accredited laboratory as a result of receiving a complaint, receiving a self-reported deficiency from someone within the laboratory, from media coverage, from a routine inspection, from failed proficiency testing performance, or from some other source. When the CAP has reason to believe that an accredited laboratory may not be in compliance with CAP accreditation standards, the College will conduct an investigation to collect additional information. This investigation may involve an exchange of documents or an on-site inspection. If the CAP believes a deficiency exists, the College will notify laboratory management that the laboratory must demonstrate it has brought practices back into compliance with standards. Management is normally given 30 days to bring the laboratory into conformance. A demonstration of compliance may be made through further document exchange between the laboratory and CAP or after a follow-up on-site inspection, depending on the nature of the deficiency. Laboratories may be charged additional fees to support the cost of involved investigations.

For laboratories certified as CLIA-compliant by CMS or its state agent, the process of investigating and correcting deficiencies is similar to the process used by the CAP. When CMS or its agent becomes aware that a laboratory may not be in compliance with a key ("condition-level") CLIA regulation, CMS or its agent will investigate. This investigation may involve an inspection. Once a condition-level deficiency has been documented, a laboratory is normally given 30 days to provide a "credible allegation of compliance," which consists of documentation provided by a reliable individual that the problem has been resolved. For both the CAP and CMS, shorter time frames may be involved if the deficiency poses an immediate threat to the public health.

If a laboratory accredited by the CAP does not correct a deficiency, the CAP will remove or otherwise restrict the laboratory's accreditation and will notify CMS within 30 days (or sooner for critical deficiencies). CMS and its agents will then take whatever action CMS deems necessary to bring the laboratory into compliance, or will revoke the laboratory's CLIA license and bar the laboratory from serving patients in federal insurance programs, such as Medicare and Medicaid.

If laboratories are found to be in violation of HIPAA or FDA regulations, the laboratory's owner may be fined. Additional measures may be taken by HHS, CMS, or the FDA for infractions of HIPAA, biologics, or medical device regulations, as prescribed by law.

Regulatory Context of CAP Programs

The College of American Pathologists maintains a proficiency testing (PT) program (Surveys) along with its Laboratory Accreditation Program (LAP). These programs serve both an educational and regulatory function, and it is helpful for laboratory managers who participate in either program to keep these dual functions in mind.

The CAP launched its first chemistry survey in 1949, just two years after the College was incorporated. This survey was promoted as an educational tool, with the goal of improving laboratory quality. Clinical chemistry testing at the time was performed manually, and pathologists recognized a need for interlaboratory surveys to improve consistency and accuracy. Subscription to College surveys was entirely voluntary; federal regulatory requirements for survey participation would not be written for several decades. Over the ensuing years, the CAP added additional survey offerings. The CAP conducted a blood bank survey with the AMA in the late 1940s and began microbiology surveys in 1958.

The early CAP Laboratory Accreditation Program was also a voluntary educational undertaking designed to promote laboratory improvement and the sharing of best practices. The CAP published its first set of requirements for a hospital-based clinical pathology department in 1950, and introduced its formal accreditation program in 1961. The founding principle of the accreditation program was "to improve the quality of clinical laboratory services through voluntary participation, professional peer review, education, and compliance with established performance standards."

Over time, both the PT and LAP programs began to play a quasi-public regulatory role in addition to serving their educational objectives. In 1978, JCAHO, which was charged by Congress to evaluate hospitals, "deemed" authority to the CAP Laboratory Inspection and Accreditation Program to accredit laboratories on JCAHO's behalf. When the Clinical Laboratory Improvement Amendments of 1988 were enacted, the CAP PT program was recognized to fulfill CLIA PT requirements, and in 1994 the federal government recognized the CAP Laboratory Accreditation Program as fulfilling CLIA accreditation requirements.

With the new role for the College's PT and LAP programs came new responsibilities. No longer could the CAP be satisfied with improving laboratory performance among agreeable volunteers; the College had now assumed a formal role, protecting the public from substandard laboratory practices.

Participants in the CAP PT and LAP programs are best served when they keep the CAP's two complementary objectives in mind. On the one hand, the CAP encourages a participatory atmosphere in which local laboratorians are actively engaged in the performance improvement process. Laboratories that participate in CAP PT programs receive educational materials to improve performance, and LAP participants are encouraged to share best practices with other laboratories.

At the same time, the CAP PT and LAP programs serve an important public regulatory function. Laboratories that do not process PT specimens in the same manner as clinical specimens will be sanctioned. Laboratories that do not respond to CAP inquiries on a timely basis or do not remedy known deficiencies will have their accreditation limited or withdrawn entirely. The College has come to recognize that methods historically used to assess laboratory performance among agreeable quality-conscious volunteers are not sufficient for all laboratories, and procedures to detect fraud, malfeasance, and laboratory cover-ups have been introduced into College programs.[68]

In the chapter that follows, important individual risks to laboratory quality and patient safety are enumerated along with measures that can be adopted to mitigate these hazards. The CAP is prepared to help laboratory directors and other laboratory managers address these risks through its proficiency testing, laboratory improvement, educational, and laboratory accreditation programs. However, the CAP is also charged with protecting the public's interest when laboratories consistently fail to meet regulatory standards. The College is committed to fulfilling this obligation even if doing so causes embarrassment to a laboratory director or sanctions against a clinical laboratory.

Specific Quality and Patient Safety Risks

This chapter details specific threats to quality and patient safety found in clinical laboratories. We discuss the importance of individual risks, what we know about the magnitude of each risk within the laboratory industry, and control measures that managers may apply to mitigate particular hazards.

Most individual processes within clinical laboratories are reliable. Instruments generally function properly, clerks usually enter orders accurately, technologists typically execute procedures faithfully. Yet laboratory errors are common. The frequency of laboratory errors has been reported to range from 1 error per 164 laboratory results[69] to 1 per 8030 results.[70] Hemolytic transfusion reactions are reported to occur once every 19,000 transfusions.[71] Second review of surgical pathology cases discloses diagnostic discrepancies in 6.7% of cases.[72] Most of the American public would prefer that the clinical laboratory industry operate with fewer errors; certainly most laboratory managers are not satisfied with this level of performance.[73]

What can the laboratory manager do to reduce errors and promote quality? Clinical laboratories are complex environments and engage in complex interactions with patients and caregivers. Not every aspect of laboratory service can be monitored and managed economically. Where should the laboratory manager begin?

Identifying Important Risks

Quality and patient safety risks worth managing have the characteristics listed in Exhibit 7, which has been adapted from the National Quality Forum. Risks worth managing should be important. They should be linked to patient outcome or customer needs, and there should be variation in quality among laboratories, reagent lots, analytic platforms, human operators, or test runs. There is little point in managing a process that does not impact care or which never goes awry.[74]

Risks worth managing must also be measurable. Instructions for how to measure performance must be clearly specified so that two institutions measuring the same risk use the same measurement process; repeated measurements made of the same operation should be reproducible; the characteristic being measured should have a valid causal connection to patient outcome (not a spurious statistical association); the

> ### Exhibit 7. Risks Worth Managing
>
> **Important**
> - Linked to patient outcome or customer needs
> - Variation among laboratories, reagent lots, analytic platforms, operators, test runs
>
> **Measurable**
> - Precisely specified
> - Reproducible
> - Valid
> - Adaptable
> - Economically applied
>
> **Actionable**
> - Subject to mitigation by control measures

Exhibit 8. Major Risks to Laboratory Quality and Patient Safety

Preanalytic Operations
❖ Patient and specimen identification
❖ Order communication
❖ Specimen collection and handling
❖ Appropriate ordering of laboratory services

Analytic Operations
❖ Introducing new tests
❖ Ongoing quality management of tests
❖ Establishing reference ranges
❖ Reference laboratories

Postanalytic Operations
❖ Reporting results
❖ Administration of blood products
❖ Interpretation of results
❖ Correcting errors

General Laboratory Systems
❖ Personnel
❖ Information management
❖ Turnaround time
❖ Laboratory organization

---

measurement process should be field-tested and adaptable to different laboratory settings; and it should be possible to measure quality economically. Finally, managers should focus on aspects of operations that are "actionable." There should be some concrete, positive, affordable steps that an organization may take to improve performance and reduce the risk of errors.

Specific risks we believe important to manage are listed in Exhibit 8 and discussed in this chapter. These hazards frequently are divided into *preanalytic, analytic,* and *postanalytic* categories, although some hazards do not fit neatly into this taxonomy and are grouped under the category *general laboratory systems.*

Exhibit 8 is not an encyclopedic compendium of everything that can go wrong in a laboratory. We have constructed Exhibit 8 from our knowledge of particular laboratory failures (such as those described in chapter 2), published literature about quality management (referenced in chapter 3), and applicable regulations pertaining to laboratory quality and patient safety (reviewed in chapter 4). Unique circumstances present in individual laboratories may cause laboratory directors to focus on a different configuration of risks.

The hazards listed in Exhibit 8 generally meet the criteria listed in Exhibit 7 for risks that are worth managing. A few hazards must be managed not because they are especially important to patients, but because there is a regulatory requirement to do so. It is fortunate that the United States clinical laboratory industry benefits from constructive interaction with regulators, and most of the risks that are required to be managed by statute or regulation are also worth managing from a patient care perspective.

The remainder of this chapter is divided into four sections that correspond to the groups in Exhibit 8: preanalytic risks, analytic risks, postanalytic risks, and risks to general laboratory systems.

Preanalytic Operations: Risks and Control Measures

Patient and Specimen Identification

There is little doubt that misidentification of patients and specimens represents an important risk to patient safety. Approximately 25 deaths per year occur in the United States from hemolytic transfusion reactions caused by preanalytic identification errors. Each year, several patients undergo a disfiguring resection for a tumor that was diagnosed in the wrong patient due to an identification error. Based on data from a study of 110 laboratories, it has been estimated that 1 in 18 identification errors cause some type of adverse patient event. More than 160,000 adverse events occur yearly in the United States as a result of laboratories testing misidentified specimens.[75]

The College of American Pathologists has made patient and sample identification a national patient safety goal (Exhibit 9), as has the Joint Commission on Accreditation of Healthcare Organizations. Both the CAP and JCAHO require that at least two patient identifiers (neither to be the patient's room number) be used whenever drawing blood samples or administering blood products.

In this section, we discuss procedures for detecting identification errors, their frequency, and control measures that can be applied to minimize their occurrence and impact upon patients.

Exhibit 9. CAP National Laboratory Patient Safety Goals

1. Improve patient and sample identification
   a. At the time of specimen collection
   b. At the time of analysis
   c. At the time of results delivery
2. Improve verification and communication of life-threatening or life-altering information regarding
   a. Malignancies
   b. HIV and other infections
   c. Cytogenetic abnormalities
   d. Critical values
3. Improve the identification, communication, and correction of errors
4. Improve coordination of the laboratory patient safety role within health care organizations

---

Detecting Identification Errors

Any result that is reported for the wrong specimen (or would have been reported for the wrong specimen without some intervention) can be considered an identification error. It is immaterial whether the error resulted from the actions of laboratory staff or nonlaboratory staff, or was the result of some other failure. A mix-up of two specimens from the same patient collected from different body sites or at different times should still be considered an identification error, because the site or time of collection may be important in interpreting results and planning subsequent care.

Case-finding of identification errors in normal laboratory practice underestimates the true frequency with which errors occur. Most identification errors go undetected. Approximately 85% of identification errors that come to light surface before test results are released to caregivers.[75] Therefore, an approach to detecting errors that relies exclusively on complaints from caregivers will be particularly unreliable.

Exhibit 10. Systems for Classifying Identification Errors
❖ Setting in which error occurred (labeling, order entry, etc)
❖ Impact on the patient (none, change in management, morbidity, etc)
❖ Type of error (patient vs specimen misidentification)
❖ Cause of the error (human slip, instrument failure, defective procedure, etc)

Exhibit 11. Causes of 4852 Identification Errors in 110 Laboratories [75]

Cause	Number (%)
Primary specimen label error	2691 (55.5)
Initial registration/order entry error	1088 (22.4)
Other clerical error	604 (12.4)
Other reason for error	205 (4.2)
Aliquot/block/slide label error	184 (3.8)
Result entry error	80 (1.7)

There are a number of methods for detecting identification errors before results are released. Improperly labeled specimens (eg, incorrectly spelled name or missing information) may alert laboratory staff to the possibility of an identification error, as may specimen labels that do not match accompanying requisitions, the receipt of a specimen from a patient who is not on file in a laboratory database, a blood specimen that types for a different ABO group than the group on file for the patient, or a practice of routinely comparing demographic information entered into a computer to demographic information on a test requisition. In anatomic pathology, identification errors frequently are detected because the type of tissue seen under the microscope by a pathologist does not correspond to the biopsy site specified in the clinical history. Delta checks of clinical chemistry and hematology values have been suggested as a means to detect specimen identification errors,[76] although this detection method is difficult to apply in practice[77] and was not associated with increased error detection rates in a recent study.[75]

Errors identified after the release of results are usually detected by caregivers and not laboratory staff. A provider may contact the laboratory because a test result is inconsistent with the patient's clinical picture or a repeat test result, or because the provider knows that the patient named in the report did not, in fact, have the test performed at all. Sometimes an adverse event, such as a transfusion reaction, alerts the laboratory to an identification error.

There is no generally accepted taxonomy of identification errors. Four taxonomic systems have appeared in the literature (Exhibit 10), but it is not clear that any of these classification schemes are particularly useful. One study that examined the cause of 4852 identification errors found the majority of errors to be caused by improper specimen labeling. A large fraction of the remainder were caused by improper initial registration or order entry (Exhibit 11).[75]

Frequency of Identification Errors

Identification errors are usually quantified as a rate. Incorrect identifying information on patient wristbands is expressed as an error rate per patient. Incorrectly identified specimens destined for chemistry, hematology, or microbiology sections are expressed as an error rate per million billable tests.[78] In surgical pathology, identification errors are usually reported per case (accession number); in transfusion medicine, the frequency of identification errors is expressed as the number of errors per transfused patient or per transfused unit. In this section, we review identification error rates in different areas of laboratory medicine. Managers may use any of these rates to benchmark their laboratory's own performance.

Exhibit 12. Types of Patient Wristband Errors Observed in 217 Hospitals, 1993 [79]

Type of Error	All Participants Percentiles (% of wristbands with errors)		
	10th	50th (median)	90th
Any error type	18.8	6.5*	1.4
Missing wristbands	13.1	4.1	0.8
Multiple wristbands with different information	2.9	0.1	0.0
Missing information	2.7	0.2	0.0
Erroneous information	1.5	0.1	0.0
Illegible wristbands	0.6	0.0	0.0
Wearing another patient's wristband	0.1	0.0	0.0

* For example, in this study the median hospital reported that 6.5% of patients had one or more wristband errors. The most common error type was a missing wristband.

Exhibit 13. Total Wristband Errors Observed in 154 Hospitals, 2004 [81]

		All Institutions Percentiles (% of wristbands with errors)				
	N	10th	25th	50th (median)	75th	90th
Any wristband error (%)	154	0.13	0.40	1.02	2.61	4.36

Patient Identification Errors

Accurate identification of specimens begins with accurate identification of patients. In the early 1990s, the CAP conducted several one-time Q-Probes studies of wristband identification errors.[79] For one month, laboratory phlebotomists checked inpatients for the presence of a legible wristband with complete and correct identifying information. Wristband identification errors were defined as patients missing wristbands entirely, wristbands with illegible information, those with missing information, those with a different patient's identifying information, and patients with more than one wristband with conflicting identifying information. Error rates were calculated by dividing the number of errors by the number of wristbands checked. In a study of 451,436 wristbands, 25,800 errors were detected. The all-participant error rate (wristbands with one or more errors) was 5.5%; the median hospital recorded an error rate of 6.5%. The distribution of errors by type is shown in Exhibit 12. Recently, the CAP has given laboratories the opportunity to continuously monitor wristband errors as part of the CAP Q-Tracks program.[80] The 2004 wristband error rates for Q-Tracks participants is lower than was observed in earlier Q-Probes studies, probably as a result of systematic improvement, and is shown in Exhibit 13.[81]

Identification Errors in Transfusion Medicine

The transfusion medicine community has gone the furthest in quantifying the frequency of identification errors. In a review of serious transfusion errors in New York State, ABO incompatible transfusion was identified in 1 in 33,000 transfusions.[82] Of the 54 incompatible transfusions, 22% (or 1 in 150,000) of the events were the result of phlebotomist or preanalytic identification errors. Correcting for under-reporting (due to the fact that approximately 2 in 3 misidentified specimens will by chance be of the same ABO type),[83] the fraction of misidentified specimens arriving in New York State blood banks was estimated to be 1 in 54,000. Expressed as errors per million, this equates to 19 identification errors per million specimens.

A higher incidence of specimen identification errors was reported in a prospective study by the International Society of Blood Transfusion (ISBT) Biomedical Excellence for Safer Transfusion (BEST) Committee.[84] In the United Kingdom, 85 hospitals provided data on the number of ABO discrepancies found by comparing samples received by the transfusion service to a patient's historical ABO record. After correcting for chance coincidence of ABO type and other factors, the authors calculated that 45 of 133,600 (0.03%) samples were misidentified. Among the individual study participants, the discrepancy rate varied from 1 in 238 to 1 in 3303 samples. The median institution had a specimen misidentification rate of 1 in 1786 specimens, which is equivalent to 560 identification errors per million specimens. The BEST estimate of identification errors is probably more accurate than the New York State figure, which relied on reporting of transfusion errors as the initial case-finding method.

Identification Errors in Chemistry, Hematology, and Microbiology

Identification error rates found in transfusion medicine cannot be extrapolated to general clinical laboratory specimens because the care with which blood bank specimens are identified exceeds that of other laboratory specimens. For example, criteria for accepting specimens are less stringent in chemistry and hematology than in transfusion medicine. Minor spelling discrepancies in patient names on specimen labels or the absence of phlebotomist initials on a collection tube commonly leads to specimen rejection in transfusion medicine, but not in other laboratory disciplines. Specimens with one or more minor labeling errors are 40 times more likely to contain someone else's blood than specimens that meet strict labeling standards.[85]

In a recent survey of specimens bound for all sections of the laboratory, the rate of identification errors that involved results which had already been released to caregivers was reported by the median hospital to be 60 per million billable tests.[75] Interlaboratory variation was wide (Exhibit 14). Since 85% of identification errors are detected before results are released, the incidence of misidentified specimens arriving in the laboratory was probably closer to 400 per million tests. This higher figure is itself likely to be an underestimate, since many identification errors are never detected.

A study conducted in Australia examined errors transcribing a patient's name from pathology requisitions to computer systems.[86] The median institution made transcription errors involving patient identity in 1% of cases, whereas the worst performer made identification errors in 9% of cases. The study did not indicate how many of these errors were detected before results were verified.

Exhibit 14. Frequency of Identification Errors Observed in 120 Laboratories, 2005 [75]

Quality Indicator	Mean	All Institutions Percentiles*				
		10th	25th	50th (median)	75th	90th
Rate of identification errors detected after release of results (per million tests)	60	340	130	60*	20	0
Percent of identification errors detected before release of results	85%	44%	70%	86%	95%	100%

* For example, the median of 120 laboratories reported that staff subsequently became aware of identification errors in .006% of results that had already been released (a rate of 60 errors per million results). Higher percentile ranks indicate better relative performance (lower postverification error rates).

In addition to comparing the *rate* of identification errors among laboratories, laboratories may be compared according to the *proportion* of misidentified specimens identified before results are verified. Some facilities are much better than others in detecting identification errors before results are sent to caregivers (Exhibit 14).[75] One-quarter of laboratories identify at least 19 of 20 errors before result verification, whereas another quarter identify fewer than 2 in 3. Laboratories that identify a higher percentage of results before verification have lower postverification error rates, which underscores the importance of early detection.

Identification Errors in Anatomic Pathology

Identification errors in anatomic pathology have the potential to cause great patient harm because anatomic pathology diagnoses play a pivotal role in patient management. In 1995, 417 laboratories studied identification and accessioning deficiencies and found errors in 60,042 (5.9%) of 1,004,115 surgical pathology cases.[87] Errors related to specimen identification accounted for 9.6% of these deficiencies, for an overall identification error rate of 0.57% or 5740 identification errors per million accessions. Most of these errors were detected at the time of order entry and were therefore unlikely to cause a diagnosis to be rendered for the wrong patient.

Control Measures to Reduce Identification Errors

What control measures can be applied to reduce the frequency of patient and specimen identification errors? Several practices and technologies have been associated with lower error rates in clinical laboratories. Techniques that have been successfully used to address similar problems in other industries may also be applicable to laboratory medicine.[88]

Monitoring

Continuous monitoring of identification errors is associated with a lower frequency of errors. In a one-time Q-Probes study of identification errors, institutions that had established programs for monitoring errors before the study began showed a significantly lower rate of identification errors.[75] In an ongoing CAP Q-Tracks study that focuses on wristband errors, continuous program enrollment has been associated with progressive within-institution

Exhibit 15. Reduction in Wristband Error Rates with Continuous Monitoring of Errors [80]

Years of Continuous Error Rate Monitoring	Mean Reduction In Wristband Error Rate*
1	1.0%
2	3.3%
3	3.3%
4	3.9%
5	4.9%
6	6.8%

* This percentage represents the absolute reduction in error rates observed for the typical participant. For example, after one year of monitoring, a laboratory with an initial wristband error rate of 5% would record a wristband error rate of 4% (a reduction in the laboratory's error rate of 1%).

reduction in error rates; by the end of the sixth year of participation, error rates for individual institutions are less, on average, than a third of their starting value (Exhibit 15).[81] This reduction has been carefully analyzed and been shown not to be due to selective drop-out of poorly performing institutions.

Other Laboratory Practices

The rate of wristband identification errors is significantly lower in hospitals that require written orders before removal of wristbands or require the notification of nursing staff when wristband errors are discovered. Rates are also lower in institutions that file incident reports when wristband errors are discovered. Lower wristband error rates are found in institutions that monitor patients for wristband errors upon transfer from one location to another, in hospitals where non-nursing staff initially place wristbands on patients, in institutions where emergency department patients routinely receive wristbands, and in facilities where laboratories are inspected by the CAP.[79,80] These simple control measures to reduce identification errors may be adopted by any hospital. In a Q-Probes study of specimen identification accuracy, errors were found to be less frequent when the accuracy of order entry was investigated whenever a specimen was drawn from a patient who was new to the laboratory database. Identification errors were also lower when every identifier on a specimen label was required to be correct before accepting specimens into the transfusion medicine service.[75]

Check Digit Technology

Check digits were introduced by International Business Machines in the 1950s to reduce the rate at which numbers are incorrectly transcribed. An extra digit (the "check digit") is added to an identification number and calculated uniquely from the other digits in the number, using a rule that is too complex for humans to perform mentally. Since there are 10 potential values for the check digit (0 through 9), only 1 in 10 incorrectly entered identification numbers will "check" correctly. The check digit calculation rule is designed to detect almost all errors involving single-digit changes or substitution of two adjacent digits—two of the more common errors made by humans when transcribing numbers. Check digits are commonly incorporated into the patient identification numbers (sometimes called history or unit numbers) used by many health systems. Inclusion of check digits in specimen accession numbers might reduce the frequency with which case numbers are incorrectly transcribed or entered into computer systems. Only a few laboratory information systems offer this option.

Machine-readable Bar Code Technology

Bar codes have significantly reduced identification errors within the clinical laboratory. Bar coding technology was developed in the 1930s and entered the retail market in the early

1970s. While manual entry of identifying information is associated with an error rate of 1 per 300 characters entered, modern bar codes have a substitution error rate of 1 per million characters. Newer bar code symbologies, such as multi-row two-dimensional bar codes, allow information to be stored in a more compact form so that bar codes can be placed on small containers, such as the front of plastic cassettes that hold tissue during paraffin embedding.

Most bar codes are printed on labels that are then applied to specimens. The use of bar codes does not prevent bar coded labels from being misapplied to the wrong collection tube or container—an occurrence that is all too frequent in clinical care settings where groups of specimen labels are printed together as a batch, in advance of specimen collection. Similarly, the use of bar coded wristbands does not prevent wristbands from being applied to the incorrect patient. While bar code technology reduces transcription errors, the technology by itself does not guarantee accurate specimen or patient identification. In fact, transition to bar codes without deployment of an adequate number of bar code printers may paradoxically increase identification errors, because already-collected specimens tend to queue up in a batch near the closest available bar code printer, while labels print.

Positive Patient Identification Systems

The emergence of point-of-care bar code label printers and bar code scanners offers the potential to capture the high read-reliability of bar codes in clinical settings, while minimizing the likelihood that labels will be applied to the incorrect specimen container. Portable bar code label printers generate specimen labels at the time of venipuncture, after a patient's bar coded identification bracelet is scanned. Some systems make use of portable scanners in which collection tubes that have been bar coded by the manufacturer are associated with a particular patient by scanning both the patient's identification bracelet and the specimen container, one after the other. In some implementations, the phlebotomist's identification badge is also scanned in order to capture the identity of the phlebotomist. Several identification systems that use point-of-care bar code printing and scanning technologies are available commercially, although the systems are expensive, and real-world data demonstrating the effectiveness of these systems is disappointingly sparse.

Radio Frequency Identification

Radio frequency identification (RFID) systems are made up of readers and "tags" that consist of a microchip attached to a micro-antenna. When the tag comes in proximity to a reader, the tag broadcasts the information contained in its chip. Recently, the cost of tags has plunged from 2 dollars to 20 cents each, and is likely to fall to 5 cents or less in the next several years. RFID tags are made in the millions and used to track livestock, parts in car factories, razor blade packages on store shelves, and luggage at airports.[89] The principal advantage of RFID tags in the health care industry is that they do not need to be physically scanned—they signal their presence when in the proximity of a reader. RFID chips can be affixed to patient wristbands and to specimen tubes at the time of manufacture. The patient and tube identification numbers can be positively associated with one another when both come within proximity of a single reader, obviating the need for labeling tubes and the problems that occur when nursing staff print labels in batches prior to specimen collection.

Process Redundancy

In the absence of a technical system to prevent identification errors, the application of redundancy to critical steps in the identification process has the potential to reduce errors. The College of American Pathologists and JCAHO currently require that two different data elements be used to positively identify patients (such as name and medical record or unit number). During the patient registration process, this requirement is often met by having registrars pick patients off of computer screens that include two or more identifying elements. Unfortunately, registrars do not faithfully check all of the elements before selecting patients from the list. A system which first requires that patients be picked from a list by name, followed by separate confirmation of birth date or medical record number, creates a more robust double-check that is more likely to decrease identification errors.

Order Communication

The goal of order communication is to accurately transmit a provider's request for specific laboratory services, along with any special information necessary to carry out the provider's request. Inaccurate order communication may cause a laboratory to perform tests that a physician did not order, or to not perform tests that a physician requested. At a minimum, order communication errors waste resources. More seriously, order communication failures may delay diagnosis, cause results to be inaccurate (when required ancillary information is garbled), or deny patients timely delivery of blood products or other treatments.

CLIA regulations specify certain standards that must be followed to ensure accurate order communication:

> The laboratory must have a written or electronic request for patient testing from an authorized person. The laboratory may accept oral requests for laboratory tests if it solicits a written or electronic authorization within 30 days of the oral request and maintains the authorization or documentation of its efforts to obtain the authorization. The laboratory must ensure the test requisition solicits the following information: (1) The name and address or other suitable identifiers of the authorized person requesting the test and, if appropriate, the individual responsible for using the test results, or the name and address of the laboratory submitting the specimen, including, as applicable, a contact person to enable the reporting of imminently life threatening laboratory results or panic or alert values. (2) The patient's name or unique patient identifier. (3) The sex and age or date of birth of the patient. (4) The test(s) to be performed. (5) The source of the specimen, when appropriate. (6) The date and, if appropriate, time of specimen collection. (7) For Pap smears, the patient's last menstrual period, and indication of whether the patient had a previous abnormal report, treatment, or biopsy. (8) Any additional information relevant and necessary for a specific test to ensure accurate and timely testing and reporting of results, including interpretation, if applicable.
>
> If the laboratory transcribes or enters test requisition or authorization information into a record system or a laboratory information system, the laboratory must ensure the information is transcribed or entered accurately.[90]

This section discusses the magnitude of order communication problems and the control measures that have proven to be effective in reducing communication errors.

Exhibit 16. Accuracy of Order Communication During First 2 Days of Hospitalization [94]

| | Institution Percentiles (N=577) Orders or tests without any errors (percent) | | | | |
	10th	25th	50th (median)	75th	90th
Ordered tests that were performed (%)	92.9	96.2	98.1*	99.3	100.0
Performed tests that were ordered (%)	93.5	97.1	99.3	100.0	100.0
Orders present in medical record (%)	80.5	93.2	98.9	100.0	100.0

* For example, at the median facility of the 577 laboratories that participated in this study, 98.1% of ordered tests were performed (and 1.9% were not). Tests that could not be completed because of specimen collection difficulties were not counted. Higher percentiles indicate better relative performance.

Magnitude of Order Communication Risks

Most laboratories attempt to collect information required by CLIA, although 2.2% of laboratories inspected by the CAP in 2004 were cited for not capturing the date of specimen collection as part of the order entry process.[91] Accurate order communication appears to be a problem at a number of institutions. Finn and colleagues[92] studied orders for thyroid function studies at two academic centers and found that more than half of all orders for thyroid function tests were communicated inaccurately. In a study of 502 institutions, 19% of duplicate TSH tests had apparently never been ordered and were performed in error.[93]

Multi-institutional studies have been carried out to assess the frequency of order entry errors in both inpatients and outpatients. In a study of 225,000 test orders on inpatients at 577 institutions, staff at each facility compared a list of performed tests to tests ordered in the patient's medical record.[94] Tests which could not be performed because of specimen collection problems were excluded from the analysis. Approximately 2.5% of tests performed by laboratories were never ordered, and 2.9% of tests that were ordered were never performed. Variation in performance among laboratories is shown in Exhibit 16. When a reason for an order communication problem could be determined, two-thirds were attributed to computer order entry errors.

A parallel study of outpatient order entry errors involved 115,000 orders placed at 660 institutions.[95] Staff at each facility compared performed tests to test actually requested on 100 outpatient requisition forms. Overall, 4.8% of requisitions were associated with at least one order entry error, the most common being incorrectly entering the ordering physician's name. Variation in outpatient order accuracy among laboratories is shown in Exhibit 17.

Communication of clinical information necessary for rendering an anatomic pathology diagnosis was studied in 341 laboratories.[96] Inadequate information was defined as a requirement by the interpreting pathologist for additional, unsupplied, clinical information before a diagnosis could be rendered. Cases that had no clinical information on a requisition slip were not considered to have inadequate clinical history if the absence of history did not hinder diagnosis. Overall, 0.73% of cases required additional information; the rate was lower in larger institutions. Reports were delayed by a day or more in approximately one-third of

Exhibit 17. Accuracy of Order Communication for Outpatients [95]

	Institution Percentiles (N=603) Errors per requisitions (percent)		
	10th	50th (median)	90th
Overall error rate (any type)	18.0	6.0*	1.0
Order error rate (specific type)			
Tests ordered but not performed	6.0	1.0	0.0
Tests performed but not ordered	5.0	1.0	0.0
Physician name discrepancies	8.0	1.9	0.0
Test priority errors	3.9	0.0	0.0

* For example, at the median facility of the 603 laboratories that participated in this study, 6% of requisitions had at least one order entry error. Tests that could not be completed because of specimen collection difficulties were not counted. Higher percentiles indicate better relative performance.

Exhibit 18. Communication of Required Clinical Information in Surgical Pathology [96]

	Institution Percentiles (N=341)				
	10th	25th	50th (median)	75th	90th
Cases requiring additional clinical information (%)	3.01	1.57	0.62*	0.22	0.08

* For example, at the median facility of the 341 laboratories that participated in this study, 0.62% of surgical pathology requisitions were lacking information the interpreting pathologist believed necessary to provide a diagnosis.

cases in which additional information was required. Variation in performance among institutions is shown in Exhibit 18.

Control Measures to Improve Order Communication

The practice of checking computer orders against written orders was associated significantly with lower order error rates in studies of both inpatient and outpatient order entry errors. For inpatients, unit staff typically perform this check using the patient's medical record. For outpatients, laboratory staff perform this check using the test requisition.

In addition to checking orders, institutions that monitor order entry errors on a regular basis demonstrate lower error rates. These two control measures—double-checking computer orders and ongoing monitoring of error rates—should be seriously considered by every laboratory manager because they are easily implemented and require no special equipment or computer software.

The two multi-institutional order entry error studies are noteworthy for factors that were not found to have any significant association with order entry errors: use of test panels and profiles, use of laboratory requisition forms that contain order mnemonics or code numbers, use of order entry computer screens that match the layout of test requisitions, interfacing hospital and laboratory information systems, and preprinted order forms for common medical problems or surgical procedures. Either these practices are ineffective in reducing errors, or the studies were inadequately powered to detect a beneficial effect.

Since the CAP order entry error studies were conducted, a number of hospitals have instituted computerized physician order entry (CPOE) systems in which physicians directly enter orders into clinical computers. When integrated into an order communication system that ensures electronic transmission of orders to the laboratory information system, CPOE bypasses ward clerks and other ancillary staff who might otherwise change orders as they transfer information from paper documents to computer systems.[92] CPOE has improved the accuracy of pharmacy order communication in a number of studies; it has not been examined in multi-institutional studies of laboratory order communication.

In the study of surgical pathology requisitions with inadequate clinical information, no policies or procedures were found to be significantly associated with more complete requisitions, and we have no control measures to recommend for addressing order communication problems in anatomic pathology. The use of special requisition slips for certain anatomic sites or organs, provision of sufficient space on requisition slips for clinical history, and adoption of policies requiring clinical information before sign-out were not associated with a reduction in the number of requisitions requiring supplementary clinical information.

Specimen Collection and Handling

Clinical specimens collected for analysis should be suited to the test systems for which they are destined. This means that specimens should be collected in appropriate containers, at appropriate times, and with patients in the appropriate state (eg, prior to receiving antibiotics, fasting). Specimens should meet applicable standards for acceptability (eg, no hemolysis, clotting) and should be transported to the laboratory in a time frame and under conditions that do not interfere with analysis.

Since some specimens are collected by clinical caregivers and others by laboratory staff, responsibility for appropriate collection and handling is shared by clinicians and the laboratory. CLIA regulations stipulate that the laboratory must make available collection instructions for each assay the laboratory offers and provide a clinical consultant to answer questions about specimen collection.

Magnitude of Specimen Collection and Handling Risks

Most institutions appear to take specimen collection and handling seriously, although some laboratories need to apply more attention to this area. During 2004, CAP inspectors cited 1.5% of microbiology facilities for failing to check the quality of sputum specimens or notify caregivers when unacceptable specimens were received.[91] Multi-institutional studies that have focused on specimen collection risks are summarized below, along with data that can be used to benchmark the performance of individual facilities.

Exhibit 19. Rejected Specimens

Laboratory Test	Number of Institutions	Institution Percentiles (percent rejected specimens)		
		10th	50th (median)	90th
Complete blood count[97]	703	1.25*	0.38	0.12
Blood chemistry specimens[98]	453	1.35	0.31	0.06

* For example, among 703 laboratories that studied rejection of complete blood count specimens, 10% of laboratories rejected at least 1.25% of specimens. Higher percentiles indicate better relative performance (lower rejection rates).

Specimen Acceptability

A study of almost 8 million complete blood count (CBC) specimens in 703 institutions disclosed that 0.45% did not meet local institutional criteria for acceptability.[97] Variation among laboratories is shown in Exhibit 19. Ten percent of institutions had rejection rates 3 times the mean and 10 times the rate of the top 10% of institutions. Reasons for rejection of more than 35,000 CBC specimens are shown in Exhibit 20. Clotted specimens accounted for the majority of rejections (65%), but inadequate specimen quantity accounted for 10%.

A study of more than 10 million chemistry specimens in 453 laboratories disclosed results similar to those of the CBC study (Exhibit 19).[98] In aggregate, 0.35% of specimens were rejected; there was more than a 20-fold difference in the rejection rates of the top and bottom

Exhibit 20. Reasons for Rejected Complete Blood Count Specimens [97]

Reason	Number	(%)
Specimen clotted	22,901	(64.8)
Insufficient specimen quantity	3554	(10.1)
Unacceptable variance (delta check)	1886	(5.3)
Inadequately identified	1816	(5.1)
Specimen lost/not received	1041	(2.9)
Platelets clumped	772	(2.2)
Specimen hemolyzed	691	(2.0)
IV line fluid contamination	577	(1.6)
Improper collection container	497	(1.4)
Delayed transport	301	(0.9)
Laboratory accident	200	(0.6)
Damage in transit	146	(0.4)
Other	943	(2.7)

Exhibit 21. Reasons for Rejected Blood Chemistry Specimens [98]

Reason	Number	(%)
Specimen hemolyzed	22,531	(59.6)
Quantity insufficient	4313	(11.4)
Inadequately identified	2549	(6.7)
Specimen lost/not received	1516	(4.0)
Improper collection container	1337	(3.5)
Specimen clotted	621	(1.6)
Excessive delay	503	(1.3)
Laboratory accident	419	(1.1)
Incorrect storage	330	(0.9)
Inadequate separation	230	(0.6)
Specimen damaged in transit	144	(0.4)
Other	3340	(8.8)

Exhibit 22. Blood Culture Contamination [99]

Patient Population	Number of Institutions	Assessment of Contamination	Institution Percentiles (percent contaminated culture sets)				
			10th	25th	50th (median)	75th	90th
Inpatient	589	Laboratory	5.4*	3.8	2.5	1.5	0.9
Inpatient	560	Clinical	5.2	3.6	2.1	1.2	0.9
Outpatient	365	Laboratory	5.8	4.1	2.4	1.1	0.4
Outpatient	316	Clinical	5.6	3.9	2.1	1.1	0.4

* For example, among 589 laboratories in which the assessment of contamination was performed by the laboratory, at least 5.4% of inpatient blood culture sets were considered contaminated in 10% of laboratories. Higher percentiles equal better performance (lower contamination rates).

decile laboratories. Reasons for rejection of more than 38,000 chemistry specimens are shown in Exhibit 21. Hemolysis and inadequate specimen quantity were the two most common reasons for rejection.

Specimen Contamination

Contamination rates can be used as a measure of the quality of specimens collected for microbiologic culture. Although some contamination is unavoidable, specimen contamination rates vary significantly among laboratories. A study of blood culture contamination involving 640 institutions and 497,134 blood cultures showed the median laboratory to have a contamination rate of 2.1% to 2.5%, depending on whether the specimens were from inpatients or outpatients and whether contamination was assessed by the laboratory or clinical staff (Exhibit 22).[99] Regardless of the population being tested and the individuals responsible for assessing contamination, there was more than a 5-fold difference in the contamination rate of the top and bottom decile laboratories.

Urine culture contamination rates were explored in a study of 630 institutions that collectively cultured 155,037 urine specimens.[100] Because there is a marked difference in the contamination rates of urine specimens from males and females, only sex-specific contamination rates should be compared among institutions to ensure that differences are not due to a different mix of specimens from males and females (Exhibit 23). The median institution reported that 9.5% of male and 20.6% of female urine culture specimens were contaminated.

It is important to make a distinction between the definition of specimen contamination used to assess specimen quality and the definition of contamination used to guide clinical decision making. The definition of blood culture contamination used to assess specimen quality (isolation of coagulase-negative staphylococci, diphtheroid organisms, or *Bacillus* species from single blood culture bottles) is not suitable for clinical decision making because a small number of cultures classified as contaminates will actually represent clinical infection.[101] Similarly, the definition of urine specimen contamination used to benchmark urine specimen

Exhibit 23. Urine Culture Contamination in Outpatients [100]						
		Institution Percentiles (percent contaminated specimens)				
Patient Population	**Number of Institutions**	**10th**	**25th**	**50th (median)**	**75th**	**90th**
Male	593	22.0*	14.5	9.5	5.2	2.3
Female	590	41.7	32.0	20.6	11.8	6.4
Emergency Department	524	33.3	25.3	15.7	8.1	4.4
Other Adjacent Site	523	40.8	28.0	16.5	7.8	3.3
Non-Adjacent Site	532	42.3	31.0	19.3	10.9	5.5

* For example, at least 22% of male urine culture specimens met the study definition of contamination in the bottom 10% of 593 laboratories. Higher percentiles equal better performance (lower contamination rates).

quality (specimens that yield at least 10,000 colony-forming units (CFU)/mL of two or more organism types) is not suitable for determining which patients to treat, because a small fraction of specimens classified as contaminated will actually be from patients with polymicrobial urinary tract infections.

Timing of Specimen Collection

In some circumstances, such as the measurement of digoxin levels, the timing of specimen collection has important implications for the interpretation of results. More than 600 laboratories that collectively performed more than 280,000 digoxin measurements studied issues with timing of collection.[102] Of the 15,155 toxic levels reported by laboratories, 1346 (9%) were collected between 6 and 8 hours from the patient's last dose of digoxin, and 3705 (24%) were obtained less than 6 hours from the patient's last dose. These intervals are generally considered too short to produce interpretable results. This is because physiologic equilibrium after digoxin ingestion is not established for 6 to 8 hours after ingestion, and serum digoxin levels measured before this time will not accurately reflect tissue levels. The failure to adequately time digoxin specimen collection has important patient safety implications because values that appear to be "toxic" may actually reflect the timing of collection and not a patient's physiological state. A more recent study[103] of digoxin level collection timing in 59 laboratories (Exhibit 24) showed that the median facility collected 22.2% of digoxin levels at an inappropriate time (less than 6 hours after the patient's last digoxin dose).

Unsuccessful Specimen Collection

A global measure of blood specimen collection quality in the outpatient setting is the fraction of patients who must be turned away from a phlebotomy service area because of one or more problems. A study of 833,289 outpatient phlebotomy encounters at 210 institutions disclosed that the vast majority (99.6%) resulted in successful specimen collection (Exhibit 25).[104]

Exhibit 24. Digoxin Collection Timing [103]

Interval from Patient's Last Digoxin Dose	Institution Percentiles (N=59) (percent of specimens collected)				
	10th	25th	50th (median)	75th	90th
Less than 6 hours	66.7	44.4	22.2*	14.3	1.2
Less than 8 hours	80.0	55.6	34.3	20.0	1.2

* For example, among 59 laboratories, the median facility reported that 22.2% of outpatients had blood collected for digoxin determination less than 6 hours from the time patients received their last dose.

Exhibit 25. Outpatient Phlebotomy Success [104]

Quality Indicator	Institution Percentiles (N=210)		
	10th	50th (median)	90th
Successful encounters (%)	98.05	99.61*	99.96
Recollection rate (%)	0.90	0.26	0.05

* For example, among 210 facilities, the median laboratory reported that 99.61% of phlebotomies resulted in successful specimen collection. A "successful encounter" resulted in an acceptable specimen. "Recollection rate" indicates the number of specimens requiring recollection divided by the number of outpatient phlebotomy encounters. Higher percentiles indicate better relative performance (more successful encounters and lower recollection rates).

Phlebotomies were unsuccessful because patients were not fasting as directed (32.2% of failed collections), test orders were missing information (22.5% of failures), patients' specimens were difficult to draw (13.0%), patients left the collection area before specimens could be collected (11.8%), patients were improperly prepared for reasons other than fasting (6.3%), patients presented at the wrong time (3.1%), or for other reasons (11.8%). Of the specimens that were collected, 0.3% were later found to be unsuitable. These samples were hemolyzed (18.1% of unsuitable specimens), of insufficient quantity (16.0%), clotted (13.4%), lost or not received in the testing laboratory (11.5%), inadequately labeled (5.8%), at variance with previous or expected results (4.8%), or unacceptable for other reasons (31.1%).

Volume of Specimen Collection

Collection of excess blood volumes may cause iatrogenic (care-induced) anemia.[105] A study of blood volumes collected in 140 facilities showed that the average laboratory's blood collection volume for complete blood counts (2.76 mL) was 8.5 times the volume required by the laboratory's CBC testing instrument. On average, the volume collected for electrolyte panels (1.75 mL) was 12 times the volume required by the electrolyte testing instrument in use.[106] Performance among institutions showed considerable variation (Exhibit 26).

Exhibit 26. Blood Collection Volume [106]

Blood Volume Collected (mL)	Institution Percentiles (N=140)				
	10th	25th	50th (median)	75th	90th
Complete Blood Counts					
Standard volume	5.00	4.00	3.00*	2.00	1.00
Reduced volume	2.50	1.90	1.00	0.50	0.25
Electrolytes					
Standard volume	4.10	3.00	2.00	1.00	0.50
Reduced volume	2.00	1.00	0.50	0.30	0.20
Overcollection Ratio					
Complete Blood Counts					
Standard volume	21.6	16.7	8.5*	4.5	2.5
Reduced volume	10.0	6.7	3.0	1.7	1.0
Electrolytes					
Standard volume	60.0	29.0	12.0	5.4	2.8
Reduced volume	20.0	10.0	4.2	2.0	1.3

* For example, the median facility collected 3 mL for a standard CBC, which was 8.5 times more than required by the facility's analytic instrument. Overcollection ratio equals requested volume divided by minimum analytic volume. "Reduced volume" refers to an institution's pediatric tube size. Higher percentiles indicate better relative performance.

Exhibit 27. Longitudinal Tracking of Specimen Collection Quality (2004 Q-Tracks Data) [107,108]

	Number of Institutions	Institution Percentiles				
		10th	25th	50th (median)	75th	90th
Blood culture contamination (%)	151	1.59	2.03	2.65	3.41	4.27
Specimen rejection rate (%)	147	0.12	0.26	0.56	1.02	1.51

Specimen Collection Quality Over Time

Participants in CAP Q-Tracks programs have the opportunity to track two indicators of specimen collection over time: blood culture contamination rate[107] and the chemistry/hematology specimen acceptance rate.[108] Performance data from 2004 are shown in Exhibit 27 and can be used by managers to benchmark quality locally.

Control Measures to Improve Specimen Collection

A number of procedures can be applied to mitigate the risk of inadequate or improper specimen collection. In the previously cited study of hematology specimen rejection,[97] rejection was

Exhibit 28. Reduction in Specimen Collection Errors with Continuous Monitoring of Errors [107,108]		
Years of Continuous Monitoring	Mean Reduction in Specimen Rejection Rate*	Mean Reduction in Blood Culture Contamination Rate*
1 – 2	0.13%	N/S
3 – 4	0.26%	0.24%
5 – 6	0.44%	0.93%

* Figures represent the absolute reduction in the percentage of inadequate specimens experienced by the average participant. For example, after 1-2 years of monitoring specimen rejection, a laboratory near the median (with an initial specimen rejection rate of 0.56%) would on average have reduced its rejection rate to 0.43% (a reduction in the overall rejection rate of 0.13%). Similarly, after 5-6 years of monitoring blood culture contamination, a laboratory near the median (with an initial blood culture contamination rate of 2.65%) would record on average a contamination rate of 1.72% (a reduction in the contamination rate of 0.93%). Of course, some laboratories did not improve by the amount shown in the exhibit, while others enjoyed more pronounced improvement. Some laboratories began the study with better baseline performance, and others with worse. N/S = no significant change.

significantly more common when microtube containers were used (4.4 times the rejection rate reported with standard tubes), when specimens were collected by in-hospital nonlaboratory phlebotomy personnel (2.5 times the rejection rate of laboratory phlebotomists), and when specimens were collected by in-hospital, nonlaboratory, nonphlebotomy staff (4.0 times the rejection rate of laboratory phlebotomists). The previously cited study of chemistry specimen acceptability drew similar conclusions.[98]

In a study of blood culture contamination,[99] the use of a dedicated phlebotomy service was also associated with significantly lower contamination rates, as were the use of tincture of iodine (versus iodophor) as a topical disinfectant and the application of antiseptic to the top of blood culture collection bottles prior to inoculation. In the previously cited urine culture contamination study,[100] no control measures were found effective in reducing urine contamination, although specimens transported over greater distances showed a trend towards more frequent contamination.

In studies of digoxin level collection timing, significantly worse performance (higher fraction of inappropriately timed specimens) was more common with stat specimens, outpatient specimens, and the absence of a written policy to check the timing of the last digoxin dose before collecting blood.[102] Institutions that tracked the timing of therapeutic drug monitoring as a quality indicator prior to the onset of the study also demonstrated better performance.[103]

In the outpatient arena, blood collection facilities that are staffed by laboratory-administered phlebotomists are also more likely to successfully collect blood, and less likely to collect specimens that will later be rejected, than facilities that are staffed by others.[104] Overcollection of blood volumes appears to be primarily a function of the type of specimen collection tube (microtube versus other) employed by a facility and is not influenced by the analytic platform used to test specimens.[106] Microtube containers are associated with lower over-collection ratios (although they are also associated with more frequent hemolysis).

Finally, monitoring specimen collection quality on an ongoing basis is associated with improved performance over time. Data from the two Q-Tracks studies that focus on specimen collection have both demonstrated progressive improvement in performance with more lengthy program enrollment (Exhibit 28).[107,108]

Appropriate Ordering of Laboratory Services

A physician's decision to order a laboratory test or blood product represents the first step in the laboratory value stream—the initial request by a customer for service. Promoting the thoughtful use of laboratory services is where laboratory quality management properly begins. There is little point to ensuring the accuracy and timeliness of an examination that never needed to be ordered in the first place.

The responsibility for ordering laboratory services appropriately is divided between the clinical caregiver and the clinical laboratory. An authorized caregiver (the customer) makes the final decision about what services to order and generally does not communicate to the laboratory his or her reasons for ordering a particular test or blood product. However, a laboratory (the supplier) may also become involved in ordering decisions, particularly when expensive or esoteric services are involved. Most laboratories receive periodic inquiries from caregivers who wish to know what test to order, usually in complex or unusual clinical situations. CLIA requires that laboratories which perform nonwaived testing engage a "clinical consultant" who is available to assist laboratory clients in ensuring that appropriate services are ordered.

Many laboratories have taken a newfound interest in ensuring appropriate use of services in order to control expenses. Blood products have become increasingly costly,[109] and charges for some molecular diagnostic tests may reach several thousand dollars. Inappropriate use of laboratory services can divert resources from quality management and other productive activities. In the case of blood products, inappropriate use also exposes patients to unnecessary clinical risk.

How Appropriately are Laboratory Services Ordered?

Global Laboratory Utilization Ratios

Early investigations showed that many laboratory tests are not used productively by physicians, and that test use could be reduced without causing under-utilization.[110] As cost containment efforts spread throughout medicine, four ratios emerged as global top-down measures of laboratory test utilization (Exhibit 29).[111] In the outpatient setting, the number of tests per person per month and the number of tests per requisition were used as overall measures of laboratory utilization; while on the inpatient side, the number of tests per discharge and number of tests per day became the most popular measures of utilization.

> **Exhibit 29. Global Laboratory Utilization Rates**
>
> ❖ Tests per person per month
>
> ❖ Tests per requisition
>
> ❖ Tests per discharge
>
> ❖ Tests per inpatient day

There is wide variation among laboratories in these four measures. Nevertheless, we are not enamored with these ratios as quality indicators. In the first place, they are subject to confounding by a number of other variables. Different laboratories count tests differently. In the outpatient setting, the number of tests ordered per person per month is impacted by insurance benefit structure, population age, and the inclusion or exclusion of anatomic pathology testing, physician-office testing, reference testing, and out-of-network testing. In the inpatient setting, utilization ratios are influenced by the Medicare case mix index, length of stay,

		Institution Percentiles				
Monitor	**Number of Institutions**	**10th**	**25th**	**50th (median)**	**75th**	**90th**
aPTT or anti–factor Xa level obtained within 12 h of first heparin dose	140	85.5*	93.3	98.3	100.0	100.0
Platelet count obtained within 72 h of first dose	140	66.7	81.7	93.3	100.0	100.0

Exhibit 30. Monitoring Patients Receiving Unfractionated Heparin [114]

* For example, in 10% of 140 laboratories, 85.5% or fewer patients who were receiving unfractionated heparin had an aPTT or anti-factor Xa assay performed within 12 hours of the first heparin dose. Higher percentiles indicate better performance (a higher proportion of monitored patients). aPTT = activated partial thromboplastin time.

hospital size, physiological status of patients in intensive care units, surgical/medical service mix, hospital teaching status, and the inclusion or exclusion of point-of-care test counts.[112]

More fundamentally, it is not clear to us what laboratory directors should do if they find that their hospital-based laboratory has a high test per discharge ratio or a high number of tests being ordered per inpatient day. Global utilization ratios, adjusted for confounding co-factors, may indicate that a health plan, capitated outreach laboratory, or inpatient laboratory has an opportunity for improvement, but these utilization ratios do not suggest where opportunity lies or a specific course of action that can be pursued to correct a problem.

Specific Indicators of Appropriate Laboratory Use

For promoting the appropriate use of laboratory services, we find most useful specific indicators of proper laboratory use that can be readily measured and impacted by concrete management initiatives. Any number of clinical practice guidelines can be adapted as a measure of appropriate laboratory use. For example, when the National Cholesterol Education Project (NCEP) recommends that cholesterol in adults be assayed every five years,[113] a laboratory manager may construct an indicator of appropriate laboratory use based on the frequency with which patients receive NCEP-recommended cholesterol screening. In this section, we list indicators of appropriate laboratory use that have been studied in multiple laboratories, so that managers may compare local performance with peer institutions and determine where utilization management efforts can be most fruitfully directed.

Anticoagulant Monitoring. Patients receiving unfractionated heparin should be monitored for anticoagulant and antiplatelet effects and have their dose adjusted in response to monitoring results. A study of heparin monitoring practices at 140 institutions showed significant variation in compliance with recommended heparin monitoring practices (Exhibit 30).[114] Since the clinical risks from under- and over-anticoagulation with heparin are significant, this indicator of laboratory utilization has important patient safety implications.

Blood Product Wastage. Blood product wastage signals inappropriate use of laboratory services and represents a significant expense at some facilities. At the time of this writing, the CAP has been measuring wasted allogenic blood products in a longitudinal Q-Tracks study

Exhibit 31. Blood Product Wastage Rate [115]

Blood Product	Number of Institutions	Institution Percentiles				
		10th	25th	50th (median)	75th	90th
Overall rate (%)	92	3.89	2.56	1.65	1.11	0.64
Red blood cell rate (%)	92	1.05*	0.65	0.36	0.21	0.10
Fresh frozen plasma rate (%)	92	9.37	7.03	4.85	2.94	1.24
Platelet concentrates rate (%)	62	16.13	6.33	1.58	0.00	0.00
Single donor platelets rate (%)	89	10.42	4.44	0.97	0.15	0.00
Cryoprecipitate rate (%)	81	13.00	7.82	4.52	0.41	0.00

* For example, among 92 laboratories, 10% of facilities wasted at least 1.05% of allogenic red blood cells units. Outdated units are not included in these figures. Higher percentiles indicate better performance (lower wastage rates).

Exhibit 32. Type and Screen Completion Prior to Start of Elective Surgery [117]

Type and Screen Completion	Number of Institutions	Institution Percentiles				
		10th	25th	50th (median)	75th	90th
Completed at least 1 d prior to surgery	106	21.0*	42.4	68.9	86.0	94.0
Completed after start of surgery	103	75.0	46.2	22.6	2.9	0.0

* For example, among 106 laboratories, 10% of facilities has only 21% of the requested type and screen examinations completed one day prior to surgery. Higher percentiles indicate better relative performance.

for six years (Exhibit 31)[115] and has measured blood product wastage in several one-time Q-Probes studies.[116] Outdated units are not counted as wasted products; only allogenic units that were ordered but never used are tabulated by study participants. Cancelled orders are the most common reason for product wastage (45% of units), followed by improper handling and/or breakage (26%).

Type and Screen Completion Prior to Surgery. Exhibit 32 shows data from a multi-institutional study of how frequently blood type and screen (T&S) procedures were completed prior to the start of elective scheduled surgery.[117] This indicator measures whether laboratory services are ordered at an appropriate interval before surgery, so that surgeons can count on the availability of blood. (The indicator also measures whether the collection and testing of specimens is timely.) Failure to complete T&S prior to the onset of surgery may pose risks for

Exhibit 33. Solitary Blood Cultures in Adults [118]

Solitary Blood Cultures	Number of Institutions	Institution Percentiles		
		10th	50th (median)	90th
Adult inpatients (study #1)	521	39.3	10.1*	2.0
Adult inpatients (study #2)	673	44.4	12.1	2.5
Adult outpatients (study #1)	475	71.9	25.4	4.3
Adult outpatients (study #2)	637	83.3	33.3	7.1

* For example, among 475 laboratories in the first study of inpatient solitary blood cultures, 10.1% of blood culture sets were solitary. Higher percentiles indicate better relative performance (lower fraction of solitary blood cultures).

patients if blood is required emergently, particularly when unexpected antibodies are detected during the rush to find compatible blood.

Solitary Blood Cultures. Outside of pediatrics, there are few indications for performing solitary blood cultures (ie, ordering a single set of cultures to detect bacteremia). Solitary blood cultures do not allow infection caused by skin flora (such as coagulase-negative *Staphylococcus* species) to be reliably distinguished from blood culture contamination, and the smaller total blood volume obtained with a solitary blood culture decreases culture sensitivity. The frequency of solitary blood cultures at a large number of hospital-based laboratories is shown in Exhibit 33. Data in Exhibit 33 were drawn from two separate studies that included 289,572 blood culture sets at 909 institutions[118] and was replicated in a third study of 333 smaller-than-average hospitals.[119] These studies identified several control measures that can be applied to increase the ordering of paired sets of blood cultures in adults. Solitary blood culture rates were lower in institutions that used dedicated laboratory phlebotomists to collect blood culture specimens, where internal policies required drawing at least two blood culture sets, and where laboratory personnel contacted clinicians to clarify orders for solitary blood culture sets.

Glycohemoglobin Monitoring. Measurement of glycohemoglobin A1c (HbA1c) is used to assess long-term glycemic control in patients with diabetes. The American Diabetes Association currently recommends quarterly HbA1c monitoring of patients not in reasonable glycemic control, with semiannual monitoring thereafter.[120] A study conducted in 212 institutions demonstrated wide variation in HbA1c monitoring (Exhibit 34).[121] This same study found a significant correlation between the degree of monitoring and the level of glycemic control subsequently achieved, underscoring the clinical importance of this measure.

Stool Microbiology. Although stool examination for bacteria and parasites can be pivotal in determining the etiology of infectious diarrhea, it is unusual to acquire a parasitic or bacterial enteric infection while in the hospital (other than infection with *Clostridium difficile*). Despite this fact, a study conducted at 601 institutions showed that a sizable proportion of more than 50,000 inpatient stool bacteriology specimens had been collected after the first

Exhibit 34. Glycohemoglobin Monitoring in Diabetics [120]

	Institution Percentiles (N=212)				
	10th	25th	50th (median)	75th	90th
Quarterly Monitoring					
All patients	6.7	13.8	27.7*	43.3	55.2
Patients with initial HbA1c level <7%	0.0	15.2	30.4	43.2	57.1
Patients with initial HbA1c level <9%	0.0	5.6	29.3	50.0	66.7
Patients with initial HbA1c level <11%	0.0	0.0	0.0	50.0	100.0
Semiannual or More Frequent Monitoring					
All patients	36.7	54.1	68.6	80.0	86.7
Patients with initial HbA1c level <7%	38.5	53.8	68.2	81.3	90.5
Patients with initial HbA1c level <9%	25.0	50.0	66.7	85.7	100.0
Patients with initial HbA1c level <11%	0.0	33.3	66.7	100.0	100.0

* For example, at the median facility of the 212 laboratories that participated in this study, 27.7% of diabetic patients had their glycohemoglobin monitored quarterly. Higher percentiles indicate better performance.

Exhibit 35. Use of Stool Microbiology [122]

	All Institution Percentiles (N=601)		
	10th	50th (median)	90th
Percentage of inpatient bacteriology stool specimens collected on hospital days 1–3	38.2*	63.3	81.3
Percentage of inpatient bacteriology stool specimens with *Clostridium difficile* test order	24.0	52.1	77.0
Percentage of inpatient parasitology stool specimens collected on hospital days 1–4	48.7	71.4	89.7

* For example, at 10% of 601 facilities, no more than 38.2% of inpatient bacteriology stool cultures were collected during the first three days of hospitalization. Higher percentiles indicate better relative performance.

three days of hospitalization, when the risk of acquiring bacterial enteritis was very small (Exhibit 35).[122] Further, many bacteriology specimens ordered on inpatients were ordered without an accompanying order for *C. difficile* toxin testing, the most common cause of hospital-acquired infectious diarrhea. The study also found that a sizable fraction of more than 50,000 parasitology specimens ordered on inpatients were ordered after the fourth day of hospitalization, when community-acquired parasitic infections should already have been diagnosed. Among laboratories, there was moderate variability in these indicators, any or all of which can be used to assess the appropriateness of inpatient stool microbiology testing.

Exhibit 36. Duplicate Testing [123]

	Institution Percentiles (N=501)				
	10th	**25th**	**50th (median)**	**75th**	**90th**
Percent of TSH assays that were duplicates	4.5	2.9	1.5*	0.7	0.2

* For example, among 501 laboratories, the median facility reported that 1.5% of TSH assays were duplicates (ordered within 7 days of a previous TSH order). Higher percentiles indicate better relative performance. TSH = thyroid stimulating hormone.

Duplicate Testing. Duplicate assays for thyroid stimulating hormone (TSH) were examined in 501 institutions (Exhibit 36).[123] A duplicate assay was defined as a TSH order that was received within seven days of a previous TSH assay ordered on the same patient. There are very few clinical reasons for ordering TSH with this frequency, given the biology of the thyroid disease that TSH measures. Although the financial saving from eliminating duplicate TSH testing is low, the authors of this study argued that duplicate TSH testing served as a proxy for the degree to which all test ordering is coordinated among providers.

Control Measures to Promote Appropriate Ordering of Laboratory Services

Promoting appropriate use of laboratory services requires that the behavior of providers be changed. This is no easy undertaking. There are a number of organizational and cultural determinates of test ordering that are beyond the reach of the laboratory manager. For example, different types of on-call schedules are associated with different patterns of test use.[124] Settings in which multiple physicians order tests on the same patient are associated with a higher rate of duplicate testing,[125] and physicians who practice in groups of larger size tend to order significantly more tests than physicians who work in small groups or as solo practitioners.[126] Even the nationality of providers appears to influence test ordering.[127]

The psychology of providers also seems to influence test ordering behavior. Physicians with a higher risk-taking propensity or certain personality types tend to order fewer tests.[128] Physicians with greater medical knowledge order more laboratory tests than their less knowledgeable colleagues, but those with more clinical experience order fewer.[129] While there is considerable variation among physicians in their use of tests, most providers already know whether their test use is higher or lower than peers; informing providers of their relative position does not usually change their test ordering behavior.[130] Finally, when interventions to modify test ordering behavior are first introduced, providers often change their behavior simply because they know their decision making is being observed. In time, when the novelty of being studied wears off, old patterns reassert themselves.[131]

Several reviews of techniques to change physicians' use of laboratory tests have been published.[132] We summarize the principal techniques on the following pages.

Exhibit 37. Reduction in Blood Product Wastage With Ongoing Monitoring [115]

Years of Monitoring	Mean Reduction in Overall Blood Product Wastage
1 – 2	0.09%
3 – 4	0.14%
5 – 6	0.83%*

* For example, if a laboratory began with an overall blood product wastage rate of 1.73%, after 5-6 years of ongoing monitoring, the wastage rate would have been reduced by 0.83%, resulting in a new rate of 0.90%. The figures in this column reflect reductions in product wastage experienced by the average participant. Some participants enjoyed larger reductions, while others experienced smaller benefits.

Monitoring

Ongoing monitoring is associated with improved use of laboratory services. Exhibit 37 shows the progressive reduction in blood product wastage experienced by laboratories that engaged in quarterly monitoring as part of the ongoing CAP Q-Tracks program.[115] It is doubtful that monitoring per se reduces blood product wastage. More likely, ongoing monitoring helps increase awareness and focus attention on correcting local operational issues that contribute to wastage.

Educational Interventions

Educational interventions are designed to transmit knowledge for the purpose of changing physician behavior. The literature has been reasonably consistent in demonstrating that educational interventions do not produce sustained reductions in test use.[133] This observation extends to the dissemination of clinical practice guidelines, which tend not to be adopted when presented in educational settings. We discourage reliance on education as a technique to modify test use.

Interpretive Reporting

The provision of individualized laboratory-supplied interpretations of complex coagulation tests has been reported to cause physicians to order additional tests more appropriately.[134] This type of intervention is time consuming and relies upon local expertise, which may not be present in some laboratories. Further, the cost-effectiveness of this approach has not been formally evaluated, although interpretive reporting may save money when applied to expensive tests or in resource-intensive care settings, where delayed diagnosis is likely to be costly.

Clinical Feedback

Providing feedback to clinicians about how they use tests has had mixed success in reducing laboratory utilization.[135] Reports that compare physicians' test ordering patterns to their peers generally do not influence future test ordering, although the literature is inconsistent.[136] Some studies suggest that when clinical feedback is combined with social pressure from clinical opinion leaders, behaviors are more likely to change.[137]

Financial Feedback

When physicians are supplied with information about the cost of the procedures they are ordering, utilization of laboratory services is generally reduced. This effect has been observed when cost feedback is given in the form of summary reports,[138] on laboratory requisitions,[139] and when costs are displayed on computer workstations at the time of order entry.[140] Even the provision of manuals that discuss test cost has resulted in lower laboratory utilization.[141]

Requiring Justification

A requirement that providers justify orders for specific laboratory tests has consistently been shown to reduce test demand, even when the justifications are not individually reviewed.[142]

Requirements for justification can be perceived as administratively burdensome by busy clinicians and should not be imposed without careful planning. Requirements for justification are better tolerated when they are restricted to expensive or esoteric tests or blood products, and when indications for testing have been approved by a group with broad clinical representation. Check-off boxes on computer order entry screens that allow physicians to select from an approved list of indications for testing are usually well tolerated, so long as the computer pathways do not hinder clinical productivity.

Changing the Test Requisitioning Process

Administrative interventions that change the process for ordering tests have proven to be effective techniques for reducing test use in several studies. The development of paper requisitions and computer screens that group tests within clinically meaningful categories (eg, hypothyroidism, upper respiratory infection) have improved the appropriateness of testing.[143] Listing fewer tests on requisition forms reduces test use,[144] and the display of previously ordered test results at the time of online physician order entry reduces demand for testing.[145]

Review of Testing Protocols

Some of the most successful programs aimed at reducing inpatient laboratory cost have targeted local, often unwritten testing protocols used in common clinical situations. A report from an academic intensive care unit showed a 65% reduction in laboratory test use after modification of standing laboratory testing protocols.[146] Another study reported a 25.9% reduction.[147] On a surgical service, reworking of standing orders resulted in a durable 46% reduction in arterial blood gas determinations and a 29% reduction in demand for other laboratory tests.[148]

Analytic Operations: Risks and Control Measures

Introducing New Tests

Automated testing has revolutionized the quality of clinical pathology analyses by providing a level of consistency and economy unattainable with manual methods. But the high precision of automated testing sometimes causes laboratory managers to overlook the importance of validating new test systems. When a system is improperly set up, consistency becomes a liability, as the automated analyzer turns out inaccurate results time and time again.

In this section we discuss the quality and patient safety risks that accompany the introduction of new tests, and control measures that can be applied to mitigate these risks. Failure to properly validate new tests appears to be a problem for a number of laboratories. In 2004, CAP Laboratory Accreditation Program inspectors cited 2.7% of laboratories for failing to perform one or more CLIA-mandated validation steps before placing a new test in service.[91]

Exhibit 38 provides a checklist of tasks (control measures) that laboratory management should consider before placing a new test into production.[149] This list should be referenced before introducing any new test—automated or manual, quantitative or qualitative, whether in clinical chemistry, transfusion medicine, anatomic pathology, or another laboratory section. Some of the tasks are not applicable to every test, and several of these tasks are covered in the preanalytic, postanalytic, and general laboratory systems sections of this chapter. Key tasks that involve the analytic phase of testing are discussed here.

Exhibit 38. Control Measures for Reducing the Risks Inherent in New Test Systems

- Validate analytic accuracy
- Validate analytic precision
- Establish reportable range
- Establish reference range
- Establish critical values (if any)
- Test analytical sensitivity (certain tests)
- Test analytical specificity (certain tests)
- Establish interpretive comments (if any)
- Define and test calculations (if any)
- Check interfaces with information systems
- Enroll in proficiency testing (where available)
- Alternative validation (where no PT available)
- Design specimen workflow to minimize ID errors
- Write test procedure
- Define calibration and control procedures
- Define appropriate specimens and collection methods
- Define specimen storage and transport conditions
- Specify and test autoverification rules (if any)
- Harmonize systems measuring the same analyte
- Train and test staff
- Define and test automated interpretations (if any)
- Define interfering substances and cross-reactions
- Define clinical indications for testing
- Educate caregivers about indications and interpretation
- Specify suppliers and ordering procedures
- Define backup plan when system fails
- Define ongoing instrument maintenance
- Define process for validating new reagent lots

Analytic Accuracy

Analytic accuracy should be validated for all nonwaived tests, including FDA-cleared or approved test systems and both quantitative and qualitative tests.[150]

For quantitative tests, validation of analytic accuracy means showing that the test is acceptably accurate over a range of values called the *analytical measurement range (AMR),* and verifying that the instrument has been properly calibrated. Validation of accuracy may be accomplished through a number of methods; different methods are appropriate for different test systems and different sections of the laboratory. Consult the test system manufacturer's instructions and the relevant CAP accreditation checklist to determine which methods for accuracy validation are appropriate for a particular test system. The measured analytic accuracy of a new test system should be compared with the manufacturer's stated performance to ensure that the test system has been set up and is being used properly. If there is a meaningful discrepancy between the observed accuracy and the manufacturer's stated accuracy, the test system should not be placed into clinical use until the discrepancy is resolved.

For qualitative tests (such as an automated bacterial identification system, a Gram stain, or an automated blood typing system), a representative set of specimens with known identity (such as a representative set of previously identified microorganisms or blood samples with known blood types) should be tested to ensure that the system performs accurate identifications.

Analytic accuracy is important. In surveys of clinicians, the accuracy of test results was identified as the single most important characteristic of a high-quality clinical laboratory.[151] Records of analytic accuracy validation for all new systems—quantitative or qualitative— should be maintained as documentation that the accuracy of the test system was validated before the system was placed in service.

When multiple test platforms are available to test the same analyte, the analytic accuracy of each platform must be validated separately, and results from the platforms should be harmonized (made comparable by mathematically transforming the results produced by one platform so that they correspond to results produced by the other platforms). Harmonization seems to be a particularly troubling area for some institutions. In 2004, 1.5% to 2.5% of laboratories inspected by the CAP were cited for not verifying the comparability of patient results performed on multiple analytic platforms (citation rates varied by laboratory section).[91] For interpretive tests such as Gram stains, which are performed by multiple technologists, systems must also be in place to ensure consistency of results. During 2004, 2.8% of microbiology laboratories were cited by CAP inspectors for failing to implement such systems.[91]

Analytic Precision

Analytic precision should be validated for all quantitative nonwaived tests, including FDA-cleared or approved test systems.[152] Manufacturer's inserts or the relevant CAP checklist can provide instructions about how to measure analytic precision. Precision often is determined by assaying the same patient specimen, or a pooled sample from several patients, 20 or more times over the course of successive days, and calculating the coefficient of variation of the results.[153] Analytic precision can also be determined by measuring the same control specimen repeatedly, although matrix effects from additives in control specimens may affect the observed precision of some test systems, and repeat testing of patient specimens is preferred.

The analytic precision that is measured for a new platform should be compared to the manufacturer's stated precision to ensure that the test system has been set up and is being used properly. If there is a meaningful discrepancy between the observed precision and the manufacturer's stated precision, the test system should not be placed into clinical use until the precision can be brought into control. In addition to looking for the usual type of imprecision (many of the test results obtained from the same specimen vary too much from the mean), managers should also be attuned to new instruments that sporadically produce deviant values due to some intermittent malfunction, even though most results demonstrate good precision. A high level of imprecision of any type is the single best indicator that something is wrong with a new test system or the operators using it. Inaccuracy can be masked with recalibration; imprecision is more difficult to conceal and suggests something is amiss.

Records of analytic precision testing should be maintained as documentation that the precision of the new test system was validated. When multiple test platforms are available to test the same analyte, precision should be validated for every test system.

Analytic precision of qualitative tests (eg, an automated bacterial identification system or blood typing system) is generally not validated prior to placing a test in service. Validating accuracy suffices.[154]

Reportable Range

A reportable range should be established for all new quantitative tests. *Reportable range* is the CLIA term for the interval of result values over which the laboratory can establish or verify accuracy, and which the laboratory director believes useful for clinical care. The CAP term for reportable range is the *clinically reportable range (CRR)*. The CRR is related to the analytical measurement range (AMR) but allows for specimen dilution, concentration, or other pretreatment used to extend the direct analytically measurable range. For example, if it is desired to report a result that exceeds the AMR, the specimen commonly is diluted to bring the analyte into the AMR, the diluted specimen is re-assayed, and the final result calculated using the dilution factor. Some automated instruments perform dilutions automatically when a result falls outside of the AMR. The CRR also takes into consideration the range of results that will be clinically useful. The laboratory director may decide not to report values that can be accurately measured, but which will not be used to manage care.

The reportable range or CRR is not measured directly; it is established using the medical judgment of the laboratory director and is based, in part, on the assay technology and the clinical use to which results will be put. The test manufacturer often specifies the AMR and procedures to use for dilution or concentration of specimens with values outside the AMR, but the final decision about what range of values to report rests with the laboratory director. Once the reportable range/CRR is established by the laboratory director, the range should be documented as part of the initial validation of the new test system. Analyte results that fall outside the CRR must be reported as "greater than" or "less than" the upper or lower values of the CRR.

The CRR has no meaning for qualitative tests and need not be established. Two examples of how to establish the CRR for quantitative tests are provided in Exhibit 39.

As the practice of medicine changes, the range of analyte results that is clinically useful may also change. For example, the expanding use of C-reactive protein to predict cardiovascular risk has created a need for a reportable range that extends much lower than many traditional C-reactive protein assays can accurately measure. In another example, 19% of laboratories were found in 2005 not to report international normalized ratio (INR) values all the way up to 9.0, which means that clinicians are denied information useful in the treatment of warfarin toxicity.[155] The reportable range for INR had been set too low to support contemporary standards of medical practice.

Analytic Sensitivity and Specificity

When a test system cleared or approved by the FDA is modified by a laboratory, or when the laboratory introduces a test system that is not subject to FDA clearance (such as a Gram stain or a procedure that uses analyte-specific reagents), or when a manufacturer does not provide performance specifications for a test system, then the laboratory is obligated to determine the analytic sensitivity and specificity of the assay. Exactly how this is to be done depends on the technology used in testing and the use to which test results will be put. For example, to demonstrate the analytic sensitivity and specificity of an immunoperoxidase test for the cytokeratin antigen CK907 that will be used as an adjunctive procedure in the diagnosis of prostate cancer, immunoperoxidase studies should be performed on tissue sections from known prostate cancers and known benign prostate biopsies, and the expected basement membrane staining pattern should be observed for both types of specimens. This type of testing shows that the CK907 assay is sensitive (does not stain the basement membrane of cancerous glands) as well as specific (stains basement membranes in benign prostate biopsies). For modified test systems or systems not approved by the FDA, the results of analytic sensitivity and specificity testing should be retained as part of the laboratory's documentation of new test validation.

Calculations

Calculations are commonly performed on laboratory results to generate indices useful for care management. For example, an international normalized ratio (INR) may be calculated from a prothrombin time result to guide dosage adjustment of anticoagulants. An estimated

---

Exhibit 39. Examples of Establishing Reportable Ranges

An example of a clinically reportable range (CRR) with both low and high limits for ß-HCG.
Assume that the analytically measurable range (AMR) is 3–1000 mIU/mL. A laboratory director determines that for proper patient care, the CRR should be 5–1,000,000 mIU/mL. The lower CRR limit of 5 mIU/mL is based on the director's medical decision that values below 5 mIU/mL are not diagnostic for pregnancy. The upper CRR of 1,000,000 mIU/mL is based on the director's determination that values above 1,000,000 mIU/mL are not useful for diagnostic or prognostic purposes. Therefore, patient specimens with measured results of <3, 3, or 4 mIU/mL are reported as "<5 mIU/mL"; specimens with results >1000 mIU/mL are diluted and rerun to obtain quantitative values up to 1,000,000 mIU/mL; specimens with analytic results greater than 1,000,000 mIU/mL are reported as ">1,000,000 mIU/mL."

An example of a CRR with only a low limit for aspartate aminotransferase (AST).
Assume the AMR is 4–900 IU/L. A laboratory director establishes that numeric values <4 are not clinically useful, while values >900 are clinically useful. Patient specimens with measured results of less than 4 IU/L are reported as "<4 IU/L"; specimens with analytic results >900 IU/L are diluted and re-assayed until a quantitative result is obtained. In this case, the upper CRR is not specified because specimens are diluted until a quantitative value is obtained.

---

glomerular filtration rate may be calculated from a creatinine concentration using the MDRD equation[156] to assist physicians in dosing drugs and diagnosing early renal disease. Creatinine clearance may be calculated from the serum and urine creatine concentration along with a patient's 24-hour urine volume.

Calculations are sometimes performed improperly. Errors may result because the wrong formula was chosen, a formula was not programmed properly in a laboratory information system, or because constants used in the formulas were not updated when methods were changed or new lots of reagent placed in service. Of particular concern is the observation that critically important calculations such as the INR have been performed incorrectly by a number of laboratories.[157] The miscalculation of INR values will promote the administration of excessive or insufficient amounts of oral anticoagulants, which may result in unnecessary bleeding or thrombotic complications.

Improperly setting up the formulas to calculate values such as the INR represents a *latent error*—an error that does not call attention to itself at the time the error is made. Circumstances in which latent errors can occur represent high-risk settings. Incorrect calculation of the INR by some clinical laboratories in the United States has resulted in fatal over-anticoagulation. Accordingly, we cannot advocate strongly enough that calculations need to be checked carefully before new tests are used clinically. Any question about the correct formula or constants to use in a calculation should be definitively settled before a test is placed into clinical use. For critical computations such as the INR, it may be prudent to have calculations checked by someone who was not involved in setting up the formula in the first place, to minimize the possibility of error.

Backup Plan When a Test System Fails

In our studies of quality failures, we have come to recognize that laboratories place patients at risk when they do not develop backup plans for what to do when an important test system becomes inoperable or cannot pass quality control tests.[158] Without a backup plan, technologists often are left to improvise when test systems malfunction. A technologist may chose to ignore warning signs, such as controls that fall outside of control limits, when the technologist feels pressured to produce test results and does not have an alternative plan to follow. (See the second case study in chapter 2 for an example of this sort of problem.) In our view and in the view of regulators, the written procedure for every major test system should include a section describing what to do when the test system fails. This may require that a second, backup test system be maintained on-site, that nearby laboratories agree to "cover" one another in the event of a test system failure, or that clinical care pathways include provisions for how caregivers should manage patients during periods when the laboratory cannot measure an analyte.

Integrity of Specimen Identification

Ensuring the accuracy of specimen identification at the time of analysis is one of the CAP National Laboratory Patient Safety Goals (Exhibit 9). Whenever a new test is set up, we recommend critically examining the path specimens will follow, to identify any vulnerabilities in accurate specimen identification. This is particularly important for multi-step processes that involve repeated transfers of specimen from one container to another, as in surgical pathology. Even when specimen identification is highly reliable at each individual step in the process, the cumulative potential for error in multi-step processes may leave the overall process vulnerable (see "Cumulative Effect of Vulnerabilities" in chapter 3). The ability of surgical pathologists to rapidly identify tissue types protects patients against mix-ups of biopsies from different organs, but cannot be relied upon to prevent mix-ups of tissue from the same organ—an occurrence that may be especially frequent in specialized pathology services where relatively few tissue types are examined (eg, specialized skin, gastrointestinal, and urological services).

Selecting Test Systems

We do not discuss in this manual the selection of test systems, although clearly this decision has important implications for laboratory quality. Laboratory directors should consider many factors when choosing analytic platforms: (1) the clinical needs of caregivers for analytic accuracy and precision, freedom from interferences, and timeliness of analysis; (2) expense; (3) potential of the test systems for nonanalytic error, which may include a consideration of the reputation of the manufacturer and suppliers, the quality of user interfaces, and the quality of computer interfaces; and finally (4) the capabilities and expense of alternative test systems.

Ongoing Quality Management of Established Tests

Even when new test systems are properly set up and introduced into the production environment, they may fail to perform properly after a period of time. Therefore, as part of the process of setting up a new test, the laboratory director must specify an ongoing quality management program that reasonably assures the continued accuracy of patient results.[159] This section focuses on risks and control measures that may be applied on an ongoing basis to reasonably assure that test systems continue to perform properly.

The laboratory director enjoys some discretion in determining what activities should be included in an ongoing quality management program, but CLIA regulations and manufacturers' recommendations place minimum requirements on the director. It is important for laboratory directors to recognize that while the FDA approves clinical test systems for sale in the US, and while the manufacturers of test systems often recommend ongoing quality management practices, the FDA does not approve a manufacturer's recommended quality management program, and following manufacturers' recommendations may not satisfy CLIA regulations. The laboratory director is responsible for specifying a program that takes into account both the particulars of the test system and also how the laboratory uses the system in practice. In this section, we review the most important elements of an ongoing quality management program for test systems. Quality control of human operators—the technologists and technicians who use the test system—is discussed in a subsequent section of this chapter (see "Personnel").

Calibration and Calibration Verification

Since quantitative test systems can drift out of calibration, test systems must be periodically recalibrated. Instrument calibration must be performed and verified using the manufacturer's recommended procedure. Calibration should be performed at least every six months, and more often if the manufacturer or laboratory director specify, if ongoing control testing indicates recurring problems, or if significant changes are made to the test equipment or test reagents.[160] Solutions used to verify calibration should not be the same solutions used to calibrate the instrument; the instrument's performance should not be measured with the same yardstick that was used to bring it into conformance. Since calibration solutions contain stabilizers and additives that may exert matrix effects on a test system, it is important that calibrators be appropriate for the particular instrument platform with which they are used.

Quality Control

By convention, the term *quality control* in the clinical laboratory industry refers to the regular testing of samples of known reactivity or analyte concentration to assure operators that a test system continues to function properly. The use of "quality control" in this restrictive sense is unfortunate, because all of the measures discussed in this chapter represent "controls" designed to ensure that some facet of laboratory operations is functioning properly and safely. Nevertheless, we will use the term quality control in this chapter in its conventional restrictive sense.

The laboratory director is responsible for establishing control procedures for each test and assuring that these procedures are carried out. Failure to establish or implement a quality control program appears to be a significant quality risk in laboratory medicine. In CAP Laboratory Accreditation Program inspections conducted during 2004, some aspect of quality control activities was found to be deficient in 3.5% of chemistry sections, 2.0% of transfusion services, 1.3% of hematology sections, and 1% of microbiology facilities.[91] Since deficiencies tend to be cited when there is evidence of systemic or repeated problems, the true incidence of quality control testing not being performed is likely to be higher. In the point-of-care environment, the situation is more troubling. A survey of the quality control records of 209,000 quality control events at 544 institutions demonstrated that 10% of required quality control testing was not being performed, 12.9% of laboratories did not have clearly defined quality control rejection criteria, and 32% of quality control values that were outside of the acceptable range had no evidence of corrective action.[161] Factors associated with more faithful adherence to point-of-care quality control standards included involvement of laboratory staff in training point-of-care operators, use of training videotapes and periodic retraining, storage of quality control results within the point-of-care instrument, and (somewhat embarrassingly) organizational responsibility for the point-of-care program assigned to someone other than a pathologist.

> **Exhibit 40. Elements of Analytic Quality Control Programs**
>
> 1. How should quality control testing be conducted?
> 2. How should operators use control test results to determine that a test system is in control?
> 3. What should be done when a test system is out of control?

What guidance can we offer laboratory directors about setting up an appropriate quality control program? All quality control programs must answer the three questions listed in Exhibit 40. Any program that does not address all three elements is incomplete.

Conduct of Quality Control Testing

CLIA provides guidance about the type of controls to use in a quality control program and the minimum frequency of testing. For automated quantitative tests, two controls with different levels of analyte must, at a minimum, be run once per day, with one exception described subsequently. For some specific tests, CLIA requires more frequent testing (see CLIA regulations or the applicable CAP accreditation program checklist). Beyond CLIA requirements, automated test systems that the manufacturer or laboratory director believe to be less stable than average will require that more levels of controls be run, or that controls be run more frequently. For example, the manufacturer of the test system in the case study "Reagent Failure" (chapter 2) recommended more frequent quality control testing in response to documented problems with reagent stability.

Normally, control solutions are purchased, but in certain circumstances, patient specimens may be used as control solutions. When manufactured controls are used, they must use matrix solutions appropriate for the test system. CLIA requirements for manual qualitative tests (such as Gram stains) generally specify that positive and negative controls be tested daily. Here again, CLIA requirements for particular tests vary. For example, tissue immunoperoxidase and histochemical stains must be tested with a positive and negative control with every run.

With some automated and semi-automated test systems, quality control testing may be performed less frequently than once per day. So-called "electronic quality control," which consist of performing automated system checks designed to test various facets of a test system, may be substituted for the testing of physical control specimens, under certain circumstances. (See endnote 162 for more information about alternative quality control procedures.)

Determining if a Test System is in Control

How do operators determine that a test system is in control? For quantitative assays, *control rules* that are part of basic statistical quality control should be applied. The simplest rule (and arguably the best for most tests) is that a test system should be declared out of control if one tested value of any control solution is more than 3 standard deviations from the mean value obtained with the control.[163] The standard deviation and mean value are calculated from 20 or more previous tests performed with the same control solution. The previous month's values (or the last 20 values) may be used to calculate the mean and standard deviation.

Some laboratories use a multi-rule control procedure (the most popular of which was described by Westgard et al) to determine whether a process is in control.[164] Multi-rule procedures offer greater sensitivity in detecting *assignable-cause* variation than Shewhart's simple 3-standard-deviation rule, but multi-rule procedures are less specific than Shewhart's procedure (ie, more "false alarms").

Laboratorians tend to think of quality control as an ongoing check on laboratory inaccuracy. But ongoing quality control can also serve as a check on laboratory *imprecision*. The standard deviation of month's worth of quality control testing should be compared to a maximum limit established by the laboratory director, or the standard deviation of the previous month's values, to determine whether something is amiss with the reproducibility of a test system. In 2004, 2.1% of hematology sections and 3.5% of chemistry sections were cited by CAP laboratory inspectors for not checking the imprecision of test systems on an ongoing basis.[91]

For qualitative assays, the situation is much simpler than with quantitative tests. A qualitative test is out of control if testing of any control solution does not yield the expected result (positive or negative). For all tests, quantitative and qualitative, the process of recording and evaluating control results should be simple and understandable to operators. Managers should design work processes so that it is difficult for operators to continue testing when a test system is out of control.

Corrective Action

What should technologists do when testing of a control sample does not produce the expected result (ie, when the test system is out of control)? The course of action needs to be specified clearly by the laboratory director in the laboratory's procedure manual. In general, when a test system fails control testing, testing of patient samples must stop until the system is brought back into control. This might require repair of an instrument, recalibration, or some other intervention. During 2004, 1.4% of laboratory sections examined by the CAP Laboratory Accreditation Program inspectors were cited for failing to take corrective action when control results exceeded tolerance limits.[91]

Once the test system is brought back into control, all patient specimens that were assayed after the last successful quality control test are normally retested. Results should be corrected if they are different from previously reported values. To allow for retesting, all tested clinical specimens should be saved until the next quality control test is passed.

For quantitative automated assays that have been in control and which have a failure of one level of control (but not other levels), many laboratories allow technologists to retest the control *once* without retesting patient specimens. If retesting the control produces an acceptable result, patient specimens do not need to be retested. Other laboratories do not provide technologists with this latitude. We believe it is reasonable to adopt either approach, and both are permitted by regulation, but when technologists are allowed to retest single controls without retesting specimens, this policy should be documented in the written test procedure that is approved by the laboratory director or the director's designee. When management "looks the other way" and allows procedure and practice to diverge, leadership has only itself to blame when greater liberties are taken by technologists who feel pressure to release results despite the repeated failure of control testing.

Instruments and Equipment

Release of inaccurate results is often caused by failure of instruments. Preventative maintenance recommended by manufacturers should be performed at the frequency recommended by the manufacturer. Function checks defined by the manufacturer should also be performed at the recommended frequency, and function checks must be within the manufacturer's established limits before patient testing can be conducted. For equipment, instruments, or test systems developed in-house or modified by the laboratory, or when maintenance and function check protocols are not provided by the manufacturer, the laboratory director must establish a schedule for maintenance and define a schedule for function checks.

New Reagents, Kits, or Media Lots

Failure of manufactured consumable items represents an important source of variability in analytic testing. Despite the fact that manufacturers are required to follow the FDA's Good Manufacturing Practices (GMP) / Quality System (QS) Regulation when producing reagents, kits, and media, our experience suggests that defects in consumables are relatively frequent occurrences. Because of batch processes used in the manufacture of reagents and test kits, failures tend to occur when new lots are placed in service.[165] Therefore, all new reagent lots must be validated before or concurrent with their first use for patient testing. In 2004, CAP inspectors cited 1.3% to 2.4% of laboratory sections for failing to validate new reagent lots (different types of laboratory sections had different citation rates).[91]

When new lots of reagents are used in quantitative assays, the laboratory should document that recalibration of the instrument is not necessary by demonstrating that the assay produces acceptable results with patient specimens after the new reagent lot is introduced into the test system. For qualitative tests, known positive and negative patient specimens should be tested when new reagent lots or test kits are introduced. In some circumstances, it may be necessary to validate new lots of reagents with control materials supplied by the manufacturer or with validated proficiency test materials, but validation with patient material is preferred, if feasible. For test kits that make use of multiple reactions to determine a result (such as a bacterial identification system that uses multiple biochemical reactions to identify bacteria), current regulations specify that each test reaction must be validated when a new kit lot is placed in service. This generally means that a panel of test organisms must be used to validate the new lot. Special requirements also apply to molecular procedures that test for an array of genes or gene products.

In some instances, such as the calculation of international normalized ratio (INR) values, the international sensitivity index (ISI) of the thromboplastin reagent lot used in INR calculation must be changed when a new lot of thromboplastin is introduced. Laboratories are advised to develop checklists that ensure constants used in calculations are updated when reagent lots are changed.

External Proficiency Testing

External proficiency testing (PT) measures the ability of a laboratory to use its test system proficiently. PT deficiencies can result from improper use of a test system by human operators, improper calibration of the test system, or unacceptable precision. External PT is therefore a valuable control system that checks a wide range of activities important to producing accurate test results. As discussed in the previous chapter, PT participation is required by CLIA for certain "regulated" analytes, and the CAP requires, as a condition of CAP laboratory accreditation, external PT participation for all analytes in which PT is available.

While PT performs a valuable external check on the proficiency of a laboratory, it is not a substitute for ongoing internal quality management of test systems.[166] Laboratory managers who have not successfully controlled their test systems and do not trust the capabilities of their own operations may be tempted to manipulate PT results through a variety of subterfuges. For this reason, the Clinical Laboratory Improvement Amendments of 1988 require that: (1) PT samples be tested with the laboratory's regular patient workload by personnel who routinely perform the testing in the laboratory, using the laboratory's routine methods. The individual testing or examining the samples and the laboratory director must attest to the routine integration of the samples into the patient workload using the laboratory's routine methods. (2) The laboratory must test samples the same number of times that it routinely tests patient samples. (3) Laboratories that perform tests on proficiency testing samples must not engage in any interlaboratory communications pertaining to the results of proficiency testing sample(s) until after the date by which the laboratory must report proficiency testing results to the program for the testing event in which the samples were sent. Laboratories with multiple testing sites or separate locations must not participate in any communications or discussions across sites/locations concerning proficiency testing sample results until after the date by which the laboratory must report proficiency testing results to the program. (4) The laboratory must not send PT samples or portions of samples to another laboratory for any analysis which it is certified to perform in its own laboratory. Any laboratory that intentionally refers its proficiency testing samples to another laboratory for analysis will have its certification revoked for at least one year. Further, any laboratory that receives proficiency testing samples from another laboratory for testing must notify CMS of the receipt of those samples.[167] During 2004, 1.4% of laboratories were cited by CAP Laboratory Accreditation Program inspectors for not testing PT samples using the same procedures used for patient samples.[91]

Laboratories must demonstrate successful PT performance to remain accredited by the CAP and/or other accrediting agencies, or to be certified by CLIA. The definition of successful PT performance is found in the CLIA regulations and varies by laboratory discipline. In several disciplines, such as microbiology, CAP PT programs may include ungraded educational challenges, which are not used to determine whether PT performance was acceptable for the purposes of CLIA. Many of these ungraded challenges still measure the laboratory's capabilities and provide laboratory directors with an opportunity for improvement. When a PT challenge specimen is not graded because of late submission or lack of referee consensus, laboratories still have an obligation to assess their performance on the challenge. In 2004, 3.9% of laboratories inspected by the CAP were cited for failing to evaluate their performance on ungraded PT challenges.[91] Laboratories that perform unsatisfactorily on a PT challenge should treat the failure as an *incident* (see "Learning from Incidents" in chapter 6), investigate its cause, and take corrective action. In 2004, 1.3% to 2.2% of laboratory sections inspected by the CAP were cited for failing to take corrective action as a result of PT failures. Citation rates varied by laboratory discipline.[91]

When external PT is not available for an analyte, the CAP and CLIA require that the laboratory develop an alternative method for validating the accuracy of testing and validate accuracy at least semiannually. Alternative methods include split sample analysis, the use of previously assayed specimens or pooled material, or clinical correlation. In 2004, 1.6% to 4.8% of laboratories that performed testing for which no external PT was available were cited by CAP inspectors for failing to validate the assay semiannually. Citation rates varied by laboratory discipline.[91]

External Accuracy Testing

For quantitative chemistry tests, the ongoing management of accuracy is generally accomplished through calibration verification and the quality control testing discussed above. There is no regulatory or CAP requirement to conduct external accuracy testing analogous to the requirement for external proficiency testing. Nevertheless, maintaining the accuracy of tests for certain analytes is problematic due to tight decision-limits used in particular patient care scenarios. Creatinine, neonatal bilirubin, and calcium are three of these "problem" analytes; it is difficult to perform these tests with the accuracy required for certain clinical decisions. The CAP and other vendors offer external accuracy testing programs for several analytes. Participants who subscribe to these services receive specimens that are free from matrix effects (generally, fresh frozen serum) and are graded according to the accuracy of their reported assay results, which may be determined using a reference test method or by other means.

Exhibit 41. Interlaboratory Variation in Selected Reference Ranges

Analyte	Lower Limit			Upper Limit		
	10th	50th (median)	90th	10th	50th (median)	90th
Digoxin (ng/mL)[169]	0.5	0.8*	0.9	2.0	2.0	2.0
Calcium (mg/dL)[170]	8.3	8.5	8.8	10.2	10.5	10.7
aPTT (seconds)[114]	40	50	65	65	80	116

* For example, in the multi-institutional survey cited in reference 169, the median laboratory had established a lower limit for its digoxin reference range of 0.8 ng/mL. Higher percentiles do not indicate better or worse performance.

Interactions of Test Systems and Collection Devices

Much of the ongoing quality management of testing relies upon the use of manufactured materials that come in their own containers—calibrators, controls, and proficiency test samples. These manufactured materials may be tested in the same manner as patient specimens, but they are not exposed to the needles, swabs, collection tubes, and other collection equipment that come in contact with clinical specimens. Rarely, collection devices may interact with test systems in unanticipated ways to alter clinical results, even when calibration, control, and proficiency testing material produces acceptable performance.[168] The laboratory community does not know how widely this sort of interaction takes place and what control measures are best suited to detecting problems. One approach that may be used with quantitative tests is to track the mean of all patient values from month to month. Changes in the mean may reflect a new interaction between a test system and a collection device (although a change in the mean may also result from a change in the patient population being tested or a change in instrument calibration). Collection devices may also interact with qualitative test systems (eg, a new lot of swabs may interfere with the transport of certain microorganisms). Unfortunately, practical methods that can be used by the clinical laboratory to reliably detect this sort of occurrence have not been developed.

Reference Ranges

Establishing *reference ranges* (sometimes called *reference intervals* or *normal ranges*) is part of the process of introducing most new quantitative tests (Exhibit 38). Laboratory directors frequently experience difficulty establishing reference ranges appropriately. During 2004, 1.3% of laboratories were cited by CAP inspectors for failing to validate reference ranges properly.[91] There have been few multi-institutional surveys of the reference ranges used by laboratories, and the CAP is currently conducting a large survey of reference ranges and validation methods used in laboratories. Surveys that have been completed show moderate interlaboratory variation in reference ranges for several analytes (Exhibit 41).[114,169,170]

Exhibit 42. Reference Range Regulations and Reality

Although most CLIA regulations advance the practice of laboratory medicine, CLIA requirements for establishing reference ranges are impossible to follow in practice. CLIA regulation 42 CFR 493.1253(b)(1)(ii) states that the laboratory must "verify that the manufacturer's reference intervals (normal values) are appropriate for the laboratory's patient population." Further, the current version of the CMS *Survey Procedures and Interpretive Guidelines for Laboratories and Laboratory Services* indicates the "laboratory must evaluate an appropriate number of specimens to verify the manufacturer's claims for normal values or, as applicable, the published reference ranges."

While CMS requires that laboratories verify population-based reference ranges for every analyte by testing specimens from healthy individuals, doing so is not practical for a number of reasons: (1) More than 100 specimens from "healthy" individuals must be tested to validate most published reference intervals with reasonable certainty. For some analytes the distribution of values in the healthy population is not "normal" in a statistical sense, and for these analytes, 1000 or more specimens may need to be tested to definitively validate a published reference range. (2) When age- and sex-specific reference ranges are used, this whole testing process must be repeated for each age and sex stratum. (3) In many cases, pediatric reference ranges can not be verified because children cannot legally give consent to phlebotomy, healthy children usually do not have their blood drawn, and blood volumes obtained from infants during the normal course of patient care are small and often do not contain enough blood for reference range validation studies. (4) With some analytes, such as CSF glucose, meeting the current

CMS interpretation of CLIA regulations would be unethical. It would be unconscionable for every clinical laboratory to perform lumbar punctures on 100 healthy infants to validate normal pediatric reference ranges for CSF glucose every time a new chemistry analyzer was purchased. (5) Finally, for analytes such as cholesterol, reference ranges have nothing to do with "normal" values and are based on clinical decision points established by research studies that can not be locally replicated.

Because it is not possible to satisfy current CMS interpretations of CLIA requirements, laboratories in the United States are not validating all of their reference intervals with local studies. Many laboratories make a limited "good faith" effort to validate manufacturer's adult reference ranges by testing several dozen apparently healthy individuals for common analytes. Most do not. No laboratory we know validates *all* of its reference ranges.

We believe laboratory managers can better spend their time ensuring that their test systems remain precise and true by rigorously performing periodic calibration and quality control testing, rather than becoming involved in reference range validation studies for every analyte and every age and sex stratum. In our view, only some types of tests require local reference range validation studies. The approach we recommend to establishing reference ranges is described in this section and is based on the type of reference range that will be reported. When a local validation study is not performed, "verification" of a reference interval should consist of the laboratory director making a professional determination that the range of normal values in a manufacturer's or published reference range study is likely to be similar to the range of values found in the local healthy population.

Why does the establishment of reference ranges pose such difficulties? We believe much of the confusion can be traced to CLIA regulations. It is impossible for laboratories to strictly follow CLIA requirements for establishing reference ranges, for reasons discussed in Exhibit 42. While CLIA language requires that laboratories perform reference range validation studies on normal patients for each analyte, most laboratories do not follow this requirement and obtain reference ranges from instrument manufacturers (Exhibit 43).[171] Sometimes, instrument manufacturers supply a laboratory with specimens from a "normal" population so that laboratory staff can "validate" a reference range. In other situations, representatives of

	Laboratories (Number)	Percent of Total*
Exhibit 43. Method Used by Clinical Laboratories to Establish Reference Ranges in Practice [171]		
Accept manufacturer's published values	390	78%
Manufacturer provides material/performs analysis	94	19%
Prepare and analyze material locally	62	12%
Manufacturer provides material, laboratory performs analysis	52	10%
Other methods	33	7%

* Percentages total more than 100% because multiple responses were allowed.

instrument manufacturers will conduct a "local" (on-site) validation study on behalf of the laboratory, using the laboratory's instrument and samples from the manufacturer.

An Approach to Establishing Reference Ranges

We do not recommend that laboratories perform reference range validation testing for every analyte. Instead, we recommend that the method used to establish a reference range for a particular analyte be based on the type of reference range that will be reported. In some cases, published or manufacturer-supplied reference ranges can be used without in-laboratory testing. In other cases, a local validation study is required, using the method for reference range validation described by CLSI (formerly NCCLS)[172] or by an instrument manufacturer.

Types of Reference Ranges

Reference ranges can be divided into four basic types, shown in Exhibit 44. Some types of reference ranges require local validation studies, while others (in our opinion) do not. A laboratory director should determine what type of reference range is appropriate for a particular analyte and then establish the reference range using the method appropriate for the type of range that will be reported. Practical examples of this approach are provided in the remainder of this section.

Population Based, Method Independent

Serum potassium is an example of a test that requires a population-based, method-independent reference range. Potassium determinations are used by clinicians for dozens of different purposes. Some serum

> **Exhibit 44. Types of Reference Ranges**
>
> 1. Population based, method independent (eg, serum potassium)
> 2. Population based, method dependent (eg, prothrombin time)
> 3. Decision based, method independent (eg, serum cholesterol)
> 4. Decision based, method dependent (eg, serum troponin-I)

potassium tests are ordered to monitor diuretic therapy, others to evaluate adrenal function, still others to guide potassium replacement therapy for a diabetic in ketoacidosis. Because serum potassium values are used for so many different purposes, the laboratory cannot possibly provide caregivers with specific potassium breakpoints to guide clinical decision making. Reference ranges for analytes such as potassium are accordingly "population based." The reference range is the central 95% interval of the distribution of values obtained from individuals who are presumed to be healthy. This interval is often referred to as the "normal" range. The purpose of a population-based reference range is simply to remind clinicians about the range of values found in a healthy population; the clinician must make a professional determination about whether this normal range is relevant to the clinical decision being made for a particular patient.

Laboratory-to-laboratory accuracy and precision of potassium determinations is high. So long as laboratories follow good quality control procedures, the serum potassium of a patient measured in one laboratory is likely to be very close to the value that would be determined if the same patient was tested in another laboratory, regardless of the reagent or test system in use. We can therefore think of potassium determinations as "method independent" because the technology for measuring potassium in the clinical setting has advanced to the point where different test platforms produce similar results.[173]

For population-based, method-independent analytes such as potassium, the reference range may be obtained from a textbook, a published reference range study, or a study conducted by an instrument manufacturer. When the range of "normal" values varies according to age or sex, a normal range appropriate to the patient's age and sex should be reported by the laboratory computer system. Age- and sex-specific normal ranges may also be obtained from textbooks or an instrument manufacturer.

The laboratory director is free to conduct a local study to validate population-based reference ranges obtained from the literature, but in our opinion this is usually unnecessary.[174] If no local study has been conducted, the laboratory director's decision to use a published reference interval should be documented in the test procedure. In our potassium example, the following statement would suffice: "The laboratory director has determined that the measurement of serum potassium is reasonably well standardized, and that the concentration of potassium in apparently healthy individuals described in published (manufacturer's) studies will be similar to the concentration found in healthy patients served by this laboratory. Therefore, a reference interval drawn from published (manufacturer's) studies of serum potassium levels in healthy individuals will be used in this laboratory. This reference range will be 3.3 to 5.0 mmol/L for patients over one year of age." The source of the reference range (published study or manufacturer's insert) should be cited.

Population Based, Method Dependent

Prothrombin time serves as an example of a test that requires a population-based, method-dependent reference range. As with potassium, prothrombin time tests are ordered for many different purposes. Some caregivers order prothrombin time to adjust anticoagulant therapy, others to screen for coagulation factor deficiencies. Therefore, it is appropriate to use a population-based reference range for prothrombin time, because the laboratory cannot provide caregivers with clinical decision points for every possible use of a prothrombin time assay.

In contrast to potassium determinations, however, prothrombin time results are significantly influenced by the type of reagents used for testing and the testing platform employed. The prothrombin time of a patient determined in one laboratory is likely to be different from the prothrombin time of the same patient assayed in another laboratory, due to differences in reagents and test systems used by the two laboratories. Because of these differences, the laboratory director should not obtain the "normal" range for prothrombin time from a textbook, a published study, or the manufacturer of the test system. Instead, a group of presumably healthy individuals should be tested by the laboratory, using the test platform and reagents that will be used to test patient specimens. Results from testing this population are used to create a reference value or reference range. For tests in which results depend on the reagent as well the test platform (such as prothrombin time), the laboratory should re-establish or re-verify the reference interval with each change of lot or change in reagent. When test results are method dependent, the manufacturer of a test platform will usually provide specific instructions about how to calculate a reference range using the test results obtained from a population of presumably healthy individuals.[175]

Decision Based, Method Independent

Some analytes are measured for a single purpose, or the great majority of determinations are made for a single purpose. With these analytes, the reference range serves to remind caregivers of key decision points that they should use in patient management. For example, the upper limit of the total serum cholesterol reference range (200 mg/dL) reflects the decision point at which diet and exercise are first recommended to lower cholesterol in otherwise healthy adults (by most authorities). For cholesterol, the upper limit of the reference range is not population based. The reference range does not have anything to do with the values found in the central 95% of a healthy population because (sadly) more than 5% of "healthy" American adults have cholesterol levels above 200 mg/dL.

In the case of cholesterol, the establishment of 200 mg/dL as the clinical breakpoint for initiating lifestyle changes in otherwise healthy adults involved several large-scale studies conducted over many years at a cost of many millions of dollars.[113] These studies are not repeatable by laboratory directors. The role of the laboratory director in setting the reference range for cholesterol is simply to select from the medical literature one or more decision points that reflect contemporary standards of medical practice. This determination often is done in conjunction with clinical caregivers. The following statement, or its equivalent, may be inserted into a procedure for cholesterol: "The laboratory director has determined that the measurement of total serum cholesterol is reasonably well standardized, and when assays are properly controlled, cholesterol values will not vary significantly from one laboratory to another. Clinical guidelines suggest a benefit to lowering total serum cholesterol below 200 mg/dL in otherwise healthy adults. Therefore, the reference range for cholesterol will be <200 mg/dL." The source used to establish the reference range (published study or guideline) should be cited.[176]

Decision Based, Method Dependent

Serum troponin-I serves as an example of an analyte with a decision-based, method-dependent reference range. Troponin-I is measured primarily for one purpose: to diagnose acute myocardial infarction. Therefore, a reference interval should be chosen to alert caregivers to key clinical decision points related to the management of patients with suspected acute myocardial infarction. The reference range for troponin-I is not the range of values found in healthy individuals.

Troponin-I assays are not well standardized; the serum troponin-I level in a patient determined by one manufacturer's test platform will not necessarily correspond to the serum troponin-I level determined using another manufacturer's platform. Therefore, reference intervals developed for one test system cannot be applied to another test system.

Decision-based, method-dependent reference ranges are generally obtained from the test manufacturer. In the case of troponin-I, the manufacturer of a test system will have performed a clinical validation study to determine the best breakpoint for diagnosing acute myocardial infarction with the manufacturer's test system. Often, the manufacturer will perform the study jointly with the staff from a clinical research center; or a clinical research center will conduct its own study, and the study will be published in the literature. The laboratory director may perform a local study to validate or re-establish a breakpoint if the director is concerned that the local population of patients being evaluated for myocardial infarction might differ from the population tested by the manufacturer. If no local study is conducted, the method by which the reference range was established should be documented. A statement to the following effect in the procedure manual will suffice: "The laboratory director has determined that the validation studies conducted by the manufacturer to establish a reference range for this test system are applicable to the population being tested by this laboratory. Therefore, serum troponin-I values of 0 to 0.2 ng/mL will be considered 'negative.' Values from 0.3 to 2.0 ng/mL will be considered 'intermediate.' Values above 2.0 ng/mL will be considered 'suggestive' of acute myocardial infarction. These ranges will be used only for the [manufacturer's name] test system, and only when the test system is operated in strict accordance with the manufacturer's instructions." The source of information used to establish these breakpoints (manufacturer's product insert or published study) should be cited.

Hybrid Reference Ranges

Some analytes are best served with multiple reference ranges. For example, serum estrone will have separate reference intervals for prepubertal males, prepubertal females, females in various phases of their menstrual cycle, and postmenopausal females. Each reference range should be established using the principles outlined above, as appropriate for the type of reference range that is being reported.

Reference Laboratories

The analytic accuracy of results received from reference laboratories is important to every laboratory director. However, the referring laboratory generally is not in a position to directly assess whether reference laboratory results are accurate. The best single control on the quality of reference laboratory results is the requirement that reference laboratories be appropriately accredited or certified as compliant with regulatory requirements. Feedback about reference laboratory quality can also come from clinicians, who may observe reference laboratory test results that are incompatible with a patient's clinical presentation.

The laboratory director must approve reference laboratories and may elect not to approve a facility that is CLIA certified if the director has some reason to doubt the laboratory's commitment to quality. In JCAHO-accredited hospitals, JCAHO additionally requires that the medical staff approve all reference laboratories through its elected leadership.

If a laboratory director is making the primary decision with regards to selecting referral laboratories, it may be prudent to ask a third party to determine whether the director is free of financial conflicts of interest. In theory, if a referring clinician specifies that testing should be performed at a particular referral laboratory, it may also be prudent to investigate whether the referring physician has any conflicts of interest. In practice, this issue is rarely explored.

Postanalytic Operations: Risks and Control Measures

Reporting Results

Apart from issuing biologics such as blood, the product of clinical laboratories is information. Information is delivered on paper reports or through other media, ranging from characters on a computer display to words transmitted over the telephone. In this section, we discuss quality risks and control measures related to reporting results. We discuss the content of reports, the presentation of information, and critical value reporting.

Report Elements

CLIA requires that several elements be present in all laboratory reports (Exhibit 45).[177] The laboratory report must contain either the patient's name and identification number, or a unique patient identifier and some secondary identification number, such as an accession number. The report must contain the name and address of the laboratory,[178] the date the final report was first issued (a date which must not change when reports are reprinted), the name of the test performed, the specimen source and units of measure or interpretation (as applicable), and any information regarding the condition and disposition of specimens that do not meet the laboratory's criteria for acceptability. Finally, of course, the test result itself must be reported. When a laboratory refers patient specimens to another facility for testing, CLIA prohibits the referring laboratory from revising results reported by the testing laboratory in any manner that might affect their interpretation. CAP Laboratory Accreditation Program requirements for reports differ slightly from those within CLIA, but not substantially (see Exhibit 45).

In addition to information that must appear on the laboratory report, CLIA requires that laboratories must, upon request, make available to clients the methods used for each test, any test performance specifications established locally by the laboratory, and information about test interferences. Pertinent updates about testing information are to be provided to clients whenever changes occur that affect test results or their interpretation.

Exhibit 45. Required Report Elements [a]

1. Patient identifier(s)
2. Laboratory name and address [b]
3. Ordering provider or provider of record [c]
4. Date and time of specimen collection, when appropriate [c]
5. Test report date [d]
6. Name of test performed
7. Specimen source, when appropriate
8. Test result
9. Units of measurement or interpretation, as applicable
10. Reference range, as applicable [e]
11. Condition of specimens that the laboratory deems unacceptable

a CAP requires that additional elements be reported for specific tests (eg, fetal screening, surgical pathology).
b CLIA requires that the name of the performing laboratory appear on the report. CAP requires that the reporting laboratory's name appear on the report.
c Required by CAP, but not by CLIA.
d CAP also requires report time as well as date, but does not require either be printed on the physical report.
e CLIA allows reference ranges to be distributed separately from the report. CAP discourages this practice.

The term *report* is not formally defined by CLIA regulations, and in our electronic age the question of what constitutes a "report" is worthy of some discussion. Must all of the information in Exhibit 45 be included with every laboratory report given over the telephone? Must it all appear on the same computer screen that displays test results, or should caregivers be allowed to "click" their way to less critical information, such as the address of a reference laboratory? Does Exhibit 45 apply to preliminary, addendum, or corrected reports? Should important information not listed in Exhibit 45, such as the fact that a critical result was called to the provider, be included on the printed laboratory report, or should this information simply be maintained by the laboratory? Because regulations are not specific and laboratory reports can take so many forms, it is difficult for us to provide specific counsel. We recommend that when the laboratory communicates a test result in any form—oral, written, or electronic—all of the information in Exhibit 45 be provided or the recipient be given the opportunity to obtain this information as part of the communication. For oral reports, the recipient may ask for the information. (For example, if the recipient is interested in the name of the reference laboratory, he or she can ask and the name should be provided.) For written reports, the laboratory's name and contact information should be provided so the report recipient can make further inquiries. For electronic communication, the individuals accessing the report should be given the opportunity to electronically request the information in Exhibit 45 if it is not provided as part of the initial electronic transmission.[179]

Beyond the minimum set of report elements required by CLIA, the laboratory community is beginning to standardize elements that should be included in more complex reports, such as surgical pathology reports, microbiology reports, and investigations of blood transfusion reactions. For example, over the past several years, the CAP has developed a set of cancer checklists, which specify a minimum set of elements that should be included in reports of certain malignancies. The American College of Surgeons (ACS) currently requires that ACS-accredited cancer centers use pathology reports that contain all of the required elements in the CAP cancer checklists. CAP Laboratory Accreditation Program inspection checklists provide additional information about elements that should be included in particular types of laboratory reports, as does the CAP publication, *Quality Management in Anatomic Pathology*.[1]

What control measures can be applied to reasonably assure that required data elements are included in reports? Laboratory computer systems typically are programmed to provide required report elements on printed reports of chemistry and hematology tests. Templates can be used to force the reporting of certain elements in microbiology reports. In surgical pathology, numerous studies have shown that the use of checklists at the time of case sign-out improves the consistency of reporting and the inclusion of required prognostic indicators.[180] We wonder whether the time has come to require that checklists be used by pathologists when issuing complex surgical pathology reports. Pilots are not allowed to fly without first reviewing a checklist. Should pathologists?[181]

Report Formatting

In the previous section, we discussed data elements that should be included in reports. In this section, we discuss *formatting* reports to optimize communication. Effective communication among caregivers is one of the CAP National Laboratory Patient Safety Goals (Exhibit 9) and a goal of the Joint Commission on Accreditation of Healthcare Organizations.[182] How should this goal be achieved? As is often the case in medicine, guidance can be found within the commercial aviation industry.

Shortly after World War II and up until approximately a decade ago, aircraft cockpit instruments were standardized in the so-called "six-pack" configuration, an array of six essential gauges arranged in two rows of three, directly in front of the pilot. In clockwise order from the upper left were found the airspeed indicator, artificial horizon, altimeter, turn coordinator, heading display, and vertical speed indicator. Uniform positioning of instrumentation eased pilot transition from one type of aircraft to another and minimized the amount of time required for airborne flight crews to obtain situational awareness. Over the past 50 years, human factors researchers have continuously refined the layout of cockpit avionics to optimize interactions between pilot and aircraft.[183]

In the clinical laboratory industry, the display of information is not as well standardized as in commercial aviation, to the detriment of effective communication. An office-based physician required to use several laboratories by different HMO contracts will find little similarity in the way each laboratory formats results. In some reports, the patient name appears in the upper left corner; others use this same space to list ordering and "copy-to" physicians. Some laboratories report the date and time of specimen collection in a location that other laboratories use to show the date and time of result verification. Some cumulative (longitudinal) reports list newest results at the top; others, at the bottom. Even within a single health care "system," the layout of a test result on paper may differ dramatically from the display of the same test result on a computer screen.

The laboratory director is not in a position to standardize the presentation of clinical test information for the entire laboratory industry, but some control measures can be adopted locally to reduce the potential for confusion. At a minimum, laboratory directors should review reports for content and format. In 2004, 2.4% of laboratories inspected by the CAP were cited because no review of report format had been conducted by the laboratory director or designee during the previous year.[91]

Clear formatting of information is important to effective communication.[184] Standard "zones" can be defined within a health system for the presentation of specific information (eg, patient identification information in a zone at the top right of a report or computer screen, examination results in a zone comprising the bottom half). A policy has been established within some health systems that numeric patient test results will always be shown to the left of units of measure, which in turn will always appear to the left of numeric reference intervals. In our opinion, the only date and time that should appear near a patient result on a clinical report is the date and time of specimen collection. Other dates and times (laboratory specimen receipt, report verification, report print time, date and time a laboratory called a clinician about a critical result) should be located away from patients' results or not printed on paper reports at all.[185] In computer displays, dates and times that refer to something other than specimen collection can be relegated to ancillary screens that do not contain the patient's test results, to minimize confusion.[186] See Figure 2 for examples.

The information processing capacity of humans is limited, and the potential for error omnipresent. To avoid mix-ups, we believe that all information not relevant for everyday clinical decision making should be separated as much as possible from patient test results. There is no reason to include billing codes and other administrative data on reports destined for caregivers. Before the widespread use of computers, most of the information related to a

Figure 2. Portions of Two Hospital Information System Computer Screens Used to Display Laboratory Results

A

```
   Collection  Test          Result Units      Reference    Order No.
   ----------- ------------- ------ -----      ---------    ---------
   122104 1151 Potassium        6.4 mEq/L  CH 3.5 - 5.0    23188231
Called to J. Wan on 122104 at 1207 by JXM
   122104 1151 Sodium           139 mEq/L      135 - 148    48837123
   122104 1151 Calcium          5.1 mg/dL  C  4.6 - 5.4    12399483
Calcium reported previously as 5.4 mg/mL
Corrected by JTT on 122104 at 1930
Code 31
   122104 1151 Magnesium        2.0 mg/dL      1.7 - 2.5    00930123
   122104 1151 Amphetamines     Negative                    94883823
Amphetamines                   1000 ng/mL screening decision limit
                                100 ng/mL confirmation decision limit
AMPH-S performed at Wonder Medical Laboratory, Reno, NV.
Key: C=Corrected, H=High, L=Low, A=Abnormal, CH=Critical High, CL=
   Critical Low
Reported: 122104 1930  Screen: A345773
```

B

```
                   12-21-04
                   11:51 AM      Reference Range    Notes (click)
                   --------      ---------------    -------------
   Potassium        6.4 mEq/L  H   3.5 - 5.0        Result called
   Sodium           139 mEq/L      135 - 148
   Calcium, Ionized 5.1 mg/dL  C   4.6 - 5.4        Corrected value
   Magnesium        2.0 mg/dL      1.7 - 2.5
   Amphetamines     Negative                        Interpretation

   H=High, C=Corrected
```

Both examples shown are based on computer screens in clinical use. A computer screen similar to example "A" caused a patient to be treated for drug abuse because a physician misinterpreted the report. Screen "A" contains many common presentation defects: (1) dates and times are not formatted for clarity; (2) extraneous distracting information is included, such as test order numbers; (3) commentary is interspersed with test results, rather than relegated to separate screens that viewers may optionally call up; (4) dates, times, and incorrect test results appear near numeric test results, inviting confusion. Contrast with "B," which contains all essential clinical information in "A," and an option to "click" to supplementary commentary.

Many of the presentation defects illustrated in "A" apply to printed laboratory reports as well as computer screens. If you were flying an airplane, would you want your cockpit instrument displays to be designed by the group that created screen "A" or screen "B"? Which screen would you want your harried intensive care physician to use?

Figure 3. The Diagnosis Section of Two Surgical Pathology Biopsy Reports

A

A. PROSTATE, RIGHT BASE: ATROPHY AND CHRONIC INFLAMMATION. NO NEOPLASM IDENTIFIED.

B. PROSTATE, RIGHT MID: ACUTE AND CHRONIC INFLAMMATION. NO NEOPLASM IDENTIFIED.

C. PROSTATE, RIGHT APEX: ATROPHY. NO NEOPLASM IDENTIFIED.

D. PROSTATE, LEFT BASE: ADENOCARCINOMA, CONVENTIONAL TYPE, GLEASON 3+4=7, SIZE = 7 MM, PERINEURAL INVASION PRESENT.

E. PROSTATE, LEFT MID: SINGLE FOCUS OF ADENOCARCINOMA, CONVENTIONAL TYPE, GLEASON 3+3=6, SIZE = 2 MM.

F. PROSTATE, LEFT APEX: ATROPHY AND CHRONIC INFLAMMATION. NO NEOPLASM IDENTIFIED.

B

PROSTATE: ADENOCARCINOMA

Malignant locations: left base, left mid
Benign locations: left apex, right base, right mid, right apex
Gleason score: 3 + 4 = 7
Maximum dimension: 7 mm (left base)
Histologic type: conventional prostatic adenocarcinoma
Perineural invasion is present

"A" is a narrative specimen-centered report. "B" is a synoptic patient-centered report with a newspaper-style headline. Both reports contain all elements required by the CAP cancer checklist for prostatic adenocarcinoma. Both reports are adequate for billing purposes, since individual specimens are identified in each report. Both are adequate for cancer staging purposes.

Which report is more likely to be misinterpreted by a busy practitioner? Does report "A" represent a risk to patient safety? Does the headline in report "B" clearly communicate the single most important finding? Would you purchase a newspaper that contained no headlines? Which report would your surgical pathology customers prefer, if they were given a choice?

particular examination needed to be included on one report, because the same report was routed to caregivers, the billing department, medical records staff, and the research director down the hall. Today, busy caregivers can be insulated from potentially confusing information they do not require for clinical purposes. Special reports that contain different data elements can be produced for management, research, billing, and other nonclinical purposes.

The proper formatting of lengthy laboratory reports to maximize clarity—particularly lengthy anatomic pathology reports—is the subject of lively debate. Clinician comprehension of surgical pathology reports is significantly influenced by formatting, with "newspaper" style reports that included key features in a "headline" being much better understood than rambling diagnostic narratives.[187] Some authors have advocated the use of highly formatted "synoptic" reports to improve clarity.[188] Although the earliest recommendation for synoptic reporting was published in 1991, there is still no industry consensus about how to format surgical pathology reports to communicate most effectively with clinicians. See Figure 3 for an example.

The application of computer logic to laboratory reports can improve readability and minimize the potential for human error. Some computer "intelligence" is used in reporting today. Computers print calculated values derived from other test results so that caregivers do not have to calculate ratios by hand. Computers provide age- and sex-specific reference ranges, rather than general population reference ranges, and designate results outside of reference intervals with "low" and "high" flags, bolding, and other distinctive attributes. In some computer systems (but sadly not all), interpretive comments can be triggered based on a patient's test result. For example, a narrative interpretation of a low IgG serology titer can be included only on reports that contain a low IgG titer, while interpretative comments for high titers are suppressed and reserved for reports with high titer results. More advanced systems will undoubtedly enhance our ability to conceal clinically irrelevant information, while elaborating upon data likely to be clinically important.

The Joint Commission on Accreditation of Healthcare Organizations has recognized the vulnerability of verbal reports to misinterpretation. Individuals receiving critical verbal results are required by JCAHO hospital accreditation standards to "read back" the information to ensure that it has been transmitted accurately.[189] JCAHO also requires that clinical reports be free of abbreviations, acronyms, and symbols that an institution considers ambiguous, and that trailing zeroes not be used in clinical documentation.[190]

Reporting Critical Results

Critical results are, by definition, important. Sometimes referred to as *critical values* or *panic values,* critical values comprise between 0.05% and 1% of laboratory results.[191,192] Among surveyed physicians, 95% consider calls about critical results to be helpful in management, 75% note critical results in the medical record, and two-thirds of critical results prompt some change in therapy.[191] CLIA requires that critical results be reported "immediately"[177]; CAP has identified reporting of critical results as a CAP National Laboratory Patient Safety Goal (Exhibit 9). JCAHO requires that all critical values be reported within time frames established by the laboratory (defined in cooperation with nursing and medical staff).

A consideration of how to report critical results includes a discussion of how critical results are defined, time frames for reporting, who should be notified, the quality of communication, and documentation requirements.

What Is a Critical Result?

For any particular analyte or test, a *critical value* signals a correctable life-threatening condition that requires prompt notification and intervention.[193] Not every analyte has critical values; no patient ever died precipitously from too much or too little alkaline phosphatase. Nor does every analyte with a high range of critical values have a corresponding low range. An abnormally high serum creatinine level may signal acute renal failure; an abnormally low value does not indicate any acute condition in need of attention. Qualitative tests may also have critical values. The isolation of *Escherichia coli* from a blood culture may signal a life-threatening treatable condition that requires prompt communication to caregivers.

If a laboratory value suggests the presence of a serious illness that does not require prompt intervention, it is not "critical" as the term is used in the laboratory industry. The presence of HIV antibodies in the blood of a 40-year-old man, or adenocarcinoma in a pancreatic biopsy from a 70-year-old woman, are life-altering findings that require clear, accurate, and reliable communication; but under normal circumstances, neither finding requires immediate notification or immediate clinical intervention.

The laboratory director is responsible for establishing critical values. If the laboratory is located within a hospital, critical values are generally reviewed and approved by the medical staff. Decisions about what values to consider critical should be informed by knowledge of a laboratory's normal process for reporting results. If laboratory results are normally reported electronically, and caregivers reliably monitor terminals for new results, it makes sense to have fewer critical values because the normal process of laboratory reporting will serve for all but the most urgent situations.

Critical values should be established with an eye to the patient populations served by a laboratory. If a laboratory serves a large population of chronic renal dialysis patients, it may make sense to have a different creatinine critical value range for specimens received from the dialysis unit or ordered by certain clinicians, since patients in these units or under the care of certain doctors will already be receiving treatment for renal failure. The laboratory director may establish a policy that a result is to be considered critical only when it is the patient's first result to fall outside of critical value limits. Under this rule, the results of repeat analyses within a specified time period are not to be considered critical if the initial value fell outside of critical value limits. Establishment of patient care unit, physician-specific, and time-sensitive rules for critical values generally relies upon the ability of technologists to remember a lengthy set of rules. Given human limitations with rule processing, it is unfortunate that more laboratory information systems do not allow the specification of unit, clinician, and time-sensitive rules for critical values.

There is considerable variation among laboratories in the values they consider critical, as shown in Exhibit 46 and Exhibit 47.[191,194] Some variation is expected because of local factors discussed above, but several of the extreme critical value thresholds shown in Exhibit 46 are difficult to defend clinically. Laboratory directors should have a clear rationale for establishing unusual critical value ranges. Values should not be made critical simply because the normal result reporting process is unreliable. An unreliable reporting process for routine results requires its own attention.

Exhibit 46. Interlaboratory Variation in Critical Values Among 623 Laboratories [194]

Analyte	Low Critical Value Percentile			High Critical Value Percentile		
	10th	50th (median)	90th	10th	50th (median)	90th
Chemistry						
Ammonia, mmol/L	**0.0**	**4.4***	**22.2**	**19.4**	**43.3**	**110.8**
Arterial pH	7.2	7.2	7.3	7.5	7.6	7.6
Arterial PCO2,,kPa	2.5	2.7	4	6.7	9.3	9.3
Arterial PCO2,, kPa	5.3	5.3	8.0	**7.3**	**14.8**	**33.3**
Bilirubin (neonatal), mmol/L	0.0	0.0	**17.1**	206.2	256.5	307.8
Calcium (ionized), mmol/L	**0.22**	**0.75**	**1.50**	**0.35**	**1.58**	**1.75**
Calcium (total), mmol/L	1.50	1.50	1.75	3.0	3.25	3.50
Carbon dioxide, mmol/L	10	10	15	40	40	45
Chloride, mmol/L	70	80	90	115	120	130
Creatinine, mmol/L	**0**	**18**	**44**	265	442	884
Glucose (cerebrospinal fluid), mmol/L	1.10	2.15	2.31	4.13	11.00	27.50
Glucose (serum), mmol/L	2.20	2.20	2.75	16.50	24.75	38.50
Lactic acid, mmol/L	**0.00**	**0.06**	**0.33**	**0.27**	**0.44**	**3.40**
Lecithin/sphingomyelin (L/S) ratio	**1.0**	**1.5**	**2.0**	**2.0**	**2.0**	**3.0**
Magnesium, mmol/L	0.39	0.41	0.57	1.23	1.91	2.50
Phosphorus, mmol/L	0.32	0.32	0.65	1.78	2.58	3.23
Potassium, mmol/L	2.5	2.8	3.0	6.0	6.2	6.5
Osmolality, mOsmol/kg	219	250	270	300	323	350
Sodium, mmol/L	110	120	125	150	160	170
Urea nitrogen, mmol/L	**0.0**	**1.1**	**2.1**	17.9	28.6	35.7
Uric acid, mmol/L	**0.0000**	**0.0590**	**0.1180**	**0.5990**	**0.7611**	**0.8850**
Hematology						
Activated partial thromboplastin time, s	**0**	**19**	**23**	40	78	118
Fibrinogen, mmol/L	0.50	1.00	1.50	**3.75**	**8.00**	**8.00**
Hemoglobin, g/L	50	70	80	180	200	210
Hematocrit, %	0.15	0.20	0.25	0.55	0.60	0.65
Platelet count, 3109/L	20	40	60	600	999	1000
Prothrombin time, s	**0**	**9**	**15**	17	30	40
White blood cell count, 3109/L	1.0	2.0	3.0	20.0	30.0	60.0

* For example, the median facility that reported a low critical value for ammonia set the threshold at <4.4 mmol/L.
Boldface type indicates that fewer than 100 of the 623 study participants established a low critical value for this analyte.

Exhibit 47. Interlaboratory Variation in Microbiology Critical Values Among 623 Laboratories [194]

Result	Participant (%)	Result	Participant (%)
Positive blood cultures	95.0*	Initial stool isolates of *Salmonella, Shigella, Campylobacter,* and *Yersinia*	59.7
Positive CSF cultures	91.2		
Positive AFB smear or culture	71.9	Positive latex agglutination and/or antigen detection test	50.7
Positive Gram stains of sterile body fluids	66.8	Positive CSF VDRL	25.7
		Other microbiology critical values	44.8

* For example, 95% of 623 study participants indicated that they considered positive blood cultures to be a critical value.
CSF = cerebrospinal fluid. AFB = acid-fast bacilli. VDRL = Venereal Disease Research Laboratory test.

How Quickly Should Critical Results Be Reported?

The time frame for reporting critical results should be established by the laboratory director, in consultation (as appropriate) with clinical staff. Standards should be realistic, which means they should be informed by current industry performance. Exhibit 48 shows the average time taken to complete 2270 critical value calls at several hundred institutions.[194] The average call about an inpatient critical value took 6 minutes to complete from the time the caller first picked up the telephone, and the average call about an outpatient critical value required almost 14 minutes. Since the times shown in Exhibit 48 are averages and not 90% completion rates, institutions that wish to deliver typical industry performance should set 90% completion targets at approximately twice these time frames (12 minutes for inpatients and 24 minutes for outpatients). It is also important to keep in mind that the figures shown in Exhibit 48 do not include the interval between specimen collection and the time a technician (or patient service representative) picks up the telephone to call a critical result. We do not recommend that the time frame from specimen collection to result verification be included in local standards for the timeliness of critical result notification. When a specimen drawn from an outpatient at 4:00 in the afternoon is found to have a potassium value of 7.1 mmol/L at 11:30 in the evening, it probably makes little difference how many minutes it takes a technologists to reach a caregiver.

Laboratory goals for the time to call critical results should take into account the acuity of the patient population being treated and the types of caregivers available to receive calls. Calls placed to clerical staff generally require that the clerical staff make a second call to a physician before patient therapy can be instituted. All other factors being equal, the laboratory should complete critical value calls more quickly when notification is being provided to clerical staff and not physicians, since a second call to a physician will usually be required.

Who Should Receive Calls?

Laboratories located within hospitals accredited by JCAHO are required to report critical results directly to a *licensed* caregiver or, when the patient's licensed caregiver is not available, to an alternative *responsible* caregiver. A survey of more than 13,000 critical values called at more 623 institutions showed that approximately one-third of critical results are called to clerical staff, and fewer than 10% of values are called to physicians (Exhibit 49).[194] The study authors did not determine whether licensed caregivers were unavailable when clerical staff

Exhibit 48. Time Spent Calling Critical Results [194]

	Average Minutes (No. calls)	
Time to Complete Call		
Inpatient	6.1	(1723)
Outpatient	13.7	(550)
Time to Abandon Call		
Inpatient	20.2	(70)
Outpatient	46.3	(63)

Exhibit 49. Individuals Notified About Critical Results [169]

	Inpatients No. (% of total)	Outpatients No. (% of total)
Registered nurse	4775 (37.8)	622 (21.2)
Any staff nurse	2307 (18.3)	393 (13.3)
Unit clerk/office staff	3985 (32.5)	1237 (42.1)
Medical student	21 (0.2)	3 (0.1)
Any physician on call	455 (3.6)	196 (6.7)
Physician ordering test	1090 (8.6)	490 (16.7)

were called with results, or whether clerical staff meet the JCAHO requirement of "responsible caregivers."

In the same study, 4% of inpatient calls and 10% of outpatient calls were abandoned after an average of 20 and 46 minutes spent trying to reach a caregiver. The question of what to do when a caregiver cannot be reached about a critical result troubles many laboratory directors, particularly in the outpatient setting, where it may be difficult to reach providers after hours. In some hospitals, the emergency department has agreed to receive these calls and contact the patient. This is not the norm. In most institutions, the pathologist on call assesses the situation and contacts the patient, as required. Standards of good medical practice in the United States specify that when a physician goes off duty, the physician should designate someone to care for patients in his or her absence. When no responsible caregiver is willing to receive a call, the situation should be treated as an "incident" and reported to the physician or the physician's department chair, as appropriate (see "Occurrence Management: Learning from Incidents" in chapter 6 for a discussion about incident reporting).

Quality of Communication

As with all critical information transmitted verbally, the individual receiving a critical results call should "read back" the results to ensure that they have been understood correctly.[189] In 2004, 2.2% of laboratories inspected by the CAP were cited for not having a read-back policy for verbal communication.[91] Of course, the existence of a policy is no guarantee that the policy will be followed. To our knowledge, no multi-institutional study has examined the proportion of cases in which a critical value is actually read back by the person who received a critical value call.

Documentation

The laboratory must document calls made about critical results. Documentation should include the date and time of the call and the identities of the person making and receiving the call. Documentation often consists of a nonchartable entry made in a laboratory information system. We know of no regulatory or accreditation requirement that the individual receiving a critical value call must document the time of communication, but some institutions are asking caregivers to record this information, along with the amount of time that nonphysician caregivers on patient care units took to notify a physician about the result. While the laboratory must keep an internal record of critical value calls to evidence compliance with CLIA standards, we know of no requirement that the laboratory document critical value calls on paper laboratory reports.

JCAHO hospital accreditation requirements specify that hospitals be able to show that critical value reporting is timely. One way to demonstrate compliance with this requirement is to periodically tabulate the time between critical result verification and critical result call completion, and compare the actual interval to time frames established by the laboratory director, in consultation with the medical staff.

Administration of Blood Products

Magnitude of Blood Product Administration Risks

The risks of blood product administration are widely recognized. The most serious risk—hemolytic transfusion reaction caused by ABO mismatch of blood product and patient—

occurs approximately one-third of the time a red blood cell unit is administered to the wrong patient. (Two-thirds of the time the recipient will, by chance, have the same ABO group as the transfused unit.) Transfusion of an entire unit of ABO incompatible red blood cells causes death approximately one-third to one-tenth of the time. With careful monitoring of patients during transfusion and early discontinuance of transfusion at the first sign of a reaction, the fatality rate is reduced to approximately 1 per 20 cases of ABO incompatible red blood cell transfusion.

In New York State, 1 in 33,000 transfusions of red blood cells involve ABO incompatible units, bringing the overall ABO fatality rate to approximately 1 in 600,000 red cell transfusions.[195] Seasoned transfusion medicine staff at most large hospitals can recall one or two instances of ABO incompatible transfusions that occurred in their institution during their career.

Hemolytic transfusion reactions can result from incorrect identification of a patient at the time of initial phlebotomy, incorrect typing in the laboratory, or administration of a unit to the wrong patient. Administration of red blood cells to the wrong recipient is responsible for most hemolytic reactions, approximately 38% to 49%.[195] About half of the remaining reactions are due to incorrect patient or specimen identification during phlebotomy (discussed earlier in this chapter), and the remainder are due to either incorrect laboratory typing or a combination of errors. Removal of the wrong unit of blood from the blood bank refrigerator appears to be the major source of primary error, with blood frequently taken from the blood bank without a formal identity check against the patient's case record, followed by a bedside check that fails to disclose the discrepancy.[196]

What can be done to reduce the frequency of hemolytic transfusion reactions due to administration of blood to the wrong patient?

Control Measures

Root cause analysis of 85 transfusion fatalities reported to JCAHO through the end of 2004 showed that 75% of events involved orientation/training issues, followed by failure to assess patients (58%). Procedural noncompliance and communication failure were each cited as root causes less than 30% of the time.[197] These data suggest that emphasis be placed on training transfusionists and on ensuring the monitoring of patients receiving transfusions.[198]

It is difficult to prospectively study methods to prevent hemolytic transfusion reactions, because reactions occur rarely. Most recommended practices to prevent hemolytic reactions are based on professional opinion, not empirical evidence. Because prevention of hemolytic reactions is so difficult to study, attention has been focused on minimizing more common errors and process defects that place patients at risk for hemolytic transfusion reactions. These include improper patient identification before initiating transfusion and failure to monitor patients during transfusion.

During 2004, 1.7% of transfusion services were cited by CAP laboratory inspectors for failing to establish procedures to detect transfusion reactions, and 1.2% were cited for failing to conclusively identify patients before initiating transfusion.[91] The CAP has conducted two multi-institutional studies of transfusion safety practices.[199] A study conducted in 1994 audited more than 12,000 transfusions at 519 institutions, and a study conducted in 2000 audited more than 4000 transfusions at 223 facilities. Compliance with minimal monitoring

Exhibit 50. Monitoring Vital Signs in Transfused Patients [199]

	Number of Institutions	Institution Percentiles				
		10th	25th	50th (median)	75th	90th
Vital Sign Monitoring (1994)	519	46.2*	75.0	90.2	100.0	100.0
Vital Sign Monitoring (2000)	223	63.6	84.2	95.0	100.0	100.0
Patient Identification (1994)	519	10.0	35.7	69.0	92.7	100.0
Patient Identification (2000)	223	0.0	0.0	10.0	40.0	73.7

* For example, among 519 laboratories studied in 1994, 10 percent of facilities monitored vital signs in 46.2% or fewer transfused patients. Higher percentiles indicate better performance.

Vital sign monitoring consisted of checking vital signs prior to initiating transfusion, during the first 15 min of transfusion, and after the first 15 min of transfusion. Patient identification practices consisted of ensuring that the stated patient name matched the wristband identification, wristband identification matched the blood bag compatibility label, patient's name and wristband identification matched the name on the blood request form, and that the patient's name and identification number on blood request form were compared with results of compatibility testing and with the expiration dates on the blood bag.

recommendations and patient identification practices varied widely among the facilities (Exhibit 50).

Institutional practices and policies found to be significantly associated with greater compliance with vital sign monitoring or patient identification procedures included (1) transporting units of blood directly to the patient's bedside, (2) having no more than one individual handle blood units en route, (3) checking unit labels against physicians' orders, (3) reading identification information aloud when two or more transfusionists participate in a transfusion, (4) using written checklists to guide the administration of blood, (5) instructing health care personnel in transfusion practices, and (6) routinely auditing the administration of transfusions.[199] Laboratory managers should consider adopting all of these control measures in their institutions.

In addition to reducing the risk of ABO incompatible transfusions, other types of blood-related reactions (acute lung injury, bacterial contamination of platelets, and transfusion-associated graft-versus-host disease) are considered preventable complications of blood transfusion. Measures to control these complications are beyond the scope of this manual, but have been reviewed elsewhere.[200]

Interpretation of Results

The ability of caregivers to appropriately use laboratory results in management decision making represents the final vulnerability in the laboratory value stream—the concluding "handoff" of information from the laboratory/supplier back to the clinician/customer. An accurate, timely, clearly reported test result delivered into the hands of the ill-equipped or unprepared will count for naught.

Precisely where the laboratory's responsibility for test interpretation ends and the clinical caregiver's begins is not well defined. Some responsibility for interpreting results rests with the laboratory. CLIA requires that laboratories performing nonwaived testing engage a "clinical consultant" to provide consultation to laboratory clients regarding interpretation of test results. CLIA also requires that laboratories provide clients with information that may affect interpretation of test results (eg, interferences) and updates when methodology changes affect result interpretation. On the other hand, most of the responsibility for interpreting results rests with clinicians. Physicians who order tests are expected to interpret most results on their own.

Magnitude of Result Misinterpretation Risk

There is ample evidence that clinicians have difficulty interpreting and acting on some laboratory test results. Clinical journals regularly publish review articles that provide guidelines for interpreting the results of problematic assays, such as coagulation, molecular, cardiovascular risk, and oncologic tests. At any one time, half a dozen books about clinical test interpretation are available from major publishers. New and expensive treatments, the proliferation of difficult-to-interpret tests, a greater reliance on nurse practitioners as deliverers of primary care, and patient-initiated testing all increase the demand for help in interpreting laboratory tests.[201]

Two large multi-institutional studies of laboratory test interpretation have been conducted. Laboratory directors can use data from either of these studies to benchmark performance in their own institutions against peers. In a study of 5500 hypercalcemic results from 525 different laboratories, 3.5% of abnormal results were not documented in the patients' medical records, and physicians did not respond to the elevated calcium results by writing a note (23.1% of cases) or ordering another test (13.8% of cases). These omissions occurred despite the flagging of every abnormal result on the laboratory report and the fact that more than half of the values represented new (first-time) calcium elevations.[202]

In a study of procedural follow-up after 16,132 abnormal gynecology cytology results, 12% of women with high-grade lesions had no procedural follow-up after one year.[203] Disturbingly, younger patients and pregnant patients were less likely to be followed-up than the average patient. There was wide variation among the 316 study laboratories in the rate of follow-up, as shown in Exhibit 51.

Control Measures to Improve Interpretation of Test Results

Control measures to improve interpretation of test results have not been well studied. Moreover, there are several barriers facing laboratories that wish to implement programs to improve the interpretation of test results.[204] These barriers include (1) lack of sufficient specialists in any one clinical laboratory to provide useful interpretations; (2) absence of a reimbursement model for professional activities designed to improve result interpretation; (3) conflict with nonlaboratory specialists who derive professional income from clinical consultations initiated in response to abnormal laboratory results; and (4) accounting systems that are unable to measure the benefits of improved result interpretation (eg, speedier diagnostic work-ups and treatment) or link the benefit to incremental expense within the laboratory.

Two models for improving the interpretation of results have been studied: interpretive comments attached to individual reports, and automated care management pathways that use test results to generate clinical reminders.

Exhibit 51. Procedural Follow-up of Abnormal Pap Smears from 316 Laboratories [203]

Pap Smear Lesion and Follow-up Period	Institution Percentiles (Percent of patients followed-up)		
	10th	50th (median)	90th
HSIL/Carcinoma			
within 1 y	66.7*	90.0	100.0
within 6 mo	61.1	85.7	96.7
within 3 mo	50.0	76.7	92.0
LSIL/GIL			
within 1 y	64.3	85.2	100.0
within 6 mo	48.3	73.3	93.3
within 3 mo	27.6	56.7	82.8

* For example, in 10% of institutions, 66.7% or fewer HSIL/Carcinoma diagnoses were followed-up within 1 year. HSIL = high-grade squamous intraepithelial lesion. LSIL = low-grade squamous intraepithelial lesion. GIL = glandular intraepithelial lesion.

Exhibit 52. Sample Narrative Coagulation Test Interpretations [134]

von Willebrand Evaluation in the Presence of an Acute-Phase Response	Low Antithrombin Result in a Patient on Heparin
"The PT and PTT are normal. The fibrinogen, which is an acute-phase reactant, is elevated at 545 mg/dL. The values for the von Willebrand panel values fall within normal ranges for a blood group O individual such as this patient and are not suggestive of von Willebrand disease. However, von Willebrand factor is also an acute phase reactant. Therefore, the von Willebrand panel values may be elevated above their true baseline. If indicated, repeat testing can be performed at a time when the patient is not likely to be in an acute phase reaction."	"The specimen submitted has an elevated PTT. When the sample was treated with an enzyme that degrades heparin, the PTT corrected into the normal range, indicating the prolongation is due to the presence of heparin in the sample. The antithrombin is slightly low. Heparin administration can cause slight decreases in antithrombin within several days, secondary to increased clearance. If hereditary antithrombin deficiency is strongly suspected, the assay may be repeated once the patient has been off heparin for at least 1 to 2 weeks. The results of the other requested studies are normal."

Interpretive Comments

Narrative interpretations of complex test results provided by medical laboratory professionals, sometimes combined with reflex test protocols, have been used to decrease time to diagnosis, the number of tests clinicians must order to reach a diagnosis, and the number of patient visits.[205] Two examples of narrative interpretations are shown in Exhibit 52. In surveys of ordering physicians, 80% indicated that interpretive comments provided by the laboratory saved them time and improved the diagnostic process, and 70% of clinicians indicated that laboratory interpretations helped prevent misdiagnosis or refined the differential diagnosis.[134]

Some caution must be sounded about providing result interpretations. A group of Australian pathologists was asked to generate interpretive comments for a set of laboratory results that were accompanied by brief clinical histories. The appropriateness of pathologist comments was then evaluated by an expert panel. There was considerable diversity in the range of interpretative comments received for each case report, and while the majority of comments were judged to be acceptable by the expert panel, some comments were considered inappropriate and, in a few instances, were judged to be dangerous.[206]

Automated Care Management Pathways

Clinical practice guidelines frequently make use of laboratory test results to direct management. A patient on oral anticoagulants with a high international normalized ratio (INR) will have his or her anticoagulant dose reduced, while the dose for a patient with a low INR may be increased. A diabetic with persistently elevated blood sugar will have his or her insulin dose increased, while the dose for a diabetic with consistently normal glucose will not be changed.

When clinical practice guidelines are encoded in an automated reminder system, caregivers or patients can be alerted to important results. In some implementations, management recommendations are supplied as part of the alert. Automated reminders for warfarin monitoring based on INR results have been used successfully to improve care.[207] In a review of studies that evaluated automated reminders for diabetes care, glycated hemoglobin levels were significantly lowered in trials that made use of laboratory or home glucose test results to initiate reminders to caregivers and patients.[208]

Correcting Reporting Errors

Erroneous laboratory reports are issued with some regularity. Error rates appear to be highest in the most complex tests that involve some element of subjective human interpretation, such as surgical pathology, but errors occur with all types of laboratory testing. In a study of 74 facilities, second-pathologist review of surgical pathology cases disclosed discrepancies in 5.1% of cases.[72,209] There was wide variety in the frequency of discrepancies reported by different institutions (Exhibit 53). In a single-institution study of microbiology errors, 0.3% of final reports required subsequent correction.[210] Even with automated clinical tests, approximately 0.1% to 0.01% of reports are incorrect, usually due to patient identification errors. A study of 631 clinical laboratories found error rates (expressed as errors per 10,000 tests) were highest in

Exhibit 53. Surgical Pathology Second Review Discrepancy Rates [72]

		All Institution Percentiles				
	N	10th	25th	50th (median)	75th	90th
Discrepancy rate (%)	74	21.0	10.0	5.1*	1.0	0.0

* For example, the median institution found that 5.1% of surgical pathology cases subjected to second review showed some form of diagnostic discrepancy. More difficult cases tended to be preferentially reviewed in this study.

Exhibit 54. Impact of Diagnostic Changes in 415 Surgical Pathology Cases [72]

	Specimens, No. (%)	
Discrepancy Type		
Change within same category	194	(47.8)
Change in categorical interpretation	85	(20.9)
Typographic error	75	(18.5)
Change in patient information	37	(9.1)
Change in margin status	15	(3.7)
Effect on Patient Outcome		
Harm	63	(16.6)
Marked	8	(2.1)
Moderate	12	(3.2)
Mild	43	(11.3)
Near miss	33	(8.7)
No harm	283	(74.7)

Exhibit 55. Method Used to Detect Surgical Pathology Discrepancies at 74 Institutions [72]

Case-finding Method	Reviewed Cases with Discrepancies (%)
Intradepartmental review	7.1
Request by clinician	23.0
Interdepartmental review	4.8
Selected by quality assurance review	4.3
Extradepartmental review	8.6

microbiology, followed by hematology, transfusion medicine, and chemistry.[211]

Some erroneous reports are clinically important; others are not. Exhibit 54 shows the clinical impact of diagnostic changes in 415 surgical pathology cases: 16.6% of errors were judged to have caused some patient harm, and 2.1% to have caused serious harm; the remainder had no impact on patient outcome. In a study of corrected microbiology reports, 6.7% were associated with adverse clinical impact, ranging from delayed therapy, unnecessary therapy changes, and inappropriate therapy, to unnecessarily increased level of care.[210]

Erroneous reports may be discovered in any number of ways. A laboratory may discover an error during routine internal review of results, or the error may be brought to the laboratory's attention by a clinician. Exhibit 55 shows that surgical pathology results for which clinicians requested a review were three to five times as likely to be found in error as results reviewed for other reasons. Discrepancies detected by clinicians also tended to be more likely to have caused patient harm than discrepancies detected through routine intradepartmental review.[72]

Procedures for Correcting Reporting Errors

Correcting Reporting Errors Promptly

Erroneous laboratory reports should be corrected in a timely manner, even if the cause of the error is unknown. When an error is discovered, CLIA requires that the laboratory "promptly" issue a corrected report to the ordering provider and any other caregivers who can be identified, along with notification that the previous result was in error. The laboratory must also maintain copies of the original and corrected results.[212] There is no requirement to explain the cause of the error when a report is corrected, and issuance of a corrected report should not be delayed while the cause of an error is being investigated. If a result is known to be inaccurate, but the correct result is not yet known, an amended report should be issued that indicates the previously reported result was incorrect.

Identifying Corrected Reports

When correcting an erroneous laboratory report, it should be clear to caregivers that a correction is being made. In anatomic pathology, rectified reports may be called *corrected, amended,* or *revised* reports. When a correction is made to a numeric value, the correction can be communicated in a report that is not specifically labeled "corrected" or "amended," so long as the corrected result is flagged with a footnote or other indicator that clearly identifies the result as a corrected value.

Some institutions use the term *addendum reports* to refer to corrections. This use of the word "addendum" is incorrect. An addendum report adds new information that was not included in a previous report, but does not contradict any information that has already been released. An addendum report might be issued to communicate that mycobacteria are growing from a lung biopsy previously diagnosed as "granulomatous inflammation." But a report that changes a diagnosis from "granulomatous inflammation" to "squamous cell carcinoma" is a correction, not an addendum.

Formatting Corrected Reports

Proper formatting of corrected reports is important. The recapitulation of previously reported incorrect results in the vicinity of a corrected result invites misinterpretation (see Figure 2). For example, if a diabetic's serum glucose was incorrectly reported as 273 mg/dL and later corrected to 73 mg/dL, the incorrect value of "273 mg/dL" should not appear on the corrected report anywhere near the correct test result and should be clearly labeled as being incorrect. The laboratory is legally obligated to note on the new report that "73 mg/dL" represents a corrected value. But reprinting the old incorrect value in the vicinity of the corrected result invites confusion. An argument can be advanced that incorrect results should not be included on a corrected report at all.[213] In electronic charts, incorrect results should not be viewable by caregivers using normal result retrieval pathways.[214] Contrary to a persistent legend within the laboratory community, there is no CLIA requirement that incorrect results be reprinted on corrected reports.[215]

The importance of clearly communicating corrections applies to anatomic pathology reports as well as clinical laboratory results. If the diagnosis of a breast biopsy is changed from malignant to benign, the incorrect malignant diagnosis should be removed from electronic reports that are immediately available to caregivers and should not appear on the "diagnosis line" in the corrected paper report (or in any location that could be confused with the correct benign diagnosis). The fact that the diagnosis was changed should be included in the text of the corrected report.[216]

Investigating the Cause of the Laboratory Error

All erroneous laboratory reports should be treated as incidents (see "Occurrence Management: Learning from Incidents" in chapter 6). The cause of the error should be investigated and, when possible, corrected. Some erroneous reports are caused by laboratory failures, but others are caused by failures that occurred before a specimen ever reached the laboratory, such as mislabeling in a physician's office or failure to provide pertinent clinical history. Regardless of the cause, when an erroneous report results in what JCAHO defines as a "sentinel event," and the laboratory is part of a JCAHO-accredited organization, a sentinel event investigation should be conducted (see "Appraisal of Root Cause and Failure Effects Analysis" in chapter 3).

Errors Involving Pathologists

In September 2003, the House of Delegates of the College of American Pathologists asked the CAP for guidance about how to handle errors involving a pathologist's interpretation. In response to this request, the College approved the following policy in 2004:

> The College of American Pathologists believes that it is a fundamental ethical requirement that a physician should deal honestly and openly with patients. Situations occasionally occur in which a patient suffers significant medical complications that may have resulted from the physician's mistake or judgment. In these situations, the physician is ethically required to inform the patient of the facts necessary to ensure understanding of what has occurred. The following points will guide the pathologist in this responsibility.
>
> (1) Significant errors are considered those that have had a negative impact upon the prospective health or management of the patient. When such a error contributed to the health care injury, that error must be reported to the patient in coordination with the ordering provider and within a manner consistent with the organization's disclosure policies as well as local, state, and federal regulations.
>
> (2) All inaccuracies in the medical record should be documented and communicated at the time the inaccuracy becomes known. The correct test result or diagnosis should be made clear in an amended or corrected report as soon as possible. The reason that the original result was reported incorrectly (ie, due to error or other reason) may not be known and need not be reported in the medical record.
>
> (3) When an incorrect result or diagnosis causes material injury to a patient, the correct result/diagnosis and the fact that the result has been changed must also be reported to the patient. For an inaccuracy caused by or directly involving a pathologist, the pathologist involved in the case should discuss the matter with the physician who ordered the pathology consultation. The two physicians should jointly determine how best to communicate the result to the patient.

Control Measures to Improve Report Correction Practices

To our knowledge, no one has studied how often laboratories fail to correct results known to be inaccurate, or control measures that can be applied to improve result correction practices. We have included error correction practices in this manual because published data show that erroneous reports are associated with significant patient morbidity, and because our experience suggests that laboratory directors are often unsure of their responsibilities in this area, particularly with regard to errors that involve pathologist interpretations. Failure to correct inaccurate results represents a violation of CLIA standards, places patients at additional clinical risk, and may constitute fraud. Conversely, timely correction of an error does not imply that the error occurred as a result of substandard laboratory or pathologist practice, that the error was preventable, or even that the cause of the error is known or knowable.

General Laboratory Systems: Risks and Control Measures

Personnel

To this point we have discussed quality risks and control measures that can be applied to preanalytic processes, analytic testing, and postanalytic processes. But what about the risks posed by people and the control measures we might apply to our own actions and decision making? After all, human beings account for many—perhaps most—laboratory problems. Can we apply quality management principles to our own performance?

Let us compare ourselves for a moment to the analytic equipment with which we work. Imagine that each of us came with an operating manual, similar to the operating manual that accompanies an automated analyzer we might purchase. What would our operating manual look like? It might read like this:

> Congratulations! You have chosen to lease the most powerful instrument ever created. This device has remarkable flexibility and is extraordinarily adaptable, with the capacity to learn new procedures and think for itself. Some of its capabilities, such as the ability to recognize images, are superior to the most advanced computers ever manufactured. But before you place this instrument in service, you should be aware that it has some peculiar features that make it different from other devices used in your facility:
>
> This instrument comes in several models: pathologist, medical technologist, cytotechnologist, histotechnologist, medical laboratory technician, even laboratory director. The programming this instrument has received before shipment varies with the model, but even within models the programming varies from unit to unit. Some of this programming may be defective, and as you validate your new device, you may discover that certain units require reprogramming. Whatever the model or unit, it is doubtful that your new instrument has received any programming about local laboratory procedures or workflow, so you will need to train the device before you put it to use.
>
> The maintenance requirements of this instrument are complex and have not been defined by the manufacturer. You must decide how to manage the quality of your new instrument on an ongoing basis. The good news is that there are thousands of consultants and human resource experts who can recommend quality control procedures for your instrument. The bad news is that none of the approaches recommended by experts have been validated rigorously. And since no two units are the same, it is doubtful that any one approach will work for all devices. For example, the same corrective action plan that improves the reliability of one unit may make another unit less reliable and possibly angry.
>
> This instrument is prone to error. When operating in "schematic control" mode—automatically performing routine memorized tasks—this instrument will fail approximately 0.1% to 1% of the time. When operating in "attention control" mode—performing cognitive tasks—the error rate will be much higher. This instrument's error

rate in any particular setting will vary according to the characteristics of the individual unit, the task it is performing, and environmental factors that you cannot completely control and which, in any event, are incompletely understood. You will need to use this device in a manner that causes it to make as few errors as possible, but also design systems that protect patients from errors this instrument will inevitably make.

While capable of learning, this instrument is also capable of forgetting. Sometimes the instrument will not recognize that it has forgotten instructions and will incorrectly reconstruct previous programming from its defective memory. When making complex decisions, this instrument will demonstrate several types of cognitive bias. Do not rely too heavily on this device's memory or objectivity.

While you are leasing this instrument for approximately 40 hours per week, this piece of equipment will spend more than two-thirds of its time outside the laboratory in an uncontrolled environment where it will be exposed to physical, biological, and psychological insults that may impact its performance in your facility. This instrument's self-diagnostics will not reliably detect when it is malfunctioning. You must implement systems to detect if this device becomes impaired.

When placed in certain environments that pose extreme temptation and/or pressure to perform, this instrument may take shortcuts and intentionally ignore programmed instructions. Rarely, this device may demonstrate deliberately deceptive behavior, obfuscating actions it has taken. You are responsible for creating an environment that minimizes the potential of this instrument to purposefully circumvent its programming. When creating this environment, keep in mind that you are also one of these instruments, subject to the same temptations and pressures as the other devices in your laboratory.

The FDA has not evaluated this instrument for clinical diagnostic use and has no authority to do so. This device has not received 510(k) premarket approval. If this instrument malfunctions and causes damage, the laboratory will likely be held responsible. The manufacturer will accept no responsibility or liability for any costs, expenses, claims, or damages incurred by the laboratory or any third party as a result of the failure of this instrument, or any component thereof, or any other instrument that cannot function properly when working alongside this device.

Good luck with your new instrument!

Would patients want one of these devices in a laboratory testing their specimens? Would anyone want one of these devices directing a clinical laboratory? Given our inherent limitations as human beings, what can we do to bring ourselves into reasonable quality control?

Introduction of New Employees Into the Laboratory

Exhibit 56 provides a checklist of tasks the laboratory should consider completing before placing a new employee into a production environment. The tasks listed in the exhibit all relate to the management of quality and safety; new employees typically have additional administrative and orientation requirements, which are not included in this list. Exhibit 56 should be consulted for all new employees and close business associates—pathologists, medical technologists, histotechnologists, managers, etc. Of course, some of the tasks listed are not applicable to every type of employee.

Most of the tasks in Exhibit 56 are self-explanatory or covered elsewhere, but some elaboration on the subject of new employee training is necessary here. The introduction of a new employee into the work environment represents a vulnerable period when the quality of laboratory operations is more likely to be compromised, much as the introduction of a new test represents a period of vulnerability. Humans engaged in new tasks tend to operate in *attention control mode* until the tasks are well learned and can mostly be performed automatically. Since human error rates for jobs performed in attention control mode are much higher than for jobs performed automatically (in *schematic control mode*), new employees show an increased tendency to make errors at tasks they will later perform more reliably (see "Human Error Research" in chapter 3 for a more thorough discussion).

Transitioning performance from attention to schematic control mode is accomplished through repetitive practice, not education. Therefore, as part of training a new employee for the production environment, the laboratory should make every effort to provide the employee with extensive hands-on practice in a supervised setting. Written procedures, textbooks, and didactic presentations may provide a new employee with required knowledge that he or she did not already possess, but will not substitute for repetitive physical rehearsal of the tasks the new hire will be expected to carry out. The fact that an individual can correctly complete a new task is not evidence that the employee has successfully transitioned from error-prone attention control mode to low-error schematic control mode. Only through recurring "hands-on" practice will the task become automatic so that the error rate of the new employee comes to approximate that of his or her more experienced associates.

Some individuals, such as pathologists, practice tasks such as biopsy interpretation extensively during their professional training and do not require rehearsal in biopsy interpretation when first hired. Yet even individuals who are already highly trained in some tasks may struggle with other duties, such as verification of surgical pathology results in an unfamiliar laboratory information system. Supervised practice of new tasks is as important for physicians as for other laboratory workers.

Exhibit 56. Checklist for Introducing a New Employee Into the Laboratory

- ❖ Background verification (credentials, references, education, work experience, other)

- ❖ Define employee's job responsibilities (page 152)

- ❖ Training for major tasks (technical, computer, administrative)

- ❖ Demonstration of competence (page 126)

- ❖ Secure any required local privileges (medical staff membership, etc)

- ❖ Introduction to laboratory's organizational structure (page 151)

- ❖ Introduction to laboratory's written policies and procedures (page 143)

- ❖ Introduction to laboratory's quality management program (page 167)

- ❖ Introduction to incident/safety reporting system (page 162)

- ❖ Introduction to compliance program (page 128)

- ❖ Introduction to impaired employee referral procedures (page 129)

- ❖ Provide appropriate access to computers and privacy training (page 132)

Exhibit 57. Use of Various Methods to Assess Competency [220]

Laboratory Section	N	Percentage of Laboratories					
		Test or QC Results	Direct Observation	Preventive Maintenance	Written Testing	Other	None
Chemistry	511	92.4*	90.2	80.6	55.4	23.5	1.0
Hematology	512	92.4	90.6	79.5	60.9	24.6	0.6
Microbiology	495	91.5	91.1	70.5	52.9	23.6	1.2
Transfusion medicine	477	92.5	93.3	60.8	72.1	23.5	0.4
Phlebotomy/ specimen processing	490	27.1	94.9	24.7	47.1	14.1	3.7
Surgical pathology	341	63.6	86.5	55.7	30.5	12.9	5.6
Cytopathology	275	76.7	79.6	46.5	30.9	20.4	3.6
Totals	3101	77.4	87.5	60.0	52.2	20.8	2.1

* For example, 92.4% of 511 laboratories reported that they reviewed test or quality control results as a method for assessing employee competency in the chemistry section of the laboratory. Since a given laboratory section may use multiple methods to assess competence, row totals exceed 100%.

Ongoing Quality Management of Personnel

Competency

It is difficult to argue with the sentiment that laboratory personnel should be competent to perform the work they are assigned to do. CLIA requires the laboratory technical consultant to periodically document the competency of all personnel performing nonwaived testing, and there is some evidence that employees who work for institutions that regularly measure competence perform better than employees from sites that do not faithfully assess competence.[217,218] Particular methods that must be used to assess competence are spelled out in CLIA regulations. The CLIA standards specify:

> The procedures for evaluation of the competency of the staff must include, but are not limited to- (i) Direct observations of routine patient test performance, including patient preparation, if applicable, specimen handling, processing and testing; (ii) Monitoring the recording and reporting of test results; (iii) Review of intermediate test results or worksheets, quality control records, proficiency testing results, and preventive maintenance records; (iv) Direct observation of performance of instrument maintenance and function checks; (v) Assessment of test performance through testing previously analyzed specimens, internal blind testing samples or external proficiency testing samples; and (vi) Assessment of problem solving skills.[219]

Competence must be evaluated at least semiannually during the first year in which an individual tests patient specimens using high-complexity tests. Thereafter, evaluations must be performed at least annually unless test methodology or instrumentation changes, in which case, prior to reporting patient test results, individual performance must be re-evaluated to include the use of the new test methodology or instrumentation. In 2004, 1.3% of laboratories inspected by the CAP were cited for failing to assess the competency of employees.[91]

Exhibit 58. Institutional Adherence to Written Competency Plans [220]

Institution Type	Number of Institutions	Percent of Employees Tested According to Plan All Institutions Percentiles		
		10th	50th (median)	90th
Teaching	151	58.2	87.2*	100.0
Nonteaching	290	51.9	91.7	100.0
Overall	441	54.7	89.6	100.0

* For example, in the median teaching institution, 87.2% of employees were tested for competency in accordance with that institution's written testing plan.

How does competency assessment work in practice? An early study of competency assessment at 511 clinical laboratories was conducted by Howanitz et al.[220] Almost all institutions (98%) indicated that they evaluated competence at least yearly, and 89% had a written competence assessment plan for the general laboratory. Individuals responsible for evaluating the competence of employees were usually managers. Many laboratories did not use all six of the CLIA-required assessment activities when evaluating employee competence (Exhibit 57). Moreover, sampling of actual employee records indicated that, in the median laboratory, approximately 10% of employees had not been evaluated in accordance with the institution's own written assessment plan (Exhibit 58). A more recent study that focused on point-of-care competency testing suggests that assessment of competence is now being performed more faithfully.[217] Adherence to an institution's written assessment policy was highest when assessment was included as part of an employee's annual performance appraisal, presumably because the process of completing the performance appraisal reminded managers to assess competence. Some institutions have enrolled in external competency assessment subscription programs to help manage the competency assessment process. External vendors do not perform all of the assessments required by CLIA (such as direct observation of performance), but they provide educational and testing content and help institutions track assessments of individual employees.

One problem that appears to challenge managers is what to do with the employee who does not pass a competency assessment examination. In the US aviation industry, the competence of commercial airline pilots is assessed using standardized simulators of the aircraft pilots fly. If a pilot fails his assessment, he is not allowed to fly until he passes a reassessment.[221] In contrast, most laboratories in the original Howanitz study reported that if an employee failed a competence evaluation, the individual was allowed to continue work and was retested within four weeks. At fewer than 10% of institutions, employees who failed an evaluation were removed from the work setting until they passed a second test.[220] The question of what to do with employees who fail their competency examinations has significant practical consequences; 11% of specimen processing employees failed competency testing in the Howanitz study.[220] In 2004, 1% of laboratories inspected by the CAP were cited for not having a policy to retrain and reassess employees who fail competency testing.[91]

In 2005, a new chapter in competency assessment was opened with the CMS approval of the first national proficiency testing (PT) program for cytotechnologists and pathologists performing gynecological cytology. Traditionally, PT has focused upon assessing the proficiency of a laboratory as a whole and not the individual operators within the laboratory. Competency testing—which focuses on the individual—has largely been separate from proficiency testing. The exception to this rule is gynecological cytology. CLIA regulations explicitly specify that if a gynecological cytology PT program is approved by CMS, proficiency testing must be administered to every cytotechnologist and pathologist performing testing, and that tested professionals must demonstrate certain levels of performance in order to continue examining clinical specimens. With the approval of the first national PT program in gynecological cytology in 2005, individual performance of cytotechnologists and pathologists will now be assessed by an external vendor. This development has generated considerable controversy, and it remains to be seen how this chapter in competency assessment will end. Outside of gynecological cytology, external competency testing of pathologists in anatomic pathology procedures is not required by CLIA. The CAP publication, *Quality Management in Anatomic Pathology,* provides guidance in how individual institutions can internally assess the performance of anatomic pathologists.[1]

Fraud and Malfeasance

Given sufficient pressure or temptation, employees may deliberately circumvent policy or regulation. Rules may be circumvented for financial gain, to save time, or to conceal technical or other embarrassing problems. Managers are not immune from pressure or temptation; numerous cases of malfeasance and fraud involve management at the highest levels.

Many types of fraudulent activity may occur in a laboratory, including deliberate misappropriation of confidential patient information, falsification of quality control records, fraudulent billing practices, and purposefully compromising diagnostic examinations to save labor or reagent expense. We suspect fraudulent activity in clinical laboratories is uncommon, but the incidence is not known. Examples of fraudulent behavior are found in some of the case studies presented in chapter 2 of this manual.

> ### Exhibit 59. Controls for Preventing Fraud
>
> ❖ Avoidance of undue pressure
> ❖ Restricted access to information
> ❖ Division of responsibilities
> ❖ Anonymous reporting
> ❖ Audits and inspections

In addition to maintaining an ethical organizational "tone," the potential for fraud is reduced by the controls listed in Exhibit 59. To reduce the potential for fraud, management should keep the following in mind:

- ❖ Excess pressure promotes fraudulent behavior. Productivity and sales targets should be realistic and achievable, lest shortcuts be taken to achieve organizational goals.

- ❖ Personnel should be denied access to information for which they have no work-related use. Access to information can be restricted through administrative, physical, or technical procedures (as reviewed in Exhibit 62).

❖ In situations that present strong temptation, such as the management of money, responsibilities should be divided among several individuals, who check one another's work. This recommendation applies to managers as well as nonmanagers. Key management tasks should be divided among managers to reduce the likelihood that any one manager will engage in improper behavior.

❖ Institutions should support an anonymous reporting system through which employees at any level of an organization can report behavior they believe to be dishonest or prohibited. Sometimes this is accomplished through the institution's regular incident reporting system. More commonly, a separate anonymous reporting system is established for the confidential reporting of fraudulent activity, violations of patient confidentiality, or noncompliance with standards. Reporting may be made to an institution's compliance, safety, and/or privacy officer. To help ensure that individuals within CAP-accredited laboratories do not engage in fraudulent or improper behavior, the CAP maintains a toll-free telephone number through which laboratory employees can confidentially report quality or safety concerns that are not being addressed by laboratory management (866-236-7212 in US; 847-832-7533 internationally).

❖ Finally, audits and inspections of operations may be conducted, during which records and laboratory practices are examined by inspectors on a test basis. The CAP Laboratory Accreditation Program's external inspection process, which will include unannounced inspections beginning in 2006, represents one of several types of external audits to which laboratories may be subject. The HIPAA requirement for internal audits of attempts at computer access represents another form of audit (see Exhibit 62).

Impaired Employees

The quality of employees' work may be impaired by the abuse of physical substances (alcohol, drugs), mental illness, physical illness, or severe stress. Impaired employees do not reliably identify themselves. Therefore, employers should implement systems to facilitate detection of impaired individuals and their removal from the workplace. Several measures have been shown to improve the identification of impaired employees: (1) a referral system that maintains strict anonymity, discourages retaliatory behavior for reporting associates or superiors, and encourages self-referral; (2) an employer's commitment to arrange for treatment of impaired employees and a commitment to allow recovered employees to return to work, giving referral of an impaired employee a positive therapeutic dimension; and (3) an employer's provision of reasonable paid time away from work while the impaired employee recovers, eliminating one of the strongest disincentives to removing oneself from the workplace—loss of income.

Quality Management Practices of Uncertain Benefit

Several human resources practices are required by regulation or widely recommended, even though their impact on quality and patient safety has not been convincingly demonstrated:

❖ Most authorities believe that quality is enhanced by a program of continuing employee education, although the evidence to support this seemingly sensible practice is surprisingly sparse.

❖ Many accrediting organizations require annual or biannual performance appraisals of all employees. We are not aware of compelling evidence that annual performance appraisals improve quality, and no less of an authority than Deming spoke against the annual performance appraisal.[12]

❖ Many human resource experts advocate that employees be periodically surveyed about their job satisfaction. There is strong evidence that organizations with more satisfied employees demonstrate better financial performance, and some evidence that more satisfied employees are associated with higher-quality output. But we have not seen evidence that the regular administration of satisfaction surveys leads to improved employee satisfaction or performance.

❖ Finally, the federal government places maximum workload limits on cytotechnologists to minimize errors from overwork, although data linking cytotechnologist workload to quality are not well developed. We and others have advocated that managers exercise caution when staffing at a level that requires particularly high staff productivity, because quality may be compromised.[222] Exhibit 60 shows data about staffing levels from a recent CAP study of study of 151 clinical laboratories; managers may use these data to determine whether they oversee laboratory sections with unusually high labor productivity.[222] Efforts by researchers to link high staff productivity to low quality have generally failed to show significant associations. There is no evidence to suggest that heavy workloads necessarily reduce quality, although they may in particular institutions.

Motivation

Until now, our section on personnel has followed the general format used in this chapter. We have dutifully delineated quality and patient safety risks posed by human operators and managers, discussed the magnitude of each risk, and suggested control measures that can be applied to mitigate individual hazards. Yet we would be remiss if we did not acknowledge some of the distinctive positive qualities of human beings, which can become constructive forces for quality and patient safety. We are extraordinarily complex creatures, and our unique susceptibilities to err are matched by wonderful propensities for compassion, a sense of fairness, pride in work, and imagination. Harnessing these positive attributes for the benefit of patients and caregivers is a recurring challenge to everyone who labors within a clinical laboratory. We have no formula to offer readers and doubt the applicability of any single approach to all workers and all work settings. Further, our study of high-reliability systems makes us suspicious of "touchy-feely" management consultants, who would have us believe that enthusiasm and dedication can completely make up for intrinsic human limitations or system vulnerabilities. Still, inspiration is a wondrous thing, and to the extent that commitment, compassion, and creativity can be nourished, quality and patient safety will be promoted.

Exhibit 60. Interinstitutional Variation in Staffing of Clinical Laboratory Sections [222]

Peer Group	Annual Workload Range	No. Laboratories in Peer Group	Percentiles Within Peer Group		
			10th	50th (median)	90th
Cytology Subsection					
	Number Cytology Accessions			Cytology Accessions/Non-mgmt FTE	
1	169 – 1748	16	1181	1585*	4420
2	1952 – 7877	29	1563	2789	7419
3	8200 – 18,258	28	3249	4494	10,353
4	19,115 – 113,218	27	3050	5782	12,499
Chemistry/Hematology/Immunology Section					
	Number Billable Tests			Billable Tests/Non-mgmt FTE	
1	59,113 – 370,338	30	11,233	23,457	66,125
2	374,549 – 1,421,388	82	19,047	41,334	84,191
3	1,423,725 – 6,491,344	37	27,788	55,217	105,081
Microbiology Section					
	Number Billable Tests			Billable Tests/Non-mgmt FTE	
1	2467 – 43,472	65	4017	7772	14,193
2	46,174 – 322,010	79	7011	9661	17,467
Transfusion Medicine Section					
	Number of Transfused Units			Transfused Units/Non-mgmt FTE	
1	157 – 2540	37	498	868	1796
2	2551 – 6230	37	793	1148	2739
3	6236 – 12,261	37	1052	1787	3040
4	12,810 – 70,799	36	1529	2153	3638
	Number of Crossmatches/T&S			Crossmatch and T&S/Non-mgmt FTE	
1	463 – 6513	37	818	1820	5196
2	6567 – 14,101	37	1448	2880	6803
3	14,105 – 25,794	37	2075	3968	8402
4	26,498 – 319,256	36	2306	5388	11,088

* For example, in cytology Peer Group 1, which consisted of 16 laboratories that processed between 169–1748 accessions per year, the median institution reported that the average non-management employee examined 1585 accessions per year.

Information Management

This section reviews risks and control measures related to the management of information. We define "information" broadly to include data maintained in electronic form, information on paper, undocumented but generally understood processes and practices within a laboratory, and information still locked up in clinical specimens retained by the laboratory. Information includes data about patients, policies and procedures, and records of quality management and other administrative activities.

Chapters about laboratory information management are often organized around major pieces of legislation (eg, HIPAA, CLIA) or types of information (paper, electronic, biological). Here, we organize our discussion around five broad themes: retention, security, privacy, safety, and management of procedures.

Exhibit 61. Retention of Laboratory Records and Clinical Materials

Material / Record	Period of Retention
General Laboratory	
Accession log records	2 years
Instrument/other maintenance records	2 years
Quality control/management records	2 years
Surgical Pathology / Bone Marrow	
Wet tissue	2 weeks after final report
Paraffin blocks	10 years
Slides	10 years
Reports	10 years
Cytology	
Slides (all gynecologic diagnoses)	5 years
Fine-needle aspirate slides	10 years
Reports	10 years
Autopsy (Non-Forensic)	
Wet tissue	3 months after final report
Paraffin blocks	10 years
Slides	10 years
Reports	10 years
Autopsy (Forensic)	
Wet tissue	3 years after final report
Paraffin blocks	Indefinitely
Slides	Indefinitely
Reports	Indefinitely
Gross photographs and negatives	Indefinitely
Accession log records	Indefinitely
Body fluids and tissue for toxicology	1 year
Dried blood stains or frozen tissue for DNA	Indefinitely

Retention of Information

In theory, information should be saved for as long as the benefits of retention outweigh the cost of storage. In practice, of course, it is difficult to predict when information will be wanted and how useful it will be. Exhibit 61 lists the minimum amount of time that records and clinical materials should be retained. Exhibit 61 reflects current standards of the College of American Pathologists and United States regulatory requirements, and incorporates the best estimates by technical experts about the length of time information is reasonably likely to be useful. New technologies that make better use of information or decrease the cost of storage may cause the time frames in Exhibit 61 to change.

The retention of everyday clinical specimens not listed in Exhibit 61 also deserves comment. Some clinical specimens are too labile to preserve, while others are consumed by the testing process. Everything else—leftover blood, fluids, and tissue samples—should be retained long enough to re-examine if the initial examination fails or contemporaneous quality control testing fails. Many laboratories retain blood specimens for several additional days to accommodate "add-on" test requests. It should go without saying that saved clinical material should be maintained in an environment that will retard specimen degradation.

Exhibit 61. Retention of Laboratory Records and Clinical Materials (continued)

Material / Record	Period of Retention
Clinical Pathology Records	
Patient test records	2 years
Serum / CSF / body fluids other than urine	48 hours
Urine	24 hours
Peripheral blood and body fluid smears	7 days
Permanently stained slides (Gram, trichrome)	7 days
Cytogenetics	
Permanently stained slides	3 years
Fluorochrome stained slides	Discretion of director
Fixed cell pellet	2 weeks after final report
Final report	20 years
Diagnostic images (digitized or negatives)	20 years
Wet specimen/tissue	When adequate metaphase cells obtained
Transfusion Medicine	
Donor records	10 years
Patient records	10 years
Quality control records	5 years
Specimens from transfused donor units	7 days post transfusion
Specimens from blood donor recipients	7 days post transfusion
Records of employee signatures, initials, and identification codes	10 years
Records of indefinitely deferred donors, permanently deferred donors, donors placed under surveillance for the recipient's protection (donors that are hepatitis B core positive once, donors implicated in a hepatitis positive recipient)	Indefinitely

Information Security

Information is secure when unauthorized users cannot access the information, and when authorized users can be assured of required access. Security means keeping the unwanted out, but also means keeping information intact and available to those with a right to know. The concept of security therefore includes the concepts of confidentiality, access, and integrity.

Confidentiality

Not too long ago, maintaining the confidentiality of medical information was straightforward: people kept their mouths shut, and charts not in use were stored in a locked file cabinet. Today, improperly secured computer systems can be surreptitiously raided by the unscrupulous half a world away. How is confidentiality to be maintained in a networked digital world?

Information confidentiality is a complex subject.[223] No information system can be made completely secure from unauthorized intrusion. Every complex software application has security flaws; Carnegie Mellon University estimates that a thousand lines of computer code typically contain five to fifteen defects or "bugs." Every hardware installation is vulnerable. No hospital can shield all terminals and keyboards from unauthorized viewing all of the time. Every large organization contains unwary employees who can be duped into sharing confidential information.

Are confidentiality breaches in health care common? Quantitative data are hard to come by, but anecdotal evidence abounds. Nicole Brown Simpson's medical records appeared in the press within a week of her 1994 murder. In 1995, *The Sunday Times* of London reported that the going price for anyone's medical record in England was 200 pounds.[223] Ancillary health information systems at the universities of Washington and Michigan have been accessed by unauthorized users. The first criminal conviction of a health professional for a HIPAA violation involved a laboratory phlebotomist from Seattle named Richard Gibson, who used private information from a cancer patient to fraudulently obtain credit cards in the patient's name. Hackers have camped onto outgoing phone lines from laboratory computers to intercept toxicology results destined for autodial printers. A disgruntled overseas employee from a remote medical transcription service recently threatened to post surgical pathology reports on the Internet if he was not paid $10,000. *The Wall Street Journal* reported in 2005 that hospitals are being targeted by individuals engaged in identity theft.

The standards within the Health Insurance Portability and Accountability Act of 1996 (HIPAA) specify measures that health care institutions must adopt to protect the confidentiality of medical information. The standards require that covered entities (including clinical laboratories) implement various administrative, physical, and technical safeguards to protect data. While the standards are somewhat generic, the multidimensional approach to security envisioned by HIPAA recognizes that no single control measure can be relied upon to safeguard data. Exhibit 62 lists the procedures required by HIPAA to secure data. The technical terms in Exhibit 62 are defined in the Glossary. The laboratory information system section of the CAP Laboratory Accreditation Program's *Laboratory General Checklist* contains a number of specific requirements related to information security. Satisfaction of the CAP information system requirements addresses many (but not all) of the required HIPAA controls listed in Exhibit 62.

We believe many clinical laboratories (and health care institutions in general) are vulnerable to security breaches and should take the requirements in HIPAA to heart. When performing the security risk analysis mandated by HIPAA, it is helpful to keep in mind that the three most common causes of computer confidentiality violations do not involve any technical

Exhibit 62. HIPAA Procedures to Guard Data Confidentiality, Availability, and Integrity		
Standards	**Sections**	**Implementation**
Administrative Safeguards		
Security Management Process	164.308(a)(1)	Risk Analysis (R)
		Risk Management (R)
		Sanction Policy (R)
		Information System Activity Review (R)
Assigned Security Responsibility	164.308(a)(2)	(R)
Workforce Security	164.308(a)(3)	Authorization and/or Supervision (A)
		Workforce Clearance Procedure
		Termination Procedures (A)
Information Access Management	164.308(a)(4)	Isolating Health care Clearinghouse Function (R)
		Access Authorization (A)
		Access Establishment and Modification (A)
Security Awareness and Training	164.308(a)(5)	Security Reminders (A)
		Protection from Malicious Software (A)
		Log-in Monitoring (A)
		Password Management (A)
Security Incident Procedures	164.308(a)(6)	Response and Reporting (R)
Contingency Plan	164.308(a)(7)	Data Backup Plan (R)
		Disaster Recovery Plan (R)
		Emergency Mode Operation Plan (R)
		Testing and Revision Procedure (A)
		Applications and Data Criticality Analysis (A)
Evaluation	164.308(a)(8)	(R)
Business Associate Contracts	164.308(b)(1)	Written Contract or Other Arrangement (R)
Physical Safeguards		
Facility Access Controls	164.310(a)(1)	Contingency Operations (A)
		Facility Security Plan (A)
		Access Control and Validation Procedures (A)
		Maintenance Records (A)
Workstation Use	164.310(b)	(R)
Workstation Security	164.310(c)	(R)
Device and Media Controls	164.310(d)(1)	Disposal (R)
		Media Re-use (R)
		Accountability (A)
		Data Backup and Storage (A)
Technical Safeguards		
Access Control	164.312(a)(1)	Unique User Identification (R)
		Emergency Access Procedure (R)
		Automatic Logoff (A)
		Encryption and Decryption (A)
Audit Controls	164.312(b)	(R)
Integrity	164.312(c)(1)	Authenticate Electronic Protected Health Information (A)
Person or Entity Authentication	164.312(d)	(R)
Transmission Security	164.312(e)(1)	Integrity Controls (A)
		Encryption (A)

Key: (R)=Required (A)=Addressable as applicable

Exhibit 63. Laboratory Computer Downtime Experience, 1995 and 2001 [224,225]

	All Institution Percentiles				
	10th	25th	50th (median)	75th	90th
No. of downtime instances per 30 days					
Overall (1995, N=422)	44.0	32.0	8.0*	3.0	0.0
Overall (2001, N=97)	30.0	9.0	3.0	1.0	0.0
Unscheduled (1995)	11.0	5.0	2.0	0.0	0.0
Unscheduled (2001)	4.0	1.9	0.5	0.0	0.0
Scheduled (1995)	33.0	30.0	3.0	0.0	0.0
Scheduled (2001)	30.0	5.8	1.0	0.0	0.0
Cumulative downtime per 30 days (in hours)					
Overall (1995)	77.7	39.0	14.3*	2.9	0.0
Overall (2001)	29.3	11.5	4.0	0.7	0.0
Unscheduled (1995)	38.7	12.7	2.6	0.0	0.0
Unscheduled (2001)	11.5	2.6	0.2	0.0	0.0
Scheduled (1995)	46.4	20.6	3.8	0.0	0.0
Scheduled (2001)	21.1	6.0	1.2	0.0	0.0

* For example, the 1995 the median of 422 institutions reported 8 instances of downtime during 30 days. The cumulative duration of downtime for the median institution during 1995 was 14.3 hours during 30 days.

Exhibit 64. Computer Availability in 97 Laboratories During 2001 [225]

	All Institution Percentiles				
	10th	25th	50th (median)	75th	90th
Instances per 30 days					
Unscheduled downtime	4.0*	1.9	0.5	0.0	0.0
Downtime from 8AM to 5PM, Mon–Fri	3.0	2	0.9	0.0	0.0
Scheduled downtime, not data backup	2.9	1.0	0.0	0.0	0.0
Scheduled downtime, data backup	29.1	4.0	0.0	0.0	0.0
Overall downtime	30	9.0	3.0	1.0	0.0
Downtime longer than 90 min	4.0	1.9	0.1	0.0	0.0
Cumulative downtime per 30 days (in hours)					
Unscheduled downtime	11.5*	2.6	0.2	0.0	0.0
Downtime from 8AM to 5PM, Mon–Fri	5.4	2.1	0.3	0.0	0.0
Scheduled downtime, not data backup	4.0	1.0	0.0	0.0	0.0
Scheduled downtime, data backup	20.1	4.0	0.0	0.0	0.0
Overall downtime	29.3	11.5	4.0	0.7	0.0

* For example, the 10th percentile facility experienced 4 episodes of unscheduled downtime during 30 days, with a cumulative duration of 11.5 hours.

Exhibit 65. Impact of Laboratory Computer Downtime in 422 Laboratories [224]

Impact	All Instances		Scheduled Downtime		Unscheduled Downtime		Downtime > 8 hours
	No. (%)	Median Duration (hours)	No. (%)	Median Duration (hours)	No. (%)	Median Duration (hours)	No. (%)
No impact on work	2870 (24.9)*	0.5	1295 (21.0)	0.6	1575 (29.4)	0.3	170 (26.8)
Extra work required	5524 (48.0)	0.8	3197 (51.9)	0.8	2327 (43.5)	0.7	325 (51.3)
Overtime required	144 (1.3)	3.0	29 (0.5)	6.4	115 (2.2)	2.3	32 (5.0)
Reporting delay	4771 (41.4)	0.8	2325 (37.7)	0.9	2446 (45.7)	0.5	275 (43.4)
Adverse clinical outcome	11 (0.1)	0.5	0 (0)	-	11 (0.2)	0.5	3 (0.5)
Compromised mgmt function	192 (1.7)	1.0	37 (0.6)	2.6	155 (2.9)	2.0	41 (6.5)
Inaccurate result released	23 (0.2)	1.0	1 (0.0)	8.0	22 (0.4)	1.0	4 (0.6)
Other impact	224 (1.9)	0.5	47 (0.8)	0.5	177 (3.3)	1.0	63 (9.9)

* For example, 2870 (24.9%) of downtime instances had no discernable impact on work. Since several impacts could be recorded for each instance of computer unavailability, percentages may total more than 100%.

wizardry or nefarious sophistication. The most common cause of confidentiality violation is misappropriation of information by an authorized user with a valid password. The second most common cause involves the improper sharing of a password with an acquaintance or work associate. The third most common cause involves the fraudulent acquisition of a computer password through misrepresentation to a computer help-desk operator.

Access

The "flip side" of confidentiality is access: allowing authorized users to access laboratory data they need to do their work. Computer downtime or cumbersome processes for retrieving archived records has the potential to disrupt workflow, compromise business interests, and perturb patient care.

How often do laboratory computers become unavailable? In 1995, 422 clinical laboratories participated in a 30-day study of laboratory computer system failure.[224] A follow-up study of 97 institutions was conducted in 2001.[225] The authors of the studies used a modified taxonomy developed by the American Society for Testing and Materials (ASTM) to classify downtime into one of several categories according to its potential impact on operations.[226] Comparison of the two studies suggested that performance within the industry has improved; computers were more available to users in 2001 than they were in 1995. In both studies, there was reasonably wide variation in the amount of downtime experienced by different laboratories. Exhibit 63 shows the distribution of computer downtime in the two studies, and Exhibit 64 shows the types of downtime experienced by the 2001 cohort. Managers who oversee laboratory information systems should compare their own performance to these industry norms.

Computer downtime is clinically important.[227] The impact of computer downtime on laboratory operations and patient care was evaluated in the previously cited 1995 study (Exhibit 65). Overtime and adverse clinical outcomes were more likely to be reported with unscheduled than scheduled downtime, and with extended periods of downtime compared to downtime of normal duration.

The authors of the two studies tested a number of institutional factors for associations with increased downtime. Factors significantly associated with increased downtime in one or both studies included (1) specific LIS vendors, (2) installations that that served two or more full-service laboratories with their computer, (3) laboratory staff supporting LIS operations (compared with hospital staff supporting LIS operations), and (4) less recent installation of software patches. In the 2001 study, sites that installed their most recent patch more than 12 months before the study (N=16), 6 to 12 months before the study (N=10), or within the last 6 months (N=36) reported a median of 5.0, 3.5, and 1.4 downtime events per 30 days, respectively. Each of these associations suggest management opportunities to reduce downtime, although associations do not necessarily imply a cause-and-effect relationship.

Data Integrity

Information stored in electronic form must be protected from corruption. Computer operators with the best of intentions can accidentally destroy thousands of patient records with a few ill-advised keystrokes. Software operating in unforeseen ways may improperly jumble test results or link the records of unrelated patients. Physical disasters to computer facilities may result in catastrophic loss of data. Corrupted data transmission may cause a message to change its meaning, even though the data residing in the transmitting system remains intact. The control measures outlined in Exhibit 62 address data integrity as well as confidentiality and access risks. The process of validating new software to protect against data loss and corruption is discussed subsequently and summarized in Exhibit 67.

Privacy

The concept of privacy in health care is allied to the concept of security, but is distinct. Security breaches occur when information is acquired by a third party without the permission of the organization that operates the computer system from which information was taken. Privacy is breached whenever information is acquired by a third party without the patient's permission. Usually, security and privacy violations occur at the same time. But when an organization or its representatives purposefully divulge private information to a third party without the patient's permission, a privacy violation occurs without any security breach. Patients retain certain rights to their own health care information, which providers (including clinical laboratories) must respect.

The duty to protect patient privacy is often equated with the privacy requirements contained in HIPAA legislation, but the medical profession was committed to respecting patient privacy long before HIPAA and will remain committed long after HIPAA is retired. HIPAA defines clearly some improper uses of confidential medical data, but the health professional's fiduciary duty to protect patient privacy transcends HIPAA.[228]

Clinical laboratories may use de-identified health information (information that cannot be traced back to an individual patient) without any consideration of patient privacy. A month's worth of serum sodium values, stripped of any personal identifiers, may be posted on the Internet or used freely in research studies. Privacy becomes an issue when health information is linked to information that can be used to identify an individual, such as a patient name, social security number, address, telephone number, genomic sequence, or other unique identifier.

When a clinical laboratory receives a patient specimen and test order from a caregiver, the patient has given permission for the laboratory to use the patient's confidential health information for treatment, payment, and health care operations (TPO). This permission is implied by the patient's willingness to be treated by the caregiver who ordered the test. The laboratory does not require any written permission to use patient information necessary to perform TPO.

The laboratory is also permitted to disclose protected information to public health authorities or other individuals, as required by law, without explicit patient permission. Confidential health information may be shared with other health care providers and with insurers, so long as it is required for TPO. If, in the course of carrying out TPO, the laboratory is required to share confidential health information with business associates who are not themselves health care providers, insurers, or data clearinghouses, then the laboratory must enter into an agreement with the business associate that binds the associate to use the data in a manner consistent with HIPAA provisions.[229]

We believe the risk of clinical laboratories failing to comply with HIPAA privacy provisions is not as great as the risk of noncompliance with HIPAA security requirements, if only because a respect for patient privacy has been a tradition of laboratory medicine. In our experience, the two biggest areas of privacy vulnerability for laboratories are (1) unauthorized disclosure of personal information for research and (2) unauthorized acquisition of protected information by curious individuals who have been given access to information systems, but who do not have a work-related need to access the information they retrieve.

HIPAA and Research

HIPAA defines research as "a systematic investigation designed to develop or contribute to generalizable knowledge." When patients seek health care, they do not give implicit permission for their private information to be used in research. Explicit written permission normally must be obtained. When a laboratory manager receives a request for an extract of data that includes patient-identifiable health information which is to be used for research, and written patient permission is not provided, the request should be honored only when (1) the research project has been approved by the local institutional review board (and the board has determined that patient permission is not needed) or (2) the researcher's only interest in the data is to prepare a research proposal for an institutional review board to evaluate. Rules limiting the use of identifiable data for research apply to requests that come from within the laboratory as well as requests from external parties.

It can sometimes be difficult to determine whether a request for patient-identifiable health information is intended to support an internal quality assurance activity (for which explicit patient consent is not required, because quality assurance is part of "health care operations") or is intended to support a research activity (for which patient permission may be required). Quality-assurance activities are designed to generate knowledge that will be used locally to maintain or improve health care operations, but which will not be disseminated outside of a particular care system to be applied elsewhere. Research seeks to generate knowledge that can be widely applied, as evidenced by intended publication or presentation at a national meeting. Even if patient-identifiable data will not be included in research publications or presentations, its mere *use* by researchers is restricted. HIPAA requires that specific safeguards be applied before the laboratory releases identifiable information for research purposes (explicit patient permission, institutional review board authorization, or preparation of a proposal for review board evaluation).

HIPAA and the "Curious" Employee

There are a number of reasons why individuals who have been granted computer access may choose to look up medical information not required for their jobs. These include idle curiosity about a neighbor or acquaintance, interest in a public figure or someone identified in the news, an individual's desire to check on his or her own laboratory results, or the intent to trade confidential patient information for money or some other consideration. Often, when confronted, individuals who have accessed records for private purposes indicate that they were "checking the record for accuracy," and in fact, some individuals within the laboratory do look up already familiar laboratory results to be sure they are being filed and transmitted properly, unaware that their actions raise privacy issues.

Control Measures to Protect Patient Privacy

What controls can be applied within a laboratory to promote conformance with privacy requirements? Experience with HIPAA is too fresh to draw firm conclusions about which controls work best. In addition to the security controls already discussed in Exhibit 62, most institutions have instituted one or more of the four control measures in Exhibit 66:

> **Exhibit 66. Control Measures to Protect Patient Privacy**
>
> ❖ Education about privacy rights
>
> ❖ Creation of a "privacy officer"
>
> ❖ Audits of computer access to records
>
> ❖ Formal review of requests for data extracts that involve personal health information

- ❖ An educational approach with staff and business associates, based on scenarios that simulate situations in which patient privacy may be compromised.

- ❖ The designation of a *privacy officer* or *HIPAA compliance officer* to receive and respond to staff and associates' concerns about patient privacy.

- ❖ Audits of individuals who access clinical information systems. In some installations, the name of everyone who has accessed a particular medical record is automatically included as part of the medical record, as a deterrent to those who might call up medical records to satisfy private interests.

- ❖ Formal management review of all requests for data extracts involving protected health information.

Information Management and Patient Safety

Information systems contribute to patient safety because the strengths of computers and human beings complement one another. The human operator can learn, focuses attention when required, recognizes patterns well, and demonstrates creativity. The computer has a superior short-term memory, faster processing speed, the ability to detect nonsensical input from humans, and remarkable consistency. Computers are normally so good at what they do that human beings come to rely on them; it is unusual for a human to check a computer's work.

This reticence to check computers is unfortunate. Computer programs, after all, are designed by humans and frequently contain flaws ("bugs") that cause programs to behave in unexpected and potentially harmful ways. Alexander Pope's observation that "to err is human" applies to computer engineers as well as clinical caregivers. We believe that computer systems pose a risk to patient safety, much as human operators do. The FDA recognizes blood bank software as a "medical device" and requires manufacturers of blood bank software to adhere to the FDA's Good Manufacturing Principles (GNP) / Quality System (QS) Requirement, to minimize safety risks. Despite this requirement, FDA-approved blood bank software may behave unpredictably in the field. For this reason, the FDA also requires user validation before blood bank software is placed in clinical production.

Defects in laboratory information systems are particularly dangerous because they represent latent errors—errors that do not draw attention to themselves at the time the error occurs. Patient results can be mixed up or erased days after they are entered into a computer system, and years after a software programmer or hardware manufacturer made a programming or manufacturing error. Because computers possess tremendous speed, a problem can spread to thousands of patient records before it is recognized, understood, and corrected.

Some potentially dangerous defects we have observed in the laboratory information systems supplied by major vendors include unexpected erasure of previous blood typing information; inappropriate merger of records from different patients; pathways that allow verified results to be changed without flagging the results as changed; inconsistent transmission of results to external information systems; routing of clinical specimens to incorrect testing sites due to system timing issues; assignment of the same accession number to specimens from different patients; automatic re-attachment of interfaced instruments to incorrect ports, resulting in mix-up of patient values; and deletion of information within autodial transmissions, resulting in the demographic header from one patient being joined to results from another in a printed report.

What control measures can be applied to computer systems to reduce the risk they pose to patient safety? Laboratory data management applications are very complex. A typical installation supports multiple concurrent users and detached processes that can interact with one another in ways never anticipated by system designers. Even successful commercial vendors have typically sold only 300 to 500 systems, which means that the aggregate field-testing performed by customers is limited. Since laboratory information systems can be extensively customized ("paramatized"), no two customers' information systems are exactly alike, even when purchased from the same vendor. For this reason, all new computer systems require extensive local validation before being placed in service, and ongoing quality management thereafter. In this respect, computer systems are no different from new test systems or new employees, both of which also require initial validation and ongoing quality management.

Validating New Information Systems

User validation of new computer software is difficult; even providing guidance about how to validate software is problematic. The FDA, which in September 1993 issued a document entitled, *Draft Guidelines for the Validation of Blood Establishment Computer Systems,* had not followed up with final guidelines more than a decade later, and withdrew its draft guidelines in March of 2005 with a promise to provide an update later in the year. CLSI guidelines for validating laboratory data management systems are disappointingly (but unavoidably)

Exhibit 67. Validation of New Laboratory Information Systems

Task	Description
System Specification	Define services the information system is to deliver. Concentrate on inputs and outputs (from/to users, analyzers, printers, other systems). Concentrate on process paths (path of workflow and actions to be taken at different steps).
Validation Planning	Consider all user, patient, specimen, and testing scenarios, and develop test plan to address important scenarios. Define acceptance criteria (how proper functioning will be defined). Prepare test scripts for each contemplated test.
System Configuration	Configure system to meet specifications. Define tests, testing sites, patient types, data dictionaries, interface parameters, charting parameters, collection cycles, etc.
Unit Testing	Test individual steps in a process in "static" mode (without actual interfaces). Conduct input testing and boundary testing (testing of extreme inputs). Example: Order and result a test in the laboratory system. Correct the result.
Integration Testing	Test integration of components and modules. Examples: Admit a patient in a hospital system or result a test in an interfaced analyzer, and check for the admit/result to transfer properly to the laboratory system.
System Testing	Test an entire sequence of processes as they would occur in production. Example: Admit a patient, order a test, enter the result, transfer the patient, print a chart. Use the terminals and printers that will be used in production.
Load Testing	Test modules with transaction volumes that will be found in the production environment. Example: Run a "live" feed of admissions, transfers, and discharges from a hospital system into the laboratory system "test" partition.
User Testing	After user training, test the ability of users to perform each of the functions they will carry out in the production environment. This is often done with actual patients and results, but in the new system's test environment.
Downtime Testing	Test system shutdown, system start-up, data backup, and data restore functions. Test manual procedures that will be used during partial or complete system downtime.

generic.[230] Validation of software usually includes some or all of the tasks shown in Exhibit 67. During the validation process, the successful completion of each test is documented, and a decision to activate a new system is contingent on successful completion of all tests.

Ongoing Quality Management of Information Systems

Ongoing quality management required for laboratory information systems was outlined in Exhibit 62. Special attention should be placed on properly testing new software upgrades or patches, or testing changes that database managers make in system parameters. In an FDA analysis of 3140 medical device recalls conducted between 1992 and 1998, 7.7% of recalls were attributable to software failures, and 79% of these failures were caused by software defects introduced when changes were made to the software after its initial production and distribution.[231] Our experience with laboratory information systems is similar; software failures that occur well after activation are common causes of laboratory quality failures. Many of the steps required to validate new software must be repeated when software upgrades or patches are applied, or system parameters are modified. Managers of information systems should not assume that a "patch" offered by the vendor to correct a problem will do its job or will not adversely affect other aspects of an information system. Since changes to software represent a patient safety risk, the authority to modify laboratory software and the process for validating new software should be tightly controlled.

Procedures, Policies, and Processes

Procedures, policies, and processes represent "information" and require organization, ongoing maintenance, and authoritative approval. Written procedures, processes, and policies should be managed using document control principles, such as those listed in Exhibit 68. A complete description of a document control system can be found in CLSI publication HS1-A or GP26-A3.[232] Clinical laboratories should not have difficulty meeting the requirements of Exhibit 68, but a number do. In 2004, CAP laboratory inspectors cited 6.3% of laboratories for failure to implement a document control system—one of the highest rates of citation in the CAP Laboratory Accreditation Program[91]; 1.0% to 4.5% of laboratories were cited for failing to review the procedure manual annually (citation rates varied by laboratory section), and 1.2% to 2.0% of laboratory sections were cited for failing to make a complete procedure manual available at the work bench.[91]

> **Exhibit 68. Principles of Document Control**
>
> ❖ All procedures, policies, plans, and other documents must be approved by authorized personnel prior to issue
>
> ❖ Only currently authorized versions of documents are available for active use
>
> ❖ Documents are periodically reviewed, revised when necessary, and re-approved by authorized personnel
>
> ❖ Retired documents and versions of documents are archived and quarantined

Risks Relating to Procedures, Policies, and Processes

We believe the two most significant quality risks related to procedures and policies are: (1) the steps actually performed by operators in the laboratory may diverge from steps specified in written procedures, creating distinct and separate worlds of "practice" and "paper"; and (2) many important laboratory processes are never documented at all and have never been formally reviewed or authorized. The frequency with which these two problems occur has not to our knowledge been formally studied.

We suspect both of the two risks arise from the growing burden of paperwork in clinical laboratories. A modern hospital-based laboratory may be asked to maintain a Workplace Safety Plan, a Patient Safety Plan, a Disaster Plan (for disasters that impact local communities), a Disaster Recovery Plan (for disasters that impact the hospital and its information systems), a Quality Management Plan (discussed in the final chapter of this manual), a Patient Privacy Plan, a Data Security Plan, records of employee performance and quality management testing, and several manuals full of laboratory policies and technical procedures.

Maintaining the plethora of documents taxes many managers. Procedures found in various documents are sometimes contradictory. The burden of creating required but esoteric documents leaves many important processes undocumented and unreviewed. Managers may find themselves staying late to write a procedure describing how the laboratory will respond to a smallpox bioterrorist attack, while the process for splitting urine specimens between the urinalysis and bacteriology bench remains undocumented. Adding to managers' sense of futility, documents become so complex that most work in the laboratory ends up being performed from memory, without reference to any written procedures. When an employee has a question, he or she is more apt to ask a coworker for help than consult a written procedure. Within the industry, there is a lingering suspicion that documents do little to impact real world performance. This suspicion is not without basis. In 2002, the "ethics manual" of the Enron corporation was more than a half-inch thick, but prevented none of the ethics abuses that occurred at Enron during the year.

Control Measures

Control measures to ensure the production of required documents have not been well studied. Similarly, there have been no rigorous evaluations of control measures to ensure that operators follow written procedures. In the following section, we share techniques that others have used to meet documentation requirements and keep actual laboratory practices in conformance with written documentation. While these techniques have proven helpful in some institutions, they have not been field-tested in multi-institutional studies and may not be universally applicable.

❖ Borrow procedures from others. Procedures used in other laboratories or supplied by manufacturers (often in electronic form) may require little or no modification, although local approval of procedures is still required. For example, at the end of the last chapter, we have provided three sample quality management plans that readers may borrow for their own institution's quality management plan.

❖ Assign technologists within the laboratory the responsibility for developing new procedures or performing annual procedure review, subject to management approval.

❖ Refer to external documents, such as published textbooks or authoritative web sites, rather than copy material into local procedures. When writing procedures for commercially available test systems, refer to a manufacturer's operating manual for an analyzer or a package insert for a reagent/test kit, rather than copy instructions into local procedures. Of course, any referenced external documents must be available on-site for operators to use.

❖ On a weekly basis, have two operators working together deliberately perform a procedure, carefully following the step-by-step written instructions in the procedure manual, rather than relying upon memory. This process helps ensure that everyday practices and written procedures do not diverge. Cycle through procedures so that all are checked over during the course of a year.

❖ Hire an external company to prepare procedures, reserving local staff for review and approval.

❖ Use work products from quality circles/quality teams. When quality circles or teams meet to refine a laboratory process, the team often prepares a process map that illustrates current laboratory workflow. Incorporate these process maps into documents that are formally approved. Periodic review of procedures that contain process maps helps ensure that laboratory processes are understood and remain appropriate.

❖ When preparing procedures, do not try to anticipate every contingency that can arise. Cover common situations in procedure manuals, and instruct operators to seek guidance from management or technical experts for less common problems.

❖ Scan paper documents to reduce storage space and facilitate retrieval.

❖ Use web-based versions of procedure manuals. Web-based procedure manuals allow many operators to access the same manual concurrently, while maintaining control of revisions. In addition, web-based procedure manuals may be shared by physically separate laboratories, which often reduces the number of manuals that must be maintained. Ensure that each laboratory that uses a shared procedure manual has it authorized by the local laboratory director or designee.

❖ The most efficient tool for documenting quality control at the bench is often a paper form on a clipboard. Paper is a very efficient "input/output" device when the collected data does not need to be "touched" by multiple users or electronically manipulated. Resist computerization for its own sake.

❖ Use the laboratory information system to store policies and procedures, as well as patient data and quality control data.

❖ Many of the constraints built into instruments—lock-out features, user input validation sequences, "intelligent" review of results prior to release—represent undocumented elements in laboratory processes that help ensure accurate results. Some larger laboratories choose to explicitly document these functions, so that they can be recreated when equipment or information systems are changed.

Turnaround Time

A great deal of published and anecdotal evidence underscores the importance of laboratory turnaround time. Four-fifths of hospital-based laboratories receive complaints about test turnaround time.[233] In surveys of physician customers, turnaround time of stat and esoteric tests are identified as the prime dissatisfier with laboratory service.[151] Turnaround time is the aspect of laboratory service that hospital nursing staff rate as most important, ahead of result accuracy.[269] In some emergent clinical situations, quick turnaround of stat orders will have more impact on a patient's course than a high level of accuracy.[234] Even when turnaround time is not important clinically, delayed reporting of tests tends to cause physicians to reorder the same test, often on a stat basis.[235] In one tertiary care teaching hospital, 9% of medically unnecessary hospital delays were attributed to problems obtaining routine laboratory test results.[236]

Measuring Test Turnaround Time

Measuring and summarizing turnaround time is more difficult than it appears. There is no "correct" or single best way to track turnaround time; the approach should be tailored to an

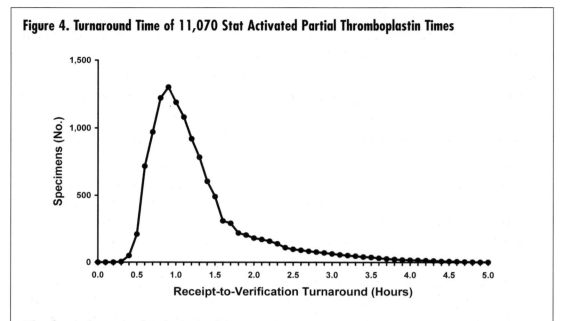

Figure 4. Turnaround Time of 11,070 Stat Activated Partial Thromboplastin Times

This figure shows the distributions of the time it took to report stat aPTT tests performed at a single institution over the course of a year. The specific interval measured was the time between specimen receipt in the laboratory and verification of results in the laboratory information system.

organization's particular requirements.[237] Laboratory managers interested in monitoring turnaround time should consider the following recommendations:

❖ Only one or two intervals in the testing cycle should be selected for monitoring. Most laboratories measure the time between order and result-verification, specimen collection and result-verification, or laboratory receipt of a specimen and result-verification.

❖ As a general rule, stat tests that have different preanalytic processing requirements should not be grouped together when summarizing turnaround time. For example, the turnaround of stat tests that require centrifugation before testing should not be mixed in with the turnaround of tests that can be performed on whole blood.

❖ Turnaround time should be recognized as a distribution, not a single number. Figure 4 shows the turnaround time of 11,070 stat activated partial thromboplastin time (aPTT) tests reported over one year at a single institution. The turnaround time of tests varied significantly. Moreover, the distribution of turnaround times was not "normal" in a statistical sense. Turnaround distributions can be divided into three segments. The first segment, comprising the first four data points in Figure 4, consists of the period during which no tests can be reported, because of the irreducible minimum time required for specimen processing and testing with the technology in use. The middle segment of the distribution (0.4 to about 1.6 hours in Figure 4) includes turnaround times that are more or less normally distributed. Most test-to-test variation in the middle segment of the distribution is due to common or "chance-cause" variation. The third segment (greater than 1.6 hours) consists of a long tail extending off to the right and includes longer turnaround times that were due to special causes of delay, such as misrouted or retested specimens.

Exhibit 69. Median Turnaround Times Desired by Caregivers				
Study Reference	240	240	241	242
Test Priority	Stat	Stat	Stat	Stat
Survey Group	Attending physicians	Laboratory directors	Laboratory directors	House officers
Turnaround Time Interval	Collection to reporting	Collection to reporting	Lab receipt to reporting	Lab receipt to reporting
CBC/Basic Hematology (min)	10 – 20	60		15
Glucose (min)	20 – 30	60		
Gram Stain (min)			60	
Basic Coagulation (min)				30
Serum Electrolytes (min)	10 – 20	60		30

❖ If the tail of a turnaround time distribution is relatively short, and caregivers are reasonably satisfied with turnaround time, the most efficient way to monitor turnaround is to follow mean turnaround time with an X-bar control chart, as described in chapter 3 of this manual (Exhibit 1). When the tail of the distribution is long, or turnaround time is perceived by caregivers to be a problem, it makes more sense to monitor the proportion of turnaround time outliers. The frequency of outliers can be summarized as the fraction of tests that were not turned around within an institution's target time frame, or the time required to complete 90% of tests.[238]

Turnaround Time Goals

Five approaches have been used to establish turnaround time goals.[237] Some facilities base their goals on customer expectations—the demands of physicians, nurses, and, in a few instances, their patients. Other institutions define goals in terms of medical necessity—responsiveness that is required by a patient's medical condition. Some facilities focus on logistical necessity— the turnaround time required to move patients through emergency departments or intensive care units expeditiously. Still others define goals in terms of what other laboratories are achieving—besting the "average" laboratory, a major competitor, or a "best performer." Finally, a philosophy of continuous quality improvement has led some facilities to concentrate on continually shortening their turnaround time, rather than focus on where their current performance stands relative to expectations or peer institutions.

We encourage laboratory directors to develop turnaround time goals in consultation with laboratory customers. The following observations should be kept in mind when working with customers to develop goals:

❖ Surveys of laboratory customers reveal considerable variation in expectations.[239] Exhibit 69 lists the results of some of the earlier published customer surveys.[240-242]

Exhibit 70. Turnaround Time of Selected General Laboratory Tests

Analyte	Summary Statistic / Interval / Priority	Number of Institutions	Percentile Rank of Institutions		
			10th	50th (median)	90th
Inpatient					
Potassium[244]	Median/order to report/stat, ED (min)	613	60*	44	30
	90% complete/order to report/stat, ED (min)	613	101*	70	50
Hemoglobin[244]	Median/order to report/stat, ED (min)	613	48	31	19
	90% complete/order to report/stat, ED (min)	613	91	56	38
Troponin[245]	Median/order to report/stat, ED (min)	158	74.5	57.8	45
	90% complete/order to report/stat, ED (min)	158	129	93	66.5
CK-MB[245]	Median/order to report/stat, ED (min)	112	82	58.0	40
	90% complete/order to report/stat, ED (min)	112	131	91.5	61
Outpatient					
CBC[246]	Percent reported in 1 day/order to report/routine	117	98.8%	100%	100%
Thyroid tests[246]	Percent reported in 1 day/order to report/routine	175	95.0%	100%	100%
Electrolytes[246]	Percent reported in 1 day/order to report/routine	117	63.8%	100%	100%

* For example, in the 10th percentile institution, the median stat potassium was completed 60 minutes after it was ordered in the emergency department (ED), and 90% were completed 101 minutes after order.

❖ Turnaround time expectations of nurses tend to be more demanding than expectations of physicians, and expectations in hospitals with faster turnaround are more demanding than expectations in hospitals with slower turnaround time, even when there are no apparent differences in patient populations.[243]

❖ The mean or median turnaround time of a procedure may be half as long as the time required to complete 90% of assays (see example in Exhibit 70 for emergency department stat tests and Exhibit 71 for cytology). Establishing a turnaround time goal for an institution based on its current mean or median performance invites frustration.

Beginning in the 1990s, the CAP conducted several large multi-institutional studies of laboratory turnaround time, using a common data collection instrument and uniform set of definitions. Laboratory managers can share data from these studies with clinicians to help frame expectations about what can realistically be achieved. Studies of turnaround time for selected chemistry and hematology procedures are shown in Exhibit 70.[244-246] Turnaround times of selected anatomic pathology procedures are shown in Exhibit 71,[247-252] for selected microbiology procedures in Exhibit 72,[240,253] and for selected transfusion medicine procedures in Exhibit 73.[254] For many analytes that have been studied on multiple separate occasions, turnaround time performance appears to have improved.[246]

Exhibit 71. Turnaround Time of Selected Anatomic Pathology Procedures

Procedure, Interval	Number of Institutions	Percentile Rank of Institutions		
		10th	50th (median)	90th
Surgical pathology routine specimen, collection to case sign-off (median, days)[247]	525	2*	1	1
Surgical pathology routine specimen, collection to report delivery, small hospitals (median, days)[248]	144	4	2	1
Surgical pathology complex specimen, collection to case sign-off (median, days)[247]	489	3	1	1
Gynecologic cytology, collection to case sign-off (median, days)[249]	371	13.6	6	2.7
Gynecologic cytology, collection to case sign-off (90th percent completion, days)[249]	371	19	8	5
Nongynecologic cytology, collection to case sign-off (median, days)[250]	180	4	2.1	1.2
Nongynecologic cytology, collection to case sign-off (90th percent completion, days)[250]	180	7	4	3
Autopsy, time of death to beginning of prosection (median, hours)[251]	452	17.1	3.5	1
Autopsy, start of prosection to preliminary report release (median, days)[252]	418	3	1	0

* For example, in 10% of institutions, the median turnaround time for surgical pathology sign-off was 2 or more days. Higher percentiles indicate better relative performance (shorter turnaround time).

Exhibit 72. Turnaround Time of Selected Microbiology Procedures

Procedure, Interval	Number of Institutions	Percentile Rank of Institutions		
		10th	50th (median)	90th
Cerebrospinal fluid Gram stain, receipt in laboratory to verification (median, minutes)[240]	492	87*	45	24
Respiratory specimen for mycobacteriology, collection to receipt (median, minutes)[253]	534	190	60	16
Mycobacterial smear, receipt to verification (median, hours)[253]	534	61.9	24.8	6.8
Mycobacterial culture, initial positive report, collection to verification (smear-positive cases, median, days)[253]	534	32	16	6
Mycobacterial culture, initial positive report, collection to verification (smear-negative cases, median, days)[253]	534	43	25	14

* For example, in 10% of institutions, the median turnaround time for cerebrospinal fluid Gram stain was 87 or more minutes. Higher percentiles indicate better relative performance (shorter turnaround time).

Exhibit 73. Turnaround Time in Transfusion Medicine					
Product	**Summary Statistic / Interval / Priority**	**Number of Institutions**	**Percentile Rank of Institutions**		
			10th	**50th (median)**	**90th**
Red blood cells[254]	Median/order to unit release/stat OR (min)	466	79*	35	14
Fresh frozen plasma[254]	Median/order to unit release/stat OR (min)	466	63	37	24
Platelets[254]	Median/order to unit release/stat OR (min)	466	115	33	12

* For example, in the 10th percentile institution, red blood cells were released from the blood bank a median of 79 minutes after being ordered in the operating room (OR). Higher percentiles indicate better relative performance (shorter turnaround time).

Control Measures to Manage Turnaround Time

There are a number of interventions that have been shown to improve turnaround time. Monitoring turnaround time is associated with improved performance. In multi-institutional studies, laboratories that prepared regular turnaround time reports enjoyed significantly shorter turnaround times. In two longitudinal Q-Tracks studies sponsored by the CAP, continued participation in an ongoing turnaround time monitoring program was associated with progressive reduction in turnaround time.[255]

Other interventions that have been associated with significantly shorter turnaround time include automated computer verification of results (so-called *auto-verification*), use of pneumatic tube transport systems, convenient location of pneumatic tube stations, automated track systems for specimen transport within the laboratory, stat laboratories, point-of-care instrumentation, use of laboratory phlebotomists (rather than other staff) to obtain blood specimens, repatriation of send-out tests back into the laboratory, and laboratory participation with managed care programs that monitor turnaround time.

Several authors have reported progress from total quality management initiatives that use Pareto diagrams and other TQM techniques to identify phases of the test cycle with the most opportunity to shorten turnaround time.[256] When laboratories adopt "lean" production techniques in phlebotomy (phlebotomists send individual specimens to the laboratory by pneumatic tube after each patient is drawn, rather than waiting for specimens to accumulate in a batch), turnaround time improves.

Some factors that are commonly thought to improve turnaround time have not had any demonstrable impact when examined formally. Computerized physician order entry is not associated with shorter turnaround time and has been associated with longer turnaround time in some studies. A low Pap smear-to-cytotechnologist ratio is not associated with shorter gynecologic cytology turnaround time.

Several factors associated with turnaround time cannot be managed. The single most important predictor of turnaround time in almost every multi-institutional study—institution size—is not easily changed. Large hospitals tend to record longer turnaround time than their smaller counterparts. In anatomic pathology, more difficult cases lengthen turnaround time, as does inclusion of pathology residents and cytotechnology students. Little can be done about these practices without fundamentally altering the character of an institution.

Laboratory Organization

Several of the case studies that opened this manual described quality failures that were exacerbated by poor laboratory organization. Clinical laboratories operate with a wide variety of organizational structures, and pathologists interact with clinical laboratories using a variety of models that range from ownership to employment.[257] It is not our purpose to review all of these structures and models, but instead to highlight certain risks to quality and patient safety that are created by poor organizational practices.

Organizational risks to quality and patient safety occur when (1) key responsibilities are not clearly vested in particular individuals, (2) delegation of duties is not clearly defined, and (3) the organization lacks a "culture" of quality and patient safety.

Assignment of Key Responsibilities

Most of the key responsibilities in a clinical laboratory are defined by CLIA. Key responsibilities of the *laboratory director* were shown in Exhibit 6. CLIA also defines responsibilities for a *clinical consultant* (Exhibit 74) and a *technical consultant* (Exhibit 75).[258] The laboratory director, clinical consultant, and technical consultant do not need to be separate individuals. The responsibilities CLIA specifies for the three roles can be assigned to one or several people, so long as the individual assigned a particular responsibility meets applicable CLIA educational, experience, and licensure requirements.

Laboratory quality and patient safety are put at risk when a key CLIA-defined responsibility is not clearly vested in a particular individual. Most commonly, problems arise when the roles of the medical director and the administrative director are not clearly mapped to key CLIA responsibilities. Probing questions that can be used to determine whether key responsibilities have been appropriately assigned in a laboratory include the following: Can the laboratory director (the person whose name

---

Exhibit 74. Responsibilities of the Clinical Consultant Under CLIA

- ❖ Ensure that reports of test results include information required for proper interpretation
- ❖ Provide consultation to laboratory clients regarding appropriateness of ordered tests
- ❖ Provide consultation to laboratory clients regarding interpretation of test results
- ❖ Provide consultation to laboratory clients regarding the quality of the test results reported

---

Exhibit 75. Responsibilities of the Technical Consultant Under CLIA

- ❖ Technical and scientific oversight of the laboratory
- ❖ Available to the laboratory on an as needed basis
- ❖ Selecting test methodology
- ❖ Validation of new tests
- ❖ Establishment of the test performance characteristics
- ❖ Participation in an approved proficiency testing program commensurate with the services offered
- ❖ Establish an appropriate quality control program from the initial receipt of the specimen through sample analysis and reporting of test results
- ❖ Resolve technical problems and ensure that remedial actions are taken
- ❖ Ensure that patient test results are not reported unless a test system is functioning properly
- ❖ Identifying training needs and ensure that testing individuals receive training and education
- ❖ Evaluate the competency of testing personnel and ensure that the staff maintain competency
- ❖ Perform certain specified cytopathology quality assurance activities

appears on the CLIA certificate) describe his or her CLIA responsibilities? Are the director's responsibilities referenced in a document (eg, a contract, job description, organizational chart, or quality management plan)? Can every laboratory employee name the laboratory director? Is it clear from laboratory documents who is vested with key responsibilities CLIA assigns to clinical and technical consultants (Exhibit 74 and Exhibit 75)? Do these individuals understand and accept their responsibilities? Are these responsibilities documented? Do other employees understand who in the laboratory is ultimately accountable for each of these key functions? Who in the laboratory is ultimately responsible for ensuring that HIPAA privacy and security controls are implemented? For ensuring compliance with FDA blood bank regulations? Are there any responsibilities spelled out in CLIA, HIPAA, or FDA requirements that have not been assigned to a particular leader within the laboratory or within the laboratory's parent organization?

Clear assignment of laboratory director responsibilities is particularly important for maintaining quality. The laboratory director represents the primary line of defense in protecting the public from the consequences of substandard laboratory practices. No external inspection system or proficiency testing program can substitute for a laboratory director who does not understand or accept CLIA responsibilities. When a laboratory director believes that the director's responsibilities end when the laboratory passes a CAP or CMS inspection, the laboratory's internal quality control system is defective and patient safety is placed at risk.

Delegation of Key Duties

Laboratory leadership typically delegate duties to qualified individuals. For example, technical consultant duties may be delegated to separate managers of chemistry, blood bank, hematology, and microbiology, and perhaps a quality manager, a safety officer, a point-of-care manager, and manager of phlebotomy and specimen processing. In large laboratories, laboratory director duties are often delegated to physician section heads, who oversee various sections of the laboratory.

Quality and safety are put at risk when duties are not delegated clearly or are delegated to individuals who lack the training, education, or qualifications required to perform a duty. Delegation of managerial and testing functions should normally be explicit and documented. It should be clear who will perform each task, and how to trace oversight of the task back to the individual who maintains ultimate responsibility to see that the function is carried out properly. In 2004, 1.4% of laboratories inspected by the CAP were cited for not explicitly specifying who could perform duties on behalf of the laboratory director.[91]

To test whether delegation is clear and explicit, the following types of probing questions can be posed to managers, technologists, and technicians in the laboratory: Is it clear who in the microbiology laboratory was responsible for performing disc diffusion quality control testing on Monday, December 15 (or some other date)? Is it clear who will review this individual's quality control activities? Is this documented on an organizational chart or in a position description? Who is authorized to enter patient results into a computer system? Is it clear who delegates this job? Do responsible individuals such as the laboratory director understand that while they can delegate duties, they must retain responsibility for ensuring that the duties are performed properly? (Thus the laboratory director who delegates the review of proficiency test evaluations to others is still responsible for overall laboratory performance on proficiency testing.) The laboratory director who is concerned about his or her responsibilities under CLIA should pay particular attention to the last chapter of this manual, which describes how a quality management plan can be used to reasonably ensure that good laboratory practices are carried out by laboratory staff.

Culture of Quality and Patient Safety

The word "culture" is used to describe a group's shared beliefs and values and, in our context, refers to a shared commitment within the laboratory to promote quality and patient safety.[259] Every organization has a unique culture, and it is easier for individuals to work within the organization's culture than at odds with it. When quality and patient safety enjoy a high priority, it becomes easier for individuals to bring up quality or safety concerns and to work as a team to address emerging issues.[260]

Culture is difficult to measure. Questions that probe an organization's cultural commitment to quality and patient safety include the following: What do employees do when they see something amiss that is not part of their normal duties? Do employees feel free to make suggestions about safety or quality concerns? To co-workers? To management? How are suggestions received? Are they viewed by co-workers and management as "more work" or as opportunities to improve? How are errors handled, particularly errors that may be embarrassing to the laboratory or individual leaders? How are "near misses" handled? Are laboratory operators and managers willing to stop producing results or send specimens elsewhere when a test system is out of control? How much time does laboratory management spend discussing quality and safety, compared with other organizational goals, such as productivity, market share, and profitability? How much time does organizational leadership and governance spend on quality and patient safety?

Cultures of safety are believed to be particularly well developed in so-called *high reliability organizations (HROs)*. HROs are organizations that manage to conduct high-risk, high-stake, error-prone activities with failure rates that are unexpectedly low. United States nuclear naval aircraft carriers and land-based nuclear power plants are often-cited examples of HROs. These organizations work under time pressure and within dynamic environments where many variables may be changing simultaneously. Yet HROs make reliability a top priority. They are preoccupied with the possibility of failure and exert extreme vigilance and systemic mindfulness about breakdowns and errors. HROs typically have flat hierarchies when it comes to safety—any member of the organization, whether high or low, is empowered to report situations that can compromise safety and has a duty to correct a problem at once if it immediately threatens safety. Where safety is concerned, there are no organizational barriers to impede the free flow of information; there is a seamless and almost automatic shift from routine activities to emergency mode. A culture of safety is reinforced by individual and team practice and by preventive analysis. The high reliability organization acknowledges inherent risk and encourages and rewards reporting of near misses as well as actual errors, viewing both as opportunities for improvement.

Control Measures to Address Organizational Risks

Unlike the situation with most other laboratory risks, we cannot quantify how often a laboratory's organizational structure poses a threat to quality and patient safety. Nor can we recommend specific control measures to mitigate organizational risks, other than the obvious exhortations to document job responsibilities and reporting relationships and ensure that they are widely understood. A laboratory's culture is an intangible, elusive quality that is influenced by the organization's history, the personality and values of leaders, and the communities from which employees are drawn. Leadership can "walk the talk"—put patients before self and quality before economy—but no one individual should expect to change a laboratory's culture alone or overnight.

Concluding Remarks

This chapter reviewed the principal threats to laboratory quality and patient safety that can be positively impacted by laboratory managers. The list of threats is not comprehensive; local factors and special circumstances may cause laboratory directors and other managers to focus on different hazards.

Even when laboratory directors confine themselves to managing the risks reviewed in this chapter, they have their work cut out for them. Configuring a laboratory to meet the challenges discussed in this chapter is not easy, especially in an economically competitive environment, where time is short and the business case for quality uncertain.

As if the tasks outlined up to this point were not enough, the next chapter will remind us that even our best efforts to anticipate and address risks will fall short. Customers and incidents will bring to light risks that have not been anticipated, needs that have not been met, and processes that have been incompletely controlled.

Quality Improvement

Managers who successfully address the risks described in the previous chapter will invariably improve the quality of their operations. Errors will be less frequent, communication more certain, and results more accurate. Experience has taught us a great deal about what can go wrong in a laboratory. The hazards identified in the previous chapter are worthy of every manager's attention.

Still, the list of risks to quality and patient safety discussed in the previous chapter is incomplete. Some customers have special requirements that will go unmet by a laboratory that addresses only common risks. Some processes will go awry for reasons that could not be anticipated. Therefore, an organization committed to continuous quality improvement should do more than attend to known hazards.[261] The organization will also be guided by feedback from laboratory clients and vulnerabilities identified through individual or recurring incidents.

In this chapter, we discuss two approaches to quality improvement that go beyond mitigation of recognized risks. The first approach involves learning from customers; the second, learning from incidents.

Learning from Customers[262]

Business periodicals remind us that the customer is king. The quality and safety risks catalogued in the previous chapter represent vulnerabilities that concern most laboratory customers, but the clients of any particular laboratory have a unique set of concerns and needs. One of the best ways to find out what a particular laboratory's customers value is by listening to them. For this reason, the major United States accrediting organizations require laboratories to periodically measure customer satisfaction.[263] In 2004, 1.5% of laboratories inspected by the CAP were cited for not having surveyed any customer about their satisfaction with laboratory services during the previous two years.[91]

Who are Laboratory Customers?

Most laboratory managers recognize patients and physicians as their customers, but the list of laboratory customers can be expanded to include nurses, administrators, insurance companies, and other third-party payors. Different customers of the laboratory have different needs. Many health maintenance organizations, for example, depend on laboratories to supply extracts of results so that health plans can calculate quality scores for health-plan accrediting agencies. A laboratory's ability to provide this information will impact a plan's satisfaction with laboratory services and may determine whether the laboratory is included in the plan's panel of laboratory providers.[264] Administrators, on the other hand, may be most interested in laboratory efficiency, regulatory compliance, and support of an institution's strategic initiatives. Nurses who work in hospitals tend to be most interested in test turnaround time.

Methods for Surveying Customers

In this section, we describe considerations that go into surveying customers about their satisfaction with laboratory services.

Types of Surveys

Apart from direct one-on-one conversations, three approaches are widely used to survey laboratory customers:

❖ Paper or electronic surveys may be sent to customers who used laboratory services during a defined period of time. The advantages of this approach are twofold: more questions may be asked (because the survey is typically completed at the customer's convenience), and subsets of customers with special characteristics can be selectively polled.

❖ Surveys may be given to customers at the time services are rendered. The principal advantage of this approach is that the survey is completed when information about the service experience is fresh in the customer's mind.

❖ Open-ended surveys, such as a focus group, may be arranged to gather feedback and impressions from laboratory users. Open-ended surveys are time consuming and difficult to analyze, but may identify opportunities or problems that laboratory management did not think to include in a more structured survey.

Development of Surveys

Customer surveys may be purchased from external vendors or developed "in-house." When surveys are purchased, the vendor may also administer the survey, tabulate results, and interpret survey findings.

Externally developed surveys tend to be validated, field-tested, and administered to statistically appropriate samples. One disadvantage of externally developed surveys is that they tend to be more expensive than surveys developed in-house. In addition, commercial surveys acquired by hospitals are sometimes so broad that they do not provide laboratory managers with sufficient detail to guide change. For example, a single question may probe physicians' satisfaction with several departments (eg, laboratory, radiology, pharmacy).

Locally developed surveys are less expensive to administer and are usually more tightly focused on laboratory-related service issues. Some of the disadvantages of locally developed surveys are that they are more likely to contain ambiguous language, may be administered to a statistically inadequate or biased group of customers, and require local resources to tabulate results. The findings from locally developed surveys do not generally contain any comparison to peer group institutions, which makes interpretation of results more difficult.

Survey Content

When designing surveys, it is important to keep in mind that the accuracy of laboratory analyses is difficult for customers to independently evaluate. The accuracy of test results is usually assumed (sometimes incorrectly!). We recommend that satisfaction surveys concentrate on preanalytic and postanalytic aspects of laboratory service, such as the timeliness of service, courtesy and responsiveness of staff, clarity of reports, accuracy of report distribution, etc. While analytic performance is important to physicians, patients, and other laboratory customers, it is best assessed using quality control and proficiency testing techniques, not through customer surveys.

Administering Surveys

As a survey is being developed, managers should begin planning what steps will be taken if satisfaction about a particular service area is found to be wanting. If low levels of satisfaction with a laboratory service will not lead to concrete action, there is no point wasting customers' valuable time with a question about the service.

Satisfaction surveys are best field-tested on a small group of customers to determine whether survey questions are clear and not open to multiple interpretations. When a group of customers cannot be recruited for field-testing, several individuals within the laboratory should be given the survey to complete before it is distributed to customers.

The target population for the survey should be carefully selected, with an eye to how survey results will be used. Sometimes, an entire population is surveyed (eg, all physician customers of a laboratory). In other circumstances, a subset of customers may be surveyed. If, for example, laboratory management is particularly concerned about the views of customers who are being solicited by competitors (eg, community dermatologists or primary care physicians affiliated with several hospitals), these individuals should be preferentially surveyed. Managers should avoid the temptation to distribute questionnaires only to "friendly" customers who are unlikely to be bothered by a survey, as their views may not be representative.

The results of surveys with low response rates are rarely representative, because individuals with extreme views are more likely than average to complete surveys. If the response rate of a survey is below 25%, the individuals who are responding are essentially self-selected.[265] The White House Office of Management and Budget requires a minimum response rate of 75% before surveys are used. Response rates can often be brought above 75% through the use of introductory letters that precede the survey, follow-up phone calls, follow-up surveys, or modest incentives for survey completion.[265]

The development and administration of surveys is an involved science. A comprehensive discussion of survey techniques lies beyond the scope of this manual.

Customer Satisfaction with Laboratory Services

Managers who survey customers about their satisfaction should be mindful of how certain groups of users tend to view laboratory services. Without this information, the laboratory manager might be inclined to conclude that the service with the lowest rating is most in need of attention, not understanding that some customer groups tend to rate certain services more highly than others. To help managers place survey results in context, we review survey response patterns from three types of laboratory customers: physicians, patients, and nurses.

Exhibit 76. Laboratory Service Rated "Most Important" by the Majority of Physicians at an Institution [151]

Laboratory Service Rated "Most Important"	Number of Institutions (%)
Quality of results	112 (76.2)
Inpatient stat test TAT	17 (11.6)
Routine test TAT	10 (6.8)
Outpatient stat test TAT	3 (2.0)
Critical value notification	2 (1.3)
Staff courtesy	1 (0.7)
Phlebotomy services	1 (0.7)
Esoteric test TAT	1 (0.7)

Physician Satisfaction

Physicians at most institutions rate "quality of test results" as the aspect of laboratory service they consider most important, with stat inpatient test turnaround time listed second most frequently (Exhibit 76).[151] Physician ratings of various laboratory services are shown in

Exhibit 77. Physician Satisfaction with Particular Laboratory Services [151]

Aspect of Service	All Institutions Percentiles (Percent of physicians rating service as "excellent/good")				
	10th	25th	50th (median)	75th	90th
Quality of results	71.4	80.6	87.5*	92.9	100.0
Staff courtesy	66.7	77.8	87.0	92.9	97.4
Test menu adequacy	61.5	75.0	81.8	90.6	95.7
Critical value notification	57.1	72.0	80.0	87.5	94.0
Phlebotomy services	52.9	69.6	79.4	89.7	100.0
Inpatient stat test TAT	50.0	63.6	76.9	88.0	96.4
Courier services	42.9	58.5	75.0	86.6	95.2
Routine test TAT	52.4	62.5	73.5	84.6	92.0
Outpatient stat test TAT	46.4	59.8	71.8	83.3	88.9
Esoteric test TAT	28.6	37.5	48.1	58.2	65.6

* For example, in the median institutions, 87.5% of physicians rate "quality of results" as "good" or "excellent".
  Higher percentile ranks indicate better relative performance.

Exhibit 77. Physicians tend to be most satisfied with "quality of results" and least satisfied with esoteric test and outpatient stat test turnaround time. Emergency department physicians have less charitable views about laboratory service than physicians in other specialties.[266] The relationship between various institutional practices and physician satisfaction is detailed in Exhibit 78. Laboratories that regularly monitor test-pending lists and telephone response time, maintain direct control of phlebotomy and courier operations, support a customer response center, and have a high fraction of outreach work enjoy more satisfied customers than facilities that do not perform these functions.

Patient Satisfaction

Patients surveyed at the time of specimen collection tend to be highly satisfied with their laboratory encounter.[267,268] Laboratory managers should be concerned if more than 5% of patients are "unsatisfied" (versus "satisfied"), or fewer than 80% of patients report being "highly satisfied" (rating of 4 or 5 on a 5-point scale), because satisfaction levels below these figures place a laboratory in the bottom quartile. Patient responses to several multi-institutional patient satisfaction surveys are shown in Exhibit 79 and Exhibit 80. Not surprisingly, patient satisfaction is higher at institutions where less time is spent waiting for phlebotomy. Drop-off in satisfaction appears to be associated with particularly long waiting times; small differences in wait times do not measurably impact satisfaction. Patient

Exhibit 78. Relationship Between Institutional Practices and Physician Satisfaction Scores [151]

Laboratory Service	Institutional Practice*	Median Percentage of Excellent/Good Ratings
Inpatient stat test TAT	Monitor pending lists	
	Yes	78.3
	No	65.0
Inpatient stat test TAT	Monitor telephone response time	
	Yes	84.6
	No	75.0
Outpatient stat test TAT	Monitor pending lists	
	Yes	76.6
	No	61.1
Outpatient stat test TAT	Percent billed tests on nonpatients	
	0–10%	68.4
	11–30%	72.2
	31–100%	80.0
Quality of results	Dedicated customer support staff	
	Yes	88.9
	No	85.9
Courier services	Off-site courier services under lab management	
	Yes	82.2
	No	70.4

* For all associations, $p < 0.05$.

Exhibit 79. Patient Satisfaction with Phlebotomy Services [267]

Factors Related to the Phlebotomy Procedure	All Institution Percentiles		
	10th	50th (median)	90th
Percentage of patients satisfied with the phlebotomy procedure	96.6	100.0	100.0
Percentage of patients who reported no bruising	71.8	82.8	94.9
Percentage of patients who reported courteous treatment	98.9	100.0	100.0
Percentage of patients who received only one venipuncture	91.9	97.7	100.0
Median patient waiting time, minutes (from registration completion to phlebotomy initiation)	13.0	6.0	4.0

Exhibit 80. Patients "Highly Satisfied" with Phlebotomy Services [268]

Aspect of Service	All Institutions Percentiles (N=86) (Percent of patients "highly satisfied")				
	10th	25th	50th (median)	75th	90th
Overall	77.9	84.5	89.3	94.0	97.1
Waiting time	65.2	73.0	82.3	89.3	93.6
Discomfort level	63.3	73.9	81.3	88.4	94.2
Courtesy	69.3	78.6	85.5*	90.3	96.4

* Higher percentile ranks indicate better relative performance; the values shown are the percentage of surveyed individuals who ranked a services as excellent or very good (4-5 on a 5-point scales). Thus, for courtesy, the median institution reported that 85.5% of patients had satisfaction ratings of excellent or very good.

Exhibit 81. Improvement in Patient Satisfaction Ratings Over Time [268]

	Years of Monitoring Satisfaction				
	1	2	3	4	5
Mean increase in overall satisfaction score*	.05	.06	.11	.11	.25

* The mean improvement in overall satisfaction score seen by the average laboratory that monitors patient satisfaction with phlebotomy on a 5-point scale. Thus, after three years of monitoring, the average laboratory has an increase in mean satisfaction of 0.11 points.

satisfaction is also significantly higher at institutions that provide employees with customer service education, and lower at facilities where phlebotomy staff tell patients that phlebotomy "will not hurt." Institutions that monitor patient satisfaction on an ongoing basis show progressive improvements in patient satisfaction (Exhibit 81).[268] This effect is not due to selective drop out of laboratories with lower-than-average satisfaction ratings and suggests that sustained attention to improving patient satisfaction can produce incremental year-over-year quality improvement.

Nursing Satisfaction

In contrast to physicians, nurses rate turnaround time of stat tests to be the most important aspect of laboratory service, with accuracy of results taking second place (Exhibit 82).[269] Nurses tend to be less satisfied than physicians with laboratory services; the lowest satisfaction scores are found among nurses who work in the emergency department and intensive care units (Exhibit 83). At the median hospital in a large multihospital survey, fewer than half of nurses were "very" or "usually" satisfied with the turnaround time of stat laboratory tests (Exhibit 84).[269]

Exhibit 82. Laboratory Service Rated as Most Important by Nurses [269]

Laboratory Service	Number of Respondents (%)
Stat test turnaround time	2432 (37.8)
Accuracy of test results	981 (15.2)
Abnormal results notification	523 (8.1)
Telephone courtesy	487 (7.6)
Phlebotomy responsiveness	455 (7.1)
Phlebotomy courtesy toward patients	404 (6.3)
Routine test turnaround time	364 (5.7)
Ability to answer telephone questions	292 (4.5)
Promptly answered phones	183 (2.8)
Phlebotomy courtesy toward nursing	94 (1.5)
Lab management responsiveness	94 (1.5)
Accessibility of lab management	71 (1.1)
Lab point-of-care testing support	55 (0.9)

Exhibit 83. Nursing Satisfaction by Service Area [269]

Nursing Service	Satisfaction Score
Intensive care	3.64
Emergency department	3.64
Obstetric	3.80
Gynecologic	3.81
Operating room	3.82
Pediatric	3.83
Medical	3.85
Surgical	3.91
Psychiatric	4.21

Exhibit 84. Laboratory Services with which Nurses are Highly Satisfied [269]

Laboratory Service	All Institutions Percentiles (Percent very/usually satisfied)		
	10th	50th (median)	90th
Accuracy of test results	79.2	90.9*	97.9
Phlebotomy courtesy toward patients	64.3	86.5	98.0
Phlebotomy courtesy toward nursing	58.5	80.4	95.5
Abnormal results notification	60.4	79.4	91.8
Lab point-of-care testing support	45.0	74.3	92.3
Telephone courtesy	51.5	74.0	88.0
Ability to answer telephone questions	48.5	73.3	89.4
Promptly answered phones	44.0	72.0	87.9
Routine test turnaround time	40.9	65.2	84.1
Phlebotomy responsiveness	35.6	64.7	90.0
Accessibility of lab management	36.1	63.9	85.0
Lab management responsiveness	35.7	62.7	83.3
Stat test turnaround time	26.0	49.0	73.7

* Higher percentile ranks indicate better relative performance; the values shown are the percentage of surveyed nurses who indicated they were "very" or "usually" satisfied with a particular service. Thus, for "accuracy of test results," 90.9% of nurses in the median laboratory indicated that they were very or usually satisfied.

Responding to Satisfaction Survey Data

How does the laboratory manager translate survey data into action? When an area of service receives particularly low ratings from customers (and national surveys do not show the area receiving low ratings nationally), the service should be carefully scrutinized for workflow or other system problems and redesigned, as required. Poor customer satisfaction is a *trailing indicator,* which typically manifests itself some time after service has deteriorated. When working to improve satisfaction scores, *leading indicators* of key service components should be monitored regularly (eg, turnaround time, percentage of rejected specimens, percentage of contaminated blood cultures, the time or number of rings before telephones are answered). Improvement in these indicators typically precedes improvement in satisfaction scores.

Laboratory directors should be aware that satisfaction problems may have as much to do with inflated expectations as deficient performance.[270] When this is the case, efforts should be focused on managing customer expectations rather than laboratory operations. Sharing information with customers about performance achieved within the industry, joint development of performance goals, and realistic communication about service capabilities (eg, turnaround time, hours of operations) keep customer expectations grounded in reality.

Finally, some organizations attempt to improve customer satisfaction by involving key customers in the design of new products and services. General Electric's medical imaging division, for example, involves a group of key clinicians (called "luminaries") in the design of new scanning devices.

Occurrence Management: Learning From Incidents

Incidents, which are sometimes called *occurrences* or *events,* can alert laboratory managers to unexpected problems. Incidents are most often brought to management's attention by customers but may also be identified by the laboratory's own employees or by suppliers.

What is an incident? Many incidents represents complaints about the quality of service delivered to a customer, but the following also are incidents: a technologist who notes that an instrument intermittently seems to stop working; a customer service representative who cannot make contact with a physician about an abnormal result; a custodian who notices that patient lab reports are being discarded in open public trash containers; an incorrect response on a proficiency testing challenge; a patient who is harmed by a transfusion reaction due to laboratory error. It is difficult to define an *incident* precisely, but a working definition might be the deviation of a process or outcome from the expected. A laboratory that is committed to continuous quality improvement uses incidents to improve laboratory performance and patient safety.

Incident Management Systems

Incidents should be approached systematically, just as the laboratory should systematically approach known laboratory risks. Laboratories are required by CLIA to maintain an *incident management system* (sometimes called an *occurrence management system* or a *complaint management system*). In 2004, 3.6% of inspected laboratories with external complaints were cited by CAP laboratory inspectors for not documenting an investigation of the complaint.[91]

An incident management system can be simple or sophisticated, but any system should include the four elements listed in Exhibit 85.

> **Exhibit 85. Elements of an Incident Management System**
>
> 1. Process to discover/collect incidents
> 2. Process to investigate incidents
> 3. Address individual incidents
> 4. Prevent recurrence of similar incidents

Process to Discover Incidents

Because individual incidents are, by definition, unexpected, laboratory management cannot set out to find them in advance. Rather, a process should be created that allows customers, employees, and suppliers to provide feedback about problems or areas of concern. This has traditionally been accomplished through the use of a paper *incident form,* although many institutions are employing web-based tools that allow individuals to enter information about incidents directly into a database. An example of a paper incident form designed for employees is shown on page 189.

Incident reporting systems that are too formal or mechanized may create unnecessary distance between the laboratory and its customers. Customers and business associates may not have incident forms handy or may not wish to complete forms. Laboratory employees should be available to receive complaints in person or over the telephone, and transfer the essence of the complaint to an incident form or data input screen.

Equally important to developing mechanisms for reporting incidents is ensuring that the mechanism is used. This usually requires employee training and a certain amount of mental discipline on the part of management, who must encourage employees to take the time to report incidents and to use the laboratory's incident reporting system. Although we are generally supportive of web-based incident reporting tools, some of the applications we have seen require the user to classify the incident in so many different ways (eg, work shift, phase of testing, location of problem, name of patient, type of problem, consequence of problem) that the complexity of the process discourages reporting. Usually, a simple free-text box is adequate for collecting essential information about an incident.

Opportunities should be provided for individuals to report incidents and concerns anonymously. Current thinking suggests that a "culture of safety" allows for anonymous reporting. Managers or coworkers may exert pressure on employees not to "cause trouble" or create extra work by reporting deviations. Providing an opportunity to report concerns anonymously helps circumvent this problem. The College of American Pathologists has created a toll-free number that laboratory employees or customers can use to anonymously report problems to the CAP if laboratory management has not addressed the issue (866-236-7212 in US; 847-832-7533 internationally). Anonymous reporting systems can capture some complaints that might not otherwise be reported, but they are often burdened with non-meritorious griping. A certain number of unfounded complaints seem to be the price paid for keeping the door open to employees who do not feel free to report an issue openly.

Process to Investigate Incidents

When an orthopedic surgeon complains that it took eight hours to receive a stat white blood cell count on a knee aspirate, some sort of investigation should be made into the cause of the problem. When and where was the specimen received? Was the test order entered correctly into the computer? Was the specimen routed properly? Did the delay result from specimen transit, testing, or result reporting?

The type of the investigation that should be conducted is dictated by the nature of the problem. For many incidents, no special investigation is required because the cause of the problem is obvious. If an employee with good eyesight complains that he or she cannot see culture plates at the urine bench because there is inadequate light, the cause of the problem is inadequate lighting. No investigation is needed. For some incidents, the process of investigating the problem and fixing the problem are one in the same. When a complex instrument stops working and a repair technician must be called, there is usually little point in launching a separate investigation into why the instrument failed. The repair technician will provide this information after the instrument is fixed (if the cause can be determined). Because many incidents do not require separate investigation, we discourage excessive formalism by requiring lengthy descriptions of causes for every incident.

Address Individual Incidents

To the extent possible, the consequences of a particular incident should be addressed. This may involve issuing a credit for a previous charge, correcting a report (see "Correcting Reporting Errors" in chapter 5), or initiating corrective action with an employee. Often, the individual who reports a problem also fixes the problem. There is no need to assign a manager to correct a problem that has already been resolved. If someone other than the incident initiator resolves the problem, follow-up communication should be provided to the person who first noted the problem. This follow-up is often neglected, which is unfortunate. Follow-up communication provides an opportunity for the laboratory to demonstrate that it cares, and encourages employees and customers to keep on the lookout for additional problems.

We caution managers about modifying a laboratory's written procedures in response to individual incidents. Since employees perform most tasks in the laboratory from memory, without consulting written documents, modifications of written procedures may not change behavior. Furthermore, instituting new procedures for "double-checking" work in response to a single slip or lapse usually makes the work environment unnecessarily complex and dilutes individual responsibility (since operators now work with the knowledge that their output will be checked over). Unless the incident involves a disastrous clinical outcome (a "sentinel event"), it is best to reserve systematic changes for recurring problems.

Prevent Recurrence of Similar Incidents

Incidents should be reviewed to identify recurring patterns. In many laboratories, incidents are tabulated by incident type, and trend reports are produced for management. We do not know if this procedure is useful or better than manually leafing through narrative reports to ascertain whether there are any recurring patterns. While it seems reasonable to search through incident reports on a monthly or quarterly basis, the specific frequency of review should be determined by the number of incidents received. Reviewing batches of approximately 50 incidents at a sitting often permits the detection of common patterns.

National Adverse Event Reporting Systems

Some authorities are of the opinion that the laboratory industry would benefit from a national *adverse event* or *near miss* reporting system, in which laboratory and clinical staff could anonymously report safety incidents, the circumstances surrounding adverse events, and their cause, when the cause is known. Commercial aviation instituted such a system in 1975 (the Aviation Safety Reporting System), and it is believed within the industry that the knowledge gained from this system has contributed to the more than 10-fold reduction in aviation injuries in the last 20 years.[271] A number of other high-risk industries, such as the nuclear power industry, maintain national incident reporting systems. Barriers to implementing national incident reporting systems in medicine have been reviewed elsewhere.[272]

A new chapter in patient safety reporting on the national level was opened on July 29, 2005, when President Bush signed into law the *Patient Safety and Quality Improvement Act,* creating the country's first national system for reporting and tracking medical errors. The law allows hospitals, doctors, nurses, and pharmacists to anonymously report errors to nonprofit "patient safety organizations" and keeps the reports private by specifically barring them from being used in civil lawsuits or in disciplinary actions against hospitals or doctors. These patient safety organizations will, in turn, feed information into a federally managed national database that will be used to house and study information on medical mistakes and "near misses" that harm patients in health care settings. At the time of this writing, it is too early to know how well this process will be received by providers or how effective it will be in improving patient safety.

Sentinel Events

One type of incident requires a special form of investigation—the *sentinel event.* A sentinel event is defined by JCAHO as an unexpected occurrence involving death or serious physical or psychological injury, or the risk thereof. Serious injury specifically includes loss of limb or function. The phrase "or the risk thereof" includes any process variation for which a recurrence would carry a significant chance of a serious adverse outcome.

The Joint Commission on the Accreditation of Healthcare Organizations and several other hospital accrediting organizations require that when a *reviewable* sentinel even occurs, a root cause analysis be conducted. Laboratory-related sentinel events that require mandatory review under JCAHO's Sentinel Event Policy are limited to clinically significant hemolytic transfusion reactions and wrong-site/wrong-patient procedures that result from laboratory operations. The FDA also requires reporting of hemolytic transfusion reactions resulting in death. In JCAHO-accredited hospitals, laboratory staff may also become involved in a root cause analysis of other "reviewable" sentinel events, including any patient death or major permanent loss of function associated with a medication error; any suicide of a patient in a setting where the patient is housed around-the-clock; any procedure on the wrong patient, wrong side of the body, or wrong organ; any intrapartum maternal death; certain perinatal deaths; certain fall-related injuries; and any assault, homicide, or other crime resulting in patient death or major permanent loss of function. The conduct of a root cause analysis is discussed in chapter 3.

The Joint Commission on Accreditation of Healthcare Organizations analyzed 2944 sentinel events that were reported to the organization between 1995 and 2004. Of these events, 74% resulted in patient death, and analysis suggested that most sentinel events involved problems with communication as a root cause (65%). Orientation/training of staff was the second most common cause (55% of events). JCAHO does not require the reporting of all sentinel event investigations to the Joint Commission. Characteristics and causes of unreported sentinel events are not known.

The Laboratory Quality Management Plan

This final chapter provides guidance in preparing and implementing a quality management plan. Sample plans from three laboratories are included, and readers should feel free to excerpt from these examples when developing plans for their own operations.

The CAP Laboratory Accreditation Program requires laboratories to maintain a written plan that describes the overall quality management program of the laboratory.[273] In 2004, 1.3% of laboratories inspected by the CAP were cited for not having an adequate quality management plan.[91]

A quality management plan spells out the specific steps that a laboratory will take to ensure that quality is being maintained. A well-constructed plan will be informed by material in the previous chapters of this manual—case studies of quality failure, approaches to quality management, regulatory and accreditation requirements, particular laboratory risks and control measures, and feedback from customers and incidents.

Throughout this manual we have emphasized that laboratory quality and safety failures may result from diverse causes, ranging from poor communication to human error and from instrument failure to fraud. The laboratory director must ultimately choose which particular quality and safety hazards a laboratory will address, and the controls that will be used to mitigate each hazard. The laboratory's quality management plan brings these decisions together in a document that spells out the approach to managing quality and patient safety that will be used in a particular organization.

Purpose

The purpose of the quality management plan is to describe the laboratory's approach to the management of quality and patient safety. A properly documented and implemented plan will provide reasonable assurance that the laboratory (1) meets defined standards of quality practice, (2) is in compliance with applicable laws and regulations related to quality and patient safety, and (3) is engaged in credible quality improvement activities. A clinical laboratory's quality management plan will be of interest to laboratory owners, laboratory users, external inspectors, and, potentially, to patients.

Some people have unrealistic expectations of what a quality management plan can accomplish. They believe a plan can absolutely ensure the quality of every laboratory operation, guarantee the accuracy of every laboratory report, and ensure complete and continuous compliance with laws and regulations. However, the quality management plan is primarily a system of controls, and all control systems have inherent limitations. Control systems rely on judgments that may be faulty. Controls may be upset by breakdowns that occur despite the existence of protective systems. Controls can be circumvented by collusion between several individuals or by managers who choose to override control systems. Finally, the design of any internal control system reflects resource constraints; controls will only be implemented when their benefits are likely to exceed their costs. Therefore, a quality management plan can provide only reasonable assurance that the laboratory substantially conforms to standards. It is not a guarantee.[274]

Authority

A quality management plan must be formally approved by the laboratory director on an annual basis.[275] This approval is normally evidenced by a signature. By approving a quality plan, the laboratory director signifies that the activities described in the plan—if faithfully executed—will reasonably ensure that the laboratory meets applicable quality and patient safety standards and is committed to a program of quality improvement. If the director knows of substantial quality deviations in laboratory operations that will not be detected or addressed by a quality plan, the director should not approve the plan.

Some organizations require that individuals besides the laboratory director approve the quality plan. Other individuals may approve quality plans, but the laboratory director must also approve the plan to satisfy regulatory requirements. In 2004, 2.2% of laboratories inspected by the CAP were cited because the quality management program had not been reviewed for effectiveness during the previous year.[91]

Relation to Other Institutional Quality Programs

In small stand-alone clinical laboratories, the laboratory quality plan usually exists on its own. In hospital-based laboratories, the laboratory quality plan may include a section that specifies information that is to be reported to a higher-level authority, such as an institution-wide quality committee. In very large operations, each section of the laboratory (eg, chemistry, anatomic pathology) may have its own quality plan, and the implementation of the plan will generate reports to a laboratory-wide quality officer or committee. In multi-site operations, each testing site may have its own quality plan. The organizational level at which quality plans are developed depends on the size and complexity of the laboratory and the nature of its corporate ownership.

Plan Elements

What should be included in a quality plan? Certain elements are required by major accrediting agencies,[276] and we believe every plan should include several additional elements that have been identified by the accounting profession as important components of management control systems.[25] We recommend the following elements be considered for inclusion in every quality management plan.

A Commitment to Quality and Patient Safety

Quality and patient safety flourish in laboratories with the proper "tone." This tone includes an acceptance of standards, controls, discipline, structure, and responsibility. Management should demonstrate that quality control and patient safety are taken seriously and create a work environment in which employees are encouraged to discuss quality and safety concerns without fear of retribution. A statement to this effect within the laboratory quality plan helps set the proper tone, although words alone are never enough.

Risk Assessment

The quality management plan should identify significant risks to quality and patient safety that could impact laboratory operations. To some extent, CLIA regulations and the CAP Laboratory Accreditation Program have already done 90% of the work required to identify risks. The CAP LAP checklists (which incorporate relevant CLIA regulations) spell out hundreds of problems that can interfere with the quality of laboratory operations, particularly in the analytic phase of testing. These risks have been identified by experts in laboratory medicine who are also familiar with the practical challenges of running a clinical laboratory. The laboratory director participating in the CAP accreditation program need only be concerned with the remaining 10%—risks that are unique to the director's organization or which local circumstances suggest require greater attention. In spelling out special local risks to quality and safety, we suggest that authors of quality management plans focus on (1) institutional priorities (perhaps the director's institution has identified cancer care or heart disease as a priority), (2) known problems with laboratory operations, (3) customer feedback, and (4) recurring incidents or sentinel events. We believe the risk of fraud and malfeasance, while small, needs to be addressed in a plan, and we suggest examples of how this risk can be mitigated in one of our sample plans. There is a regulatory requirement that the quality management plan must cover all aspects of a laboratory's scope of care, such as inpatient and outpatient services, reference laboratory services, satellite and point-of-care testing, and consultative services. Therefore, risks should be identified for each area of service. There is also a regulatory requirement that the quality management plan include all sections of the laboratory and all shifts of operation.

In some institutions, a quality management plan contains a section called *Quality Planning*, which includes the risk assessment activities discussed above as well as organized research into customers needs and the development of products and services that meet those needs.

Control Activities

Control activities (sometimes called *Quality Laboratory Practices*) are the policies, processes, procedures, and inventions that mitigate risks. For every significant risk, one or more control activities should be in place. Control activities can take a variety of forms. For example, the risk of receiving a bad lot of reagents is mitigated by a procedure to test each new lot of reagents before placing the lot into service (as well as other controls). The risk of someone misappropriating private health information is mitigated by the requirement that passwords be used to access laboratory computer systems (as well as other controls). Most control measures are spelled out in individual procedures; there is no need to repeat in the plan every control activity that is already described elsewhere. When not specified in other documents, the quality management plan should include a description of the control activities that the laboratory will follow to address a particular hazard. Controls applied to broad laboratory issues, such as turnaround time or specimen collection, often are described in quality management plans.

Information and Communication

If not described in other procedures, the quality management plan should specify how quality and safety information is to be collected and disseminated. This is particularly important for quality monitors that bridge traditional organizational boundaries. The frequency of data collection, sources of information, and any calculations should be specified in the plan or a separate procedure. If each section of a laboratory has its own quality plan, the information that will be sent "upstream" to the laboratory director or laboratory-wide quality committee should be specified. It may also be necessary to provide instructions for communicating with an institution-wide quality committee and with suppliers or customers who are to receive reports from the laboratory.

Monitoring

Internal control systems need to be monitored; that is, the performance of laboratory operations over time and the internal control system itself need to be periodically reviewed. At least three types of monitoring are performed and should be spelled out in a quality management plan:

❖ First, complaints, incidents, and sentinel events should be reviewed. There must be an organized program for documentation of external complaints and internal problems involving the laboratory. Any problem that could potentially interfere with patient care must be addressed, and the laboratory must document investigation and resolution of the problem. For JCAHO-accredited hospitals, there is a regulatory requirement that all sentinel events be investigated with a root cause analysis. The laboratory must be able to demonstrate that it has implemented any appropriate risk-reduction activities based on root cause analyses of sentinel events.

❖ Second, the results of ongoing measurement activities should be compared with internal or external benchmarks and trended over time. If performance is significantly worse than a laboratory's past performance or industry norms, it is likely that processes or procedures will need to be changed.

❖ Finally, the quality management plan itself requires regular (at least annual) review. The plan need not be changed every year but should be reviewed annually and kept current, as required. The annual review should be documented.

Continuous Improvement

A quality operation is committed to continuous improvement. At any point in time, some aspects of laboratory operations should be explicitly targeted for improvement. The actions that are planned to improve performance should be documented in the plan, and the effects of past quality improvement efforts (successful or unsuccessful) should be documented. In an organization committed to continuous improvement, small changes to operations are made daily, often without lengthy or formal planning, to make processes work better. There is no need to document these sorts of activities in an annual quality management plan. The plan should focus on major quality improvement activities that extend over longer periods of time and are more far-reaching.

Format of the Plan

There is no required format for a quality management plan. The plan may be of the laboratory's own design, or it may follow a reference resource, such as CLSI guideline GP-22, *Continuous Quality Improvement: Integrating Five Key Quality System Components,* or GP-26, *Application of a Quality Management System Model for Laboratory Services*; the ISO 9000 series; JCAHO's model for improving organizational performance; or the AABB quality program. The document need not be detailed, but it should itemize the essential aspects of the program. For a small office-based laboratory, the quality management plan may be as short as two typed pages in length; for a large laboratory, it may be several dozen pages long.

The quality management plan should contain all of the required elements listed in preceding sections of this chapter or should reference the procedures that contain the required elements. For example, the plan should either spell out the approach that will be used to investigate and address complaints that could affect patient care or should reference a separate procedure that contains this information.

The plan can exist as a separate document, or it can be a single procedure within a larger laboratory procedure manual. One advantage of making the quality management plan a procedure within a larger manual is that the plan will be reviewed automatically as part of the annual review of the laboratory procedure manual.

Some organizations maintain a separate patient safety plan. We have incorporated patient safety considerations into our sample quality management plans because combining the two reduces paperwork and is consistent with our general philosophy that assuring patient safety is part of quality management. Some organizations may prefer to address patient safety in a separate document.

Implementing the Plan

A quality management plan that is not implemented has little value. Moreover, the CAP accreditation standards require that the plan be implemented as designed.[277] In 2004, 1.6% of laboratories inspected by the CAP were cited for not implementing their quality management plans.[91] The authors of this manual share deep concerns about laboratory managers who create beautiful paper documents that never come to life. Lest we lose site of our goal, it is worth reminding ourselves that the purpose of quality management is to foster quality, not the creation of quality plans.

How do plans become practice? Often it is helpful to make specific individuals responsible for each task spelled out in the plan. Milestones and deadlines may be specified. Responsible individuals should also be given sufficient time to carry out assigned tasks. Insufficient time devoted to quality monitoring activities may result in incomplete or misleading information. Many laboratories create a quality committee that meets regularly to receive reports of ongoing measurements and to review complaints, problems, and any sentinel events. Social pressure from the quality committee helps motivate responsible individuals to complete required tasks.

Evidence of plan implementation includes the minutes of the quality committee, the results of ongoing measurement, and any documentation related to complaint investigation, problems, and adverse events. These records, along with the plan itself, should be available to external inspectors. Quality management record-keeping need not be centralized, but on the day of a CAP inspection, summaries of all QM records should be grouped and provided to the inspector.

In our experience, plans are most easily implemented when a culture of safety and quality already exists within an organization. There are many authors and consultants ready to help managers cultivate a culture of safety and quality. Unfortunately, most approaches to promoting the right culture have not been scientifically tested, and we are reluctant to recommend specific techniques, even as we acknowledge the central importance of organizational culture to successful plan implementation.

Sample Plans

Three sample quality management plans are provided. These samples are based on real plans in current use, but the names of the laboratories from which they have been borrowed and some laboratory-specific information have been changed. The samples included in this manual are significantly longer than many quality management plans. Shorter plans that are well constructed can meet regulatory requirements as well as these samples.

The first plan serves a fictitious 145-employee laboratory located within a Florida community hospital. The second plan serves a microbiology section of a large free-standing laboratory in Oklahoma, where each laboratory section maintains its own quality management plan. The third plan serves a fictitious academic medical center in California.

The three samples address all of the elements we believe should be included in a quality management plan. Yet each plan describes the laboratory's quality program in its own way. To conserve space, only the most significant portions of the sample plans are included in this manual. Readers should feel free to borrow sections from any of these examples.

Laboratory Quality Management Plan
South Florida Medical Center

Approved by

Medical Director, Clinical Laboratory
Administrative Director, Clinical Laboratory

Effective: November 1997
Revised: June 2005

Table of Contents

Quality Planning

It is the philosophy of the Clinical Laboratory to develop and implement a quality management program that encompasses all functions and testing performed in the lab. Quality is placed first in importance among management activities and in decision making. The purpose of our quality program is to provide a systematic, ongoing, and unified process for ensuring and improving the quality of laboratory services for patients and health care providers who request our service.

Quality planning for the laboratory is done by linking the mission and work of the laboratory into (1) the mission and work of South Florida Medical Center; (2) the needs of laboratory customers, as made known to the laboratory; (3) what we know generally about quality management of laboratory services; (4) knowledge of specific incidents and problems that have involved the laboratory in the past; (5) comparative information about quality performance at other organizations; and (6) regulatory requirements. From these six inputs, quality objectives and specific plans are developed.

Quality planning is done annually or more often, as needed. This document reflects the outcome of the quality planning process.

South Florida Medical Center

Quality Leadership

Responsibilities. The medical director of the laboratory serves as the chief pathologist for the laboratory. The medical directors of each functional area are qualified professionals with appropriate clinical training and experience and are responsible for the clinical direction of patient care provided by their section. The medical director of the laboratory ensures that the qualifications, authority, and duties of the medical directors of each laboratory section are defined in writing.

The medical director of the clinical laboratory, along with the medical directors of the functional areas and the chief technologists, are responsible for defining quality laboratory practices for the laboratory and for reviewing internal quality control and external proficiency test results.

The medical director of the clinical laboratory is responsible for implementing the performance improvement (PI) program. The coordination and maintenance of the PI program within the laboratory and integration of the PI activities with other hospital departments are delegated to the administrative coordinator. The medical director reviews all quality indicators and performance improvement projects. The medical director and the administrative director of the laboratory review and sign the annual quality plan and evaluation. On a periodic basis, and at least annually, the medical director reports on performance improvement activities of the Clinical Laboratory to the South Florida Medical Center Quality and Safety Committee.

The administrative director of the laboratory is responsible for initiating appropriate quality studies, reviewing all sections' PI activities, documenting and resolving all quality problems, and providing information about quality or process improvement activities to the laboratory staff.

The staff of the laboratory are responsible for following quality control (QC) and quality laboratory practices (QLP), identifying opportunities for improvement, documenting problems arising on each shift, and actively participating in performance improvement activities.

Organization. The medical and administrative director of the laboratory organize the staff into functional work groups. Each functional area of the laboratory is headed by a chief technologist and a medical director. The outline of the organizational structure is maintained in an organization chart in Appendix I *(not included in this manual)*. The chief technologists meet monthly with the laboratory medical and administrative directors to

South Florida Medical Center

share information and coordinate action regarding management and quality issues.

Awareness. The medical director and administrative director of the clinical laboratory are committed to quality, patient safety, and regulatory compliance. All employees are encouraged to discuss quality, patient safety, and regulatory compliance concerns with their superiors without fear of retribution. The leaders of the laboratory help all employees understand the vision and mission of the laboratory and the focus on serving laboratory customers. The leaders involve their staff in planning and decision making. Communication to employees about quality standards and practices is done by the use of policies and procedures, written and electronic communication, formal meetings, and informal communication.

Education/Knowledge. The leaders of the laboratory provide training and education in both technical/professional areas and also in quality principles and techniques. Laboratory leaders provide opportunities for staff development and education through courses and workshops offered by manufacturers of lab equipment and professional organizations, and by hospital or laboratory groups. Specific training goals are established for each employee as part of the performance planning process. The specific requirements for continuing education are outlined in detail in the laboratory Continuing Education policy.

Teamwork. The leaders of the laboratory support the philosophies of teams and teamwork both within the laboratory and throughout the health system. Laboratory staff participate actively as part of process improvement teams within the laboratory and the hospital. Teamwork is encouraged by sharing knowledge, giving challenges to staff, providing opportunities to get involved, and encouraging problem solving by employees. Teamwork is supported by communication from the leaders to the staff via meetings, electronic mail and bulletin boards, handouts and newsletters, etc.

Quality Control and Quality Laboratory Practices

Quality control includes the objective evaluation of test performance, comparing actual performance to established goals or ranges, and acting on the difference. Quality laboratory practices include the processes, procedures, and evaluation that provides the basis for quality laboratory services. The laboratory is committed to establishing and following

South Florida Medical Center

excellent quality control and quality laboratory practices through the following activities:

Surveys of Customers. The laboratory surveyed outpatient physicians, nurses, and medical assistants in June 2003 to assess their satisfaction with laboratory services. A follow-up survey was completed in June 2004. The CAP Inpatient Nursing Satisfaction Q-Probe was completed in February 2005.

Test Catalog. The laboratory supports the quality of the pre-analytical processes by creation of a comprehensive web-based test catalog. In the test catalog, information is provided about correct specimen collection, labeling, containers, transport, and storage; use of requisition/test order forms and on-line test ordering; and test utilization and interpretation. The on-line lab catalog is made available to all nursing units and clinics, to housestaff and staff physicians, and to outside users of laboratory services.

Phlebotomy and Capillary Puncture. The laboratory supports the quality of the pre-analytical processes by providing procedures for specimen collection in the laboratory test catalog and with training provided to nursing units or clinics, on request. Laboratory representatives attend nursing staff meetings, when requested, to discuss collection techniques and optimal specimen types for quality results and desired result turnaround times. Training material, tours, and guidelines are provided, as requested, to newly hired ancillary health technicians and new graduate nurses.

Specimen Labeling. The laboratory requires positive patient identifiers, proper specimen labeling, and submission of acceptable specimens to protect patients from adverse consequences of errors. The laboratory follows the South Florida Medical Center Specimen Integrity policy, which incorporates the JCAHO requirement for two forms of identification. All specimens are required to be labeled with the patient's first and last name and medical record number or birth date.

Appropriate Testing. The laboratory supports the quality of the pre-analytic process by establishing a plan of care for use of specific tests, such as stat antibiotic testing. In addition, laboratory staff participate in development of plans of care that define optimal sequencing and timing of tests and interventions for a particular diagnosis or procedure. The plans of care are designed to better utilize resources, maximize quality of care, and minimize delays. The laboratory also participates in development of request forms that help modify and optimize ordering

South Florida Medical Center

patterns. Customized request forms are designed for specific customers, upon request, to include their most commonly ordered tests or special tests to facilitate customers' test ordering requirements.

Referral Laboratories. The medical director, in consultation with South Florida Medical Center and client clinicians (as appropriate), selects referral laboratories based on, but not limited to, quality, methodology, and accreditation status (a high complexity CLIA license is mandatory, CAP accreditation desirable). The medical director monitors the quality of test results by annually reviewing a sampling of results as they are received in the laboratory. A complaint by a physician concerning tests sent to a reference laboratory is referred to the Clinical Laboratory Medical Director, and an investigation is initiated with the reference laboratory.

Personnel. The laboratory is committed to hiring the best possible personnel. Each job description lists job responsibilities and functions, identifies equipment and methods used, states the qualifications in terms of education and training required for the job, and describes reporting relationships. Progression through levels of technical and leadership responsibility, from medical technologist to lead technologist, specialist, shift supervisors, and chief technologist, provide career growth for laboratory professional staff.

The laboratory recognizes that quality testing comes from having a well-trained staff. The chief technologist of each area identifies training needs and ensures that each individual performing tests receives regular in-service training and education appropriate for the type and complexity of laboratory services performed. The competency of all testing personnel to perform test procedures and report test results accurately and proficiently is measured periodically using a variety of techniques that include direct observation, monitoring and review of results, worksheets, quality control, proficiency testing, and preventive maintenance records, assessment of test performance with blind or previously tested specimens, and assessment of problem-solving skills. Overall employee performance is evaluated annually using standards defined by Human Resources.

Staffing. Staffing is adjusted to achieve operational efficiency without compromising quality. The Clinical Laboratory bases its staffing plan on its typical workload pattern. This pattern shows high volumes during the weekdays and lower volumes on weekends, holidays, and off shifts. Patient census does not have a significant effect on this pattern. The lab assesses the effectiveness of staffing by monitoring turnaround times

South Florida Medical Center

(TAT) and test volumes. Laboratory errors are also monitored to determine if staffing patterns and errors are related. Staffing adjustments are made, as needed, following Human Resources policies.

Work Flow. Simplicity and consistency of work flow in the laboratory impacts the quality and efficiency of the testing process. Work flow is evaluated with turnaround time monitors or with process improvement tools and techniques.

Written Procedures. The NCCLS GP2-A4 fourth edition guidelines are used as a model for documentation of technical procedures in the laboratory. Procedures are created for all tests and for all significant processes in the laboratory. All procedures are reviewed at least annually. If significant changes are made to a procedure, it is revised and reprinted. A sign-off sheet in the front of each procedure manual provides documentation that the manual has been read by the technologists/ technicians performing the tests included the manual. As procedures are revised, previous editions of the procedure are stored according to the Document Control policy. All procedures are re-reviewed and re-approved within a reasonable timeframe by the laboratory director or designee when there is a change is directorship.

Documentation. Each laboratory section will follow good record-keeping practices for all their testing processes. Records include meeting minutes, instrument printouts, worksheets, paper forms, computer data, and database files. Meeting records include a summary of information shared and of ideas exchanged. Problem-solving activities are documented with a summary of the discussion; assignments are clearly stated. A summary of how problems are resolved is clearly documented.

For function and maintenance records, the laboratory standards for good record-keeping state: A good record includes a title, date, results of function checks, comments, a place for the technologist's/technician's initials, a place for the reviewer's initials, and established performance limits. It also has a statement as to the action to take if limits are exceeded, or a reference to a specific procedure manual in which such action is defined.

Supplies. The laboratory administrative staff, with support from the technical staff, are responsible for supporting lab operations with an uninterrupted flow of materials and services. The objective of the purchasing and materials management activities of the lab is to acquire materials of the right quality, in the right quantity, at the right time, from the right supplier, at the right price.

New Test Management. The following documentation must be provided to the Clinical Laboratory Services Committee before implementation of a new test (or before significantly changing the methodology of an existing test). The committee must approve that validation studies and procedures are completed:

❍ For tests and test methods not approved by the FDA for clinical use, studies will be completed to establish the validity (accuracy, precision, reportable range, and reference interval) for the assay. Data should be sufficient to calculate the sensitivity and specificity of the assay in the clinical population for which it is intended.

❍ For tests and test methods approved by the FDA, performance characteristics specified by CLIA will be determined.

❍ Recommendations for clinical use of the assay will be specified (e.g., Under what clinical conditions should the test be ordered? Under what clinical conditions should the test not be ordered? How does the new test compare in predictive value, utility and cost with other tests for the same conditions?).

❍ Establishment of reference ranges. Each functional area determines the method used and takes necessary action on their findings. When reference ranges are updated, the changes and dates of changes are documented in the technical procedure of the tests or a reference range history file. For significant changes to reference ranges, the laboratory sends out a notice to all attending physicians, to all nursing areas, and to applicable clients. In addition, notification of changes to reference ranges are documented in the laboratory computer, with a footnote concerning the date of change, for a minimum of one month.

Test Quality Control. It is the policy of the Clinical Laboratory to establish and use quality control procedures for all testing that is performed. No patient results are reported if reagents, equipment, methods, or test samples exceed the tolerance limits set for specific control procedures. To the extent appropriate for the matrix of quality control (QC) specimens, controls are tested identically to patient specimens.

The medical director and chief technologist of each functional area are responsible for developing quality surveillance procedures to detect, reduce, and correct deficiencies in the analytical process. QC of reagents and equipment must include verification of reagents, testing of instrument/equipment functions, and preventive maintenance procedures. Calibration procedures for measuring devices, methods, and equipment are documented. Statistical or other objective QC

South Florida Medical Center

procedures are used to validate ongoing performance characteristics of a method in terms of accuracy and precision.

For those tests performed using multiple methodologies or instruments, or at different testing sites, the chief technologist in charge of the testing is responsible for defining a mechanism to verify the comparability of results throughout the clinically appropriate ranges. This comparison testing is performed a minimum of twice yearly. If the laboratory performs test procedures for which calibration and control materials are not available, the chief technologist with responsibility for this testing defines procedures to verify the reliability of patient test results, including elements of accuracy, precision, and clinical discriminating power.

The medical director and chief technologist of each functional area or their designee are responsible for periodic review of QC records. It is the responsibility of all technologists/technicians who work in the laboratory to maintain QC records in an organized manner and to complete all record-keeping or review that is assigned. All QC checks are documented, and all QC records are kept a minimum of two years.

Reporting. Laboratory reports contain accurate demographic information, are organized for effective communication, and contain appropriate comments concerning the specimen, comments about results, reference values, and other interpretive information, as required

Annual review of the reports of all lab tests is performed to ensure clarity and accurate transmission of test results from test systems to final reports and clinical information systems. Test catalog information is also verified during this review. An annual review by the medical director of the clinical laboratory of all types of patient reports (inpatient, outpatient, and clients) is performed to ensure clinical relevance.

Procedures are established for the documentation and correction of errors on reports. Critical values are reported to a person responsible for the care of the patient. The specific policy for calling critical values is documented in the Critical Call policy.

Section-Specific Practices. QC and QLP specific to each laboratory section is described in Appendix II *(not included in this manual)*.

External Proficiency Testing. It is the policy of the Clinical Laboratory to participate in an external audit of its tests in the form of proficiency testing. The goals of proficiency testing are to identify problems that affect test accuracy and precision, to improve the methods used in the

Clinical Laboratory, and to provide education to technologists. Proficiency testing is also required to fulfill the requirements of the Clinical Laboratory Improvement Amendments of 1988 and the Final CLIA rules, effective April 24, 2003.

To the extent possible from the matrix or form in which specimens are received, all proficiency test samples are treated exactly the same as patient specimens. Proficiency testing results are reviewed on a timely basis by the medical director and by the chief technologist of the area. Review includes evaluation and documentation of all unacceptable results to determine the source of error and of corrective action taken to resolve problems. The administrative coordinator prepares a summary of external proficiency testing results. When required, the laboratory provides to the proficiency testing vendor a copy of all survey problems in the format of survey exception reports.

For analytes for which no external proficiency testing materials are available, accuracy and reliability are assessed at least semi-annually by various methods, such as comparing performance with another laboratory or test reference materials that have a known or assigned value. Clinical Laboratory chief technologists define the method used, as described in Appendix II *(not included in this manual)*.

External Ongoing Performance Benchmarking. The laboratory subscribes to an external quality benchmarking program (Q-Probes and Q-Tracks). Local laboratory data is submitted to the external service, compared to peer laboratories, and then reviewed by the laboratory. The program rotates aspects of laboratory service that are subject to benchmarking, so that over time all sections of the laboratory participate in the monitoring activities.

External Inspection and Accreditation. The laboratory participates in the College of American Pathologists Laboratory Accreditation Program. The accreditation process from CAP includes review of personnel qualifications, review of compliance with proficiency testing requirements, and verification that accreditation standards are met. The laboratory is inspected by a team of professionals from a peer organization every two years. On alternating years, the laboratory inspects itself. South Florida Medical Center is accredited by the Joint Commission on Accreditation of Healthcare Organizations (JCAHO). JCAHO accepts the CAP accreditation for the laboratory-specific portion of the standards. The laboratory supports South Florida Medical Center's efforts to comply with JCAHO hospital accreditation standards.

South Florida Medical Center

Performance Improvement

Performance improvement (PI) is the continuous study and adaptation of a health care organization's function, and processes to increase the probability of achieving desired outcomes and to better meet the needs of individuals and other users of services.

PI Method. The Performance Improvement Model of South Florida Medical Center is PDCA. The PDCA process consists of four steps: (1) Plan - design an improvement; (2) Do - implement the improvement; (3) Check - determine whether the change has improved results; and (4) Act - make the change permanent to lock-in improvement. See the PDCA procedure for more detail.

PI Initiatives. The quality program of the Clinical Laboratory currently includes a number of performance improvement initiatives for important laboratory services. PI progress is compared against an applicable benchmark. The benchmark may be a practice guideline, CAP Q-Probes data, the laboratory's own experience, or a level of service agreement made with laboratory customers.

Data sources, data collection methods, sampling methods, and frequency of collection are identified for each performance improvement process. Data collection methods may include checklists/tallies, documentation review, interview, observation, or questionnaire. Data is collected routinely with sufficient frequency to identify patterns/trends and an adequate sample size that will produce a valid indication of the practice/process being measured. Each functional area maintains the schedule of data collection. Collected data is assessed at least quarterly or semi-annually, but is often assessed monthly.

Findings from data collection are documented and displayed in a way that allows for identification of patterns, trends, or shifts. Data is displayed through the use of control charts, line graphs, bar graphs, or histograms. Depending on the type of data collected, limits, patterns, or trends are analyzed and evaluated. The assessment process includes the use of statistical process control techniques/tools, as appropriate. Performance improvement efforts continue until performance is sustained at an acceptable level.

PI Teams. Each PI initiative is assigned to a PI team that is responsible for improving performance. Team leaders submit progress reports to the laboratory performance improvement committee on a monthly or quarterly basis. Members of the teams are selected by the PI coordinator

South Florida Medical Center

and/or the chief technologist. Teams may exist informally, with meetings being held and membership changing as needed. Staff from other departments are asked to participate when their involvement is indicated. The PI coordinator may serve as the PI facilitator.

2004/2005 PI Initiatives. The following PI initiatives have been selected for the current academic year. Each initiative was selected because of past problems or known opportunities to improve. Appendix III *(not included in this manual)* describes each initiative, data collection requirements for monitoring, and the changes that the laboratory plans to make to improve performance.

1. Turnaround time of selected analytes: hematocrit, potassium, prothrombin time, glucose, troponin I, aPTT, Flow Cytometry, Coagulation testing for Heparin Level, ATIII, Hemoglobin A1C, BNP, GC by amplified probe

2. Evaluate screening tests for Streptococcus agalactiae (GBS)

3. Improve appropriateness of orders for endocervical and urethral swabs for N. gonorrhoeae and Chlamydia trachomatis

4. Evaluate automated blood banking analyzer

5. Reduce contamination of blood cultures

6. Improve test order accuracy

7. Reduce late "add test" requests

8. Improve fresh frozen plasma outdate relabeling once the product is thawed, in an attempt to decrease outdating errors

9. Improve patient wristband accuracy

10. Improve critical value reporting

Previous Initiatives. Progress made with PI initiatives that are no longer active are retained on file.

Occurrence Management. The Clinical Laboratory documents and monitors problems and customer concerns/complaints that occur in each functional area of the laboratory. These problems are documented on the

South Florida Medical Center

Clinical Laboratory Customer Concern/Problem Documentation Form and are submitted to the administrative laboratory coordinator for review.

Common problems are reported to the Laboratory Quality Assurance Committee. Recommendations for PI are determined when recurring problems are experienced. A Patient Occurrence Report is sent to Risk Management for all unacceptably labeled or misidentified samples (wrong patient name on samples or test requisition) received by the laboratory.

Near Miss and Sentinel Events

When the Clinical Laboratory is involved in a near miss or an adverse event, a Patient Occurrence Report is completed and forwarded to the Professional Risk Management Department. If the patient was treated as a direct result of an erroneous laboratory result being reported, or treatment is withheld due to delay in testing, the laboratory investigates the problem. Root cause analysis and cause-and-effect diagrams, along with corrective actions and process or policy changes, are submitted to the laboratory director and medical director for review.

Quality Program Evaluation

The objectives, organization, comprehensiveness, and effectiveness of the laboratory quality program are evaluated at least annually, and the program is revised as necessary. This evaluation is performed by the QA/PI coordinator and approved by the laboratory medical and administrative directors.

South Florida Medical Center

MICROBIOLOGY LABORATORY QUALITY MANAGEMENT PLAN
CONSOLIDATED LABORATORIES OF OKLAHOMA

PURPOSE

The purpose of the quality management plan is to provide reasonable assurance to management, physicians, and patients that laboratory operations meet defined standards for quality and patient safety, are in compliance with applicable laws and regulations, and that performance will improve in selected areas.

PROGRAM STRUCTURE

The quality management plan contains seven elements. The first element is a commitment to establish a "tone" that reinforces quality and patient safety. This tone is established as much by day-to-day action of management and staff as by policies and procedures.

Commitment to Quality, Safety, and Integrity

The laboratory is committed to a culture of quality, patient safety, and organizational integrity. Management and staff should accept established performance standards, controls, discipline, and structure. All employees are encouraged to discuss quality, patient safety, and other concerns without fear of retribution.

Risk Assessment

Management has identified risks that could cause the laboratory to fail to meet its goal of providing quality service and patient safety. These risks range from the particular (e.g., the failure of a reagent lot to perform adequately) to the more general (e.g., failure to adequately train staff to perform a certain task). They may be internal to the section (e.g., a refrigerator failing to maintain its temperature) or external (e.g., operating room staff failing to properly collect tissue for culture). All phases of testing and all laboratory shifts are included in the risk assessment.

Internal Control Activities

Control procedures have been developed to mitigate each significant risk. For example, in the case of reagents, control activities involve the use of quality control samples. In the case of employee training, control activities involve a training checklist for new employees and periodic assessment of employee competence.

External Control Activities

The laboratory participates in external proficiency testing and is inspected by the College of American Pathologists as part of the CAP Laboratory Accreditation Program. In addition, the FDA, CMS, AABB, OSHA, and JCAHO may inspect the laboratory. Agencies outside the laboratory (CAP, institution privacy officer, safety officer, compliance officer) will receive in confidence employee concerns about quality or compliance issues that are not being addressed by laboratory management.

Information and Communication

Management reviews patient safety and quality records on a regular basis, and summaries are made available to the laboratory-wide quality committee and laboratory leadership. Results are shared within and outside the laboratory, as described in this plan.

Performance Improvement

Certain aspects of operations have been targeted for improvement during the current year. The improvement efforts are documented in this plan.

Monitoring

Ongoing monitoring takes a number of forms: (1) Staff and managers assess laboratory performance over time. Performance is compared to standards, benchmarks, and past performance, as applicable. (2) Complaints, deficiencies, unusual problems, and any patient adverse events are investigated. (3) The laboratory is subject to monitoring by external agencies (see section below). (4) Finally, this quality plan itself is reviewed annually. As required, processes and procedures are changed or the quality plan is changed to reduce the frequency of poor performance, complaints, deficiencies, or adverse events.

LIMITATIONS Because resources are finite, not every process and element of service can be controlled completely. The laboratory cannot afford to have each test repeated by two technologists or backup equipment on-site for every instrument that could malfunction. Management has designed and implemented internal controls based on an analysis of cost, risk, and benefit. Even under ideal circumstances, internal controls cannot provide absolute assurance that all organizational objectives will be met. Factors outside the control or influence of management and staff can affect the laboratory's ability to achieve its goals. Therefore, the laboratory's quality management plan provides reasonable, but not absolute, assurance that the laboratory will meet its quality and patient safety objectives.

AUTHORITY The pathologist in charge of the microbiology laboratory, acting as the designate of the laboratory director, has approved this plan, as evidenced by a signature. The technical manager of the section also approves this plan.

APPROVAL Pathologist signature: Date:

Technical supervisor signature: Date:

FUNCTION AT RISK	CONTROL ACTIVITIES

Preanalytic Phase of Testing

Test Ordering	See "Test Ordering Consultation" procedure
Specimen Collection	See "Blood Culture Contamination" procedure
Order Entry	See laboratory-wide procedure on Order Entry
Lost Specimens	See "Lost Specimens" procedure

Analytic Phase of Testing

Orderable Tests	See applicable individual procedures
Reagents/Stains/Additives/Media	See applicable individual procedures
Automated/Prepackaged Tests	See applicable individual procedures
Equipment	See applicable individual procedures
Interpretive/Subjective Tests	See applicable individual procedures
Maintaining Control Strains	See "Maintaining Control Strains" procedure
New Procedures	See "New Procedure Checklist" procedure
Extramural Proficiency Testing	See "Handling PT Specimens" procedure

Postanalytic Phase of Testing

Report Quality	See "Report Review" procedure
Interpretation of Test Results	See "Test Interpretation Consultation" procedure
Reporting Critical Results	See "Critical Result Reporting" procedure

General Laboratory Systems

Personnel Initial Training	See "New Employee Training Checklist" procedure
Maintenance of Competence	See "Employee Competence Checklist" procedure
Personnel Errors	See "Tabulation of Major Errors" procedure
Staffing Plan	See "Laboratory Staffing Plan" procedure
Policy and Procedures	See "Document Control" procedure
Turnaround Time	See "Turnaround Time" procedure
Information Management	See laboratory-wide procedures on Data & Confidentiality
Customer Satisfaction	See laboratory-wide procedure on Customer Satisfaction
External Inspection and Accreditation	See "CAP Accreditation" procedure
Legal and Regulatory Noncompliance	See "Reporting Noncompliance" procedure
Complaints and Unusual Problems	See "Incident Log" procedure
Sentinel Events	See laboratory-wide procedure on Sentinel Events
Correcting Errors	See "Correcting Errors" procedure
Documentation	See "Record Keeping" procedure

ROUTINE BACTERIOLOGY TESTS – DAILY MONITORING
Quality Control Log • Microbiology Laboratory • Consolidated Laboratories of Oklahoma

TEST	LOT NUMBER	EXPIRATION DATE	CONTROLS	EXPECTED RESULT	MONDAY DATE:	TUESDAY DATE:	WEDNESDAY DATE:	THURSDAY DATE:	FRIDAY DATE:	SATURDAY DATE:	SUNDAY DATE:
CATALASE			S. epidermidis QC-7	POSITIVE							
			S. pyogenes QC-8	NEGATIVE							
COAGULASE			S. aureus QC-9	POSITIVE							
			S. epidermidis QC-7	NEGATIVE							
OXIDASE			P. aeruginosa QC-48	POSITIVE							
			E. coli QC-11	NEGATIVE							
OPTOCHIN			S. pneumoniae QC-1	POSITIVE							
			S. viridans QC-5	NEGATIVE							
BILE SOLUBILITY			S. pneumoniae QC-1	POSITIVE							
			S. viridans QC-5	NEGATIVE							
BETA-LACTAMASE			H. influenzae QC-20	POSITIVE							
			H. parainfluenzae QC-40	NEGATIVE							
GERM TUBE			H. albicans QC-31	POSITIVE							
			H. tropicalis QC-32	NEGATIVE							
GRAM STAIN — Crystal violet: / Iodine: / Safranin:			S. aureus QC-9	POSITIVE							
			E. coli QC-11	NEGATIVE							
RAPID-GROUP A			POLY + CONTROL	POSITIVE							
			NEGATIVE	NEGATIVE							
RAPID-GROUP B			POLY + CONTROL	POSITIVE							
			NEGATIVE	NEGATIVE							
RAPID STREP AG			KIT CONTROL +	POSITIVE							
			KIT CONTROL -	NEGATIVE							
			Known Positive (New Lot)	POSITIVE							
CRYPTOCOCCUS AG			KIT CONTROL +	POSITIVE							
			KIT CONTROL -	NEGATIVE							
			Known Positive (New Lot)	POSITIVE							
E. COLI 0157			KIT CONTROL +	POSITIVE							
			KIT CONTROL -	NEGATIVE							
RAPID FLU A/B *Run with each new kit **Record each day in use			A+/B- External Control*	POSITIVE							
			A-/B+ External Control*	NEGATIVE							
			Procedural Control**	POSITIVE							
RAPID RSV *Run with each new kit **Record each day in use			External Control + *	POSITIVE							
			External Control - *	NEGATIVE							
			Procedural Control + **	POSITIVE							
			Procedural Control - **	NEGATIVE							

Reviewed by: _____ Date: _____

Acceptable Results: Indicate by initialing the appropriate columns or write N.A.
Unacceptable Results: Write C.A. and fill out Corrective Action Log.

Unusual Incident Log

Microbiology Laboratory • Consolidated Laboratories of Oklahoma

INSTRUCTIONS. Employees should complete this form whenever a quality-related problem is encountered that is not detected as part of the section's normal quality monitoring program. Describe the problem and initiate corrective action (if you know how to correct the problem). Follow separate procedure for patient sentinel events. Give the form to your manager, whether or not you have corrected the problem yourself.

PROBLEM DESCRIPTION. Include date of problem and any other specific information.

Initials: _____ Date: _____

CORRECTIVE ACTION/RESOLUTION. Describe corrective action and whether the problem was resolved.

Initials: _____ Date: _____

SUPERVISORY REVIEW. Determine whether any changes to operating procedures are required.

❑ If problem was corrected by someone other than the employee who first described the problem, check here to indicate that feedback about what was done has been given to the person who first described the incident.

Manager Initials: _____ Date: _____

Pathologist Initials: _____ Date: _____

Quality Management of Specimen Collection
Microbiology Laboratory • Consolidated Laboratories of Oklahoma

Background

The laboratory has identified blood culture contamination as a specimen collection risk worth managing. Occasional contamination of blood cultures is unavoidable. Nevertheless, blood culture contamination often results from improper collection and is associated with increased length of hospital stay, excess expense, and the administration of unnecessary antibiotics. The laboratory has enrolled in a College of American Pathologists Q-Tracks product to assist in the monitoring of blood culture contamination and to provide external comparative data. In addition, local quality improvement initiatives will be applied.

Procedure

1. On a monthly basis, run the computer program "BCC," which has been written to calculate overall blood culture contamination rate and the rate for each patient care unit.
2. Plot the results on the Blood Culture Contamination control chart. Plot overall blood culture contamination on one control chart, and blood culture contamination from each major patient care unit on its own chart. If a value exceeds control limits, bring the control chart to your manager.
3. Record results in the Quality Control Log. Give the log to your manager, and send the result by e-mail to the section pathologist.
4. The manager will send data to the CAP for the Q-Tracks product. The section pathologists will disseminate results to patient care units, along with Q-Tracks reports.

Benchmark

Management has determine that at this point in time, acceptable performance is a contamination rate less than 3.6%, which is a level of contamination of the 25th percentile laboratory (worst quarter) in the CAP Q-Tracks database. The threshold will be changed if Q-Tracks data changes or a new, improved level of performance is achieved.

Quality Improvement

During the year, an effort will be made to lower blood culture contamination rates, because benchmark data suggest the laboratory currently performs at the 25th percentile level, which management considers mediocre. Improvement in performance will be attempted through: (1) education of phlebotomy staff on nursing units; (2) wide dissemination of unit-specific contamination rates; (3) elimination of povidone iodine as a disinfectant in the locations where it is still used; and (4) reduction in the number of blood cultures drawn from intravenous lines.

Reporting and Review

This measure is reviewed monthly by the manager and section pathologist. If quality does not improve, the quality improvement plan will be revisited.

This measure is reported yearly to the Laboratory Director and the laboratory-wide quality assurance committee.

Quality Management of Turnaround Time
Microbiology Laboratory • Consolidated Laboratories of Oklahoma

Background

The laboratory has identified turnaround time to first reported urine cultures to be a risk worth managing. Rapid reporting of negative vs positive urine cultures – even if definitive identification and susceptibility testing is not complete – can expedite patients' treatment, reducing discomfort and risk of complications.

Procedure

1. On a monthly basis, run the computer program "UCTAT," which has been written to calculate the percentage of urine cultures for which some report has been issued (preliminary or final) within 24 hours of receipt in the laboratory.
2. Plot the results on the Urine Culture Turnaround Time control chart. If a value exceeds control limits, bring the control chart to your manager.
3. Record results in the Quality Control Log. Give the log to your manager.

Benchmark

There are no established multi-institutional benchmarks for this quality measure. Management has determined that at this point in time, performance is acceptable so long as at least 90% of cultures have a report issued within 24 hours.

Quality Improvement

This measure is not targeted for improvement during the upcoming year. Current turnaround time is considered adequate and stable (in statistical control), but is being monitored to ensure that the process does not slip out of control.

Reporting and Review

This measure is reviewed monthly by the manager and section pathologist. If out of control, additional corrective steps will be taken.

This measure is reported yearly to the Laboratory Director and the laboratory-wide quality assurance committee.

Correcting Errors

Microbiology Laboratory • Consolidated Laboratories of Oklahoma

Background

Errors should be corrected after they are discovered. Do not wait until the cause of the error is known before correcting the error – as soon as the correct result is known, it should be reported. If the error is likely to have resulted in patient harm, patients must additionally be informed about the error.

Procedure

1. Notify your manager of the error.
2. Issue an amended report with the correct result. The computer will automatically flag the report as a "correction."
3. If the new result is a critical value or changes a previously reported critical value, call the caregiver and inform the caregiver of the new result.
4. If the manager believes patient harm has occurred as a result of the error, a pathologist will be contacted. The pathologist will ensure that the patient is informed of the error, either directly or through their primary physician. If the incident qualifies as a "sentinel event," a special investigatory procedure will be followed (root cause analysis).

Benchmark

There are no established multi-institutional benchmarks for the number of acceptable errors in microbiology. On a monthly basis, the number of errors is tabulated and divided by the number of billable tests reported during the month. Management has determined that at this point in time, performance is acceptable so long as 0.1% or fewer billable tests are associated with an error.

Quality Improvement

This measure is not targeted for improvement during the upcoming year. Current error rates are considered acceptable and stable (in statistical control), but are being monitored to ensure that the process does not slip out of control.

Reporting and Review

This measure is reviewed monthly by the manager and section pathologist. If the number of errors rises above 0.1%, additional corrective steps will be taken. Since the number of errors is not in statistical control, the error rate is not plotted on a control chart.

Reporting Non-Compliance

Microbiology Laboratory • Consolidated Laboratories of Oklahoma

Background

The laboratory is committed to a culture of quality and patient safety. Further, the laboratory intends to comply with all laws and regulations pertaining to quality, patient safety, data confidentiality and security, workplace safety, fiscal integrity, and other applicable regulations.

Procedure

All employees are encouraged to discuss quality and patient safety concerns without fear of retribution. All employees are encouraged to voice concerns about workplace safety, data privacy and security, compliance with laws related to billing and finance, and any other concern about non-compliance. This includes concern about fraud (deliberate misrepresentation) or malfeasance (illegal activity).

1. Discussions about any form of non-compliance should begin with your manager. Your manager may be able to address the problem or explain to you why the organization does, in fact, comply with the law and regulations.
2. If you do not believe your manager has addressed the problem, you should escalate your concerns. The laboratory and its corporate parent have no intention of violating the law or applicable regulations. There will be no penalty against you for taking your concerns to a higher level, so long as you act in good faith and believe your concerns to be well founded. The next level to which you should take your concerns is your manager's immediate superior (boss).
3. If your manager AND manager's superior do not address your concern, contact the appropriate party listed in the table below. The authorities listed below have indicated they will protect your confidentiality:

Type of Problem	Contact the Following
Quality or Patient Safety	College of American Pathologists 866-236-7212
Workplace Safety	Corporate Safety Officer XXX-XXX-XXXX
Patient Confidentiality & Data Security	Corporate HIPAA Officer XXX-XXX-XXXX
Billing & Financial Compliance	Corporate Compliance Officer XXX-XXX-XXXX
Other Regulations	Corporate Compliance Officer XXX-XXX-XXXX

UNIVERSITY OF WESTERN SACRAMENTO COLLEGE OF MEDICINE
DEPARTMENT OF PATHOLOGY AND LABORATORY MEDICINE
QUALITY MANAGEMENT AND PATIENT SAFETY PLAN

PURPOSE

This quality management plan provides for the continuous monitoring and evaluation of patient care activities within the Department of Pathology and Laboratory Medicine. This monitoring includes pre-analytic, analytic, and post-analytic phases of testing. The plan describes a standardized quality control system that maximizes the quality of laboratory testing to produce the accurate and timely results needed in support of quality patient care. The plan includes provisions for employee training and competency assessment, document control requirements, procedures for the monitoring of quality control, quality indicators monitored on an ongoing basis, a process for the systematic detection of errors, and a formal departmental committee structure for the documentation and reporting of internal quality improvement activities. The elements of this plan have been developed after a careful risk assessment conducted by laboratory and hospital leadership that identifies the aspects of laboratory operations most in need of quality management.

PROGRAM

New Employee Training
Employee training is section specific. Each section generates a training checklist which, when completed, is signed by the employee, trainer, and section supervisor. This checklist becomes part of the employee's personnel record. In some sections, the preceptor training model is used; in others, the employee rotates through assigned blocks and is trained by a senior technologist. Employee performance is reviewed 90 days post hire and annually as part of the performance evaluation (PE) process.

Competency Training and Evaluation
Each section has an internal program of continuing education (journal articles, teleconferences, lectures) and evaluation of competency (direct observation, worksheet review, CAP proficiency sample performance). In addition, the laboratory provides for competency training with regard to age-specific competency, as appropriate, and laboratory safety.

Document Control
Each section supervisor and director is responsible for ensuring that policies and procedures for the section are current, that appropriate revisions occur annually or more often, as needed, and that each technologist is abreast of procedural changes through a method change notification or annual technologist sign off. New method procedures require director signature prior to implementation. Procedures must be retained for 2 years after discontinuation. Each section should establish a system for such document management, review, and retention.

Procedure Quality Control
Quality Control (QC; sometimes called process control) is the analysis of materials of known composition or reactivity in conjunction with patient sample testing to verify the performance of a test. QC materials are "pseudo-samples" that are designed to detect problems in instrument, reagent, or analyst performance. QC is predominantly a measure of precision (reproducibility) and confirms that a test system has maintained proper calibration.

Department of Pathology and Laboratory Medicine   *University of Western Sacramento College of Medicine*

For some analytes, the control material is a manufactured, purchased control product supplied in either a lyophilized or liquid form; the concentration has been both gravimetrically and analytically determined prior to distribution of the product. These materials must be evaluated in-house to determine the laboratory mean, standard deviation, and coefficient of variation before placing into service. This data is collected while running in parallel with the control product currently in use. There are some analytes that are not available in commercial preparations, hence they are prepared in the laboratory to create an appropriate control for the assay method performed. These materials must be evaluated in the same fashion as commercial products prior to placing in service.

The management of quality control occurs on a real time basis and as a continuous tool in evaluating the reliability of test data. Technologists, bench supervisors, chief technologist, and lab directors all contribute to this review process on a daily, weekly, and monthly basis.

The frequency of control analysis, and the preparation, reconstitution, storage conditions, and stability of specimens and reagents are described in individual procedures for each type of test. The tolerance limits for controls are established by individual sections. Values which fall outside these ranges must be evaluated according to the internal control rules. Violation of the QC rules results in review by the supervisor and/or director and may result in rejection of the analytical run. The run must be inspected to determine the cause for error. After solving the problem that caused the QC exception, the entire run may need to be repeated, along with QC evaluation. Quality control records are maintained for a period of 2 years.

Proficiency Testing (PT)

Proficiency testing is defined as periodic testing of samples whose composition or reactivity is unknown to the laboratory. PT samples are usually provided by an external agency that "knows" what an analytic result is expected to be or establishes the "correct" answer based on aggregate results from large numbers of laboratories that are participating in the survey.

In the clinical laboratory, each section (as appropriate) is enrolled in a CAP-approved proficiency testing program. Results are evaluated by the survey provider against peer group responses. Internally, results are reviewed by the section supervisor and director, and the laboratory manager and director. Outliers are investigated, corrective action is taken, and a report is made to the QA committee based on the criteria set forth below.

Surveys samples are to be integrated within the routine laboratory workload, and the samples analyzed by personnel who routinely test patient samples, using the same primary methods as for patient samples. The educational purpose and documentation of proficiency is best served by a rotation that allows all technologists to be involved in the proficiency program. Replicate analysis of surveys samples is acceptable only if patient specimens are routinely analyzed in the same manner. If the laboratory uses multiple methods for an analyte, the survey sample should be analyzed by the primary method.

In accordance with CMS regulations, laboratories are forbidden to "engage in any inter-laboratory communications pertaining to the results of proficiency testing samples" or to "send PT samples or portions of samples to another laboratory for any analysis which it is certified to perform in its own laboratory."

For analytes where graded proficiency testing is not available, performance must be checked at least semiannually using an alternate performance assessment system. These procedures include participation in ungraded proficiency survey programs, split sample analysis with reference or other laboratories, split samples with an established in-house method, certified materials, regional pools, clinical validation by chart review, or other suitable and documented means. It is the responsibility of the laboratory section director to define such procedures, as applicable, in accordance with good clinical and scientific laboratory practice.

In the event that a PT challenge is not graded because of lack of consensus, or because the laboratory either submitted results after the cut-off date or the lab section failed to submit results, the laboratory results must still be compared and evaluated internally against the peer group statistics provided by the survey group.

If a laboratory testing of a PT challenge does not produce acceptable results, the cause of the error must be investigated and corrected. There are several types of errors: methodological (the source is within the analytic system); technical (the source is attributable to performance within the laboratory); clerical (errors made in completing the forms returned to the surveyors for processing, such as transcription errors); survey (errors attributed to the survey materials or to the directions accompanying the survey material, such as matrix effects, unstable survey samples, a validated deviation from the consensus, or survey samples that did not arrive on time); or unexplained. An error should be designated as unexplained only after a full investigation eliminating every other possibility of error.

QA Monitoring

Each laboratory section has identified indicators to monitor quality of operations. Indicators may be pre-analytic, analytic, or post-analytic. When appropriate, trends are evaluated over time to evaluate deviation from baseline. Regular reports are made to quality assurance committees with regard to performance and opportunities for improvement. The indicators currently being used by the laboratory are:

Pre-analytic
- ❏ Requisition monitoring for correct test ordering
- ❏ Requisition monitoring for correct ordering physician entry
- ❏ Correct specimen labeling (mislabeled, unlabeled)
- ❏ Identification of inpatients not wearing wristbands
- ❏ Number of unsatisfactory cervicovaginal cytology specimens (obscuring factors, poor cellularity, etc.)
- ❏ Adequacy of bone marrow (aspirate and biopsy) specimens
- ❏ Specimen delivery times
- ❏ Blood culture contamination rate
- ❏ Urine culture contamination rate

Analytic
- ❏ Cytohistologic correlation of cervicovaginal cytology cases
- ❏ Comparison of "abnormal" rates and error rates for cervicovaginal specimens by cytologist
- ❏ Instrument to instrument correlation
- ❏ Frozen section discordance
- ❏ Concordance for surgical pathology cases reviewed elsewhere
- ❏ Global quality of surgical pathology reports
- ❏ Major corrections to surgical pathology reports

- ❏ Accuracy and timeliness of bone marrow reports
- ❏ Investigation of test failures in cytogenetics
- ❏ Correlation of fine needle biopsy diagnoses with "final" diagnoses, by selected organ system
- ❏ Investigation of instrument "flagged" results
- ❏ Implementation of "rules" to detect abnormal specimens

Post-analytic
- ❏ Correlation of accession and report information in laboratory information system
- ❏ Antimicrobial susceptibility trends
- ❏ Prevalence of Influenza A and B
- ❏ Prevalence of *Clostridium difficile*
- ❏ Prevalence of Vancomycin resistant enterococci
- ❏ Prevalence of MRSA
- ❏ Critical value reporting
- ❏ Auto-verification errors

Turnaround Time
- ❏ Compliance with turnaround time standards promulgated by accrediting agencies, such as CAP, and clinical professional societies, such as the American College of Cardiology
- ❏ Compliance with internal turnaround time standards for ED stat tests
- ❏ Autopsy final report turnaround time
- ❏ Special Chemistry TAT for cardiac injury markers and alcohol levels
- ❏ Cytology turnaround time
- ❏ Frozen section turnaround time

Other
- ❏ LIS monitoring of system availability
- ❏ Blood Bank FDA reportable errors
- ❏ Blood product wastage rate
- ❏ Surgical Pathology report review for necessary data
- ❏ Review of previous negative Pap smears in cases of new abnormal Pap smears
- ❏ Employee injuries/accidents
- ❏ Point of Care Testing issues from the Hospital Point of Care Steering Committee

Error Detection and Reporting

Since laboratory errors may have adverse clinical consequences, it is necessary to search actively for mistakes and investigate their causes. On a quarterly basis, the section supervisor, QI coordinator, chief medical technologist and/or director of each laboratory is responsible for reporting identified errors to their respective QI committees. The following methods are used to detect errors:

Random Review	Error detected within lab section by predetermined internal review processes.
Laboratory Detection	Error detected by technologist by means other than a random review.
External Detection	Error reported by a physician, nurse, or other individual outside the laboratory.

Each laboratory section is responsible for developing a system for detecting errors using all three of the above methods. Each section will prepare and deliver an Error Detection Report (including observed trends) and Proficiency Testing Error Report to the appropriate QA Committee on a quarterly basis.

Interdisciplinary Activities

Committee involvement by faculty and staff demonstrates integration of laboratory and hospital quality management programs. Laboratory representatives serve on the following hospital-wide quality committees:

Accreditation Management Team	Antimicrobial Committee
Environment of Care Committee	Hospital Compliance Task Force
Patient Services Improvement Committee	Point of Care Committee
Transfusion Review Committee	Trauma Care Team
Quality and Safety Committee	

Quality Oversight

The Department of Pathology and Laboratory Medicine's quality management plan is overseen by two committees:

Clinical Laboratory Quality Committee
Chair: Chair, Department of Pathology and Laboratory Medicine
Laboratory sections included: Core Lab, Special Chemistry, Blood Bank, Microbiology Laboratory, Information Systems, Cell and Molecular Pathology, Cytogenetics, and Immuno-molecular Pathology

Anatomic Pathology Quality Committee
Chair: Director, Surgical Pathology
Laboratory sections included: Autopsy, Electron Microscopy, Neuropathology, Surgical Pathology, Cytopathology, Immunocytochemistry, Histology, Bone Marrow, Anatomic Information Systems

Each committee meets quarterly, with laboratory section representation by a laboratory supervisor and/or director or designee. Minutes are recorded, electronically transmitted, and reviewed. Complete records of minutes and QA reports are maintained by the Manager, Hospital Laboratories. The laboratory quality committees will: (1) review the routine quality control monitoring reports, proficiency testing errors, and laboratory error reports from each area; (2) review corrective action taken as a result of the quality improvement findings; (3) review other QA reports, as submitted; and (4) identify and implement programs for continuous quality improvement.

Quality Planning

On an annual basis, the Chairman and the Vice Chair for Clinical Affairs and Administration of the Department of Pathology and Laboratory Medicine and the Laboratory Manager will review the efficacy of the QA plan. Focus will placed on areas of technological change and organizational change, as well as recurring problems.

APPROVAL

Chairman, Department of Pathology and Laboratory Medicine
Manager, Hospital Laboratories
Vice Chair for Clinical Affairs

Department of Pathology and Laboratory Medicine   *University of Western Sacramento College of Medicine*

Glossary²⁷⁸

Access — as defined by HIPAA, the ability or the means necessary to read, write, modify, or communicate data/information or otherwise make use of any system resource.

Access authorization — information-use policies/procedures that establish the rules for granting and/or restricting access to a user, terminal, transaction, program, or process.

Access control — a method of restricting access to resources, allowing only privileged entities access.

Accident — an event that involves damage to a patient or defined system. Accidents are usually caused by a string of latent failures, each of which alone is relatively innocuous, but which together cause the event. Accidents are usually triggered by sets of circumstances that are unpredictable.

Accreditation — the procedure by which an authoritative body (such as the CAP in the United States) gives formal recognition that an organization meets a defined set of standards.

Accredited laboratory — in the context of CLIA, a laboratory that has voluntarily applied for and been accredited by a private, nonprofit accreditation organization approved by the Centers for Medicare and Medicaid Services (CMS), such as the CAP.

Accuracy of measurement — closeness of agreement between the result of a particular measurement and the true value of the measurand/analyte.

Action plan — the result of root cause analysis or other quality management process that (1) addresses system and process deficiencies with specific improvement strategies and (2) monitors outcome measures to determine whether deficiencies have been corrected.

Active error — an error that occurs at the level of the frontline operator and whose effects are felt almost immediately. Contrast with latent error.

Adverse event — medical intervention that results in injury or material inconvenience, or causes a patient's care to be significantly changed. Examples of adverse events that involve the laboratory include patients who were admitted unnecessarily because the patient's physician received a result that belonged to another patient or patients who received a prescription medication because of an incorrect laboratory analysis. Adverse events that cause substantial patient harm are called sentinel events.

Alarm — a signal indicating the presence of an abnormality.

Alternative sanctions — sanctions that may be imposed by the United States Department of Health and Human Services (HHS) on a laboratory for a CLIA violation in lieu of or in addition to principal sanctions.

Analyte — a substance or constituent for which the laboratory conducts testing.

Analyte-specific reagent (ASR) — as defined in FDA regulations, any antibodies, both polyclonal and monoclonal, specific receptor proteins, ligands, nucleic acid sequences, and similar reagents which, through specific binding or chemical reaction with substances in a specimen, are intended for use in a diagnostic application.

Analytic accuracy — see Trueness of measurement.

Analytical interference — the effect of a substance, either identified or unidentified, that causes a difference in the measured concentration or activity from the true value.

Analytical measurement range (AMR) — a CAP term for the range of analyte values that a method can directly measure in a specimen without any dilution, concentration, or other pretreatment not part of the usual assay process.

Analytical measurement range (AMR) validation — a CAP term for the process of confirming that an assay system will correctly measure the concentration or activity of an analyte over the AMR. The materials used for validation must be known to have matrix characteristics appropriate for the method.

Analytical sensitivity — a CLIA term that means the ability of a clinical test to accurately detect the analyte or identity of interest at a particular concentration or under particular circumstances. The purpose to which a test will be put determines how analytic sensitivity is established. The process of establishing the analytical sensitivity of a ionized calcium assay and a blood typing reagent are entirely different.

Analytical specificity — a CLIA term that means the ability of a clinical test to operate free from interference by variables other than the analyte or identity of interest. The context in which a test will be used determines the types of interference that must be investigated to establish analytic specificity. The process of establishing the analytic specificity of a blood creatinine test is different from a urine creatinine test, since creatinine concentrations in blood and urine differ, as do the concentrations of potentially interfering substances. See Specificity.

Andon board — in the Toyota Production System, a visual control device in a production area, typically a lighted overhead display, giving the current status of the production system and alerting team members to emerging problems. The authors have seen an Andon board in a clinical laboratory that displays the number of callers to the laboratory who are talking with client services staff and the number waiting "on hold." Order entry staff can stop performing order entry and assist on-hold callers when backlogs emerge.

Approved accreditation organization for laboratories — a private nonprofit accreditation organization that has received Centers for Medicare and Medicaid Services (CMS) approval based on the organization's compliance with CLIA regulations.

Approved state laboratory program — a licensure or other regulatory program for laboratories in a state, the requirements of which are imposed under state law, that has received Centers for Medicare and Medicaid Services (CMS) approval based on the state's compliance with federal standards.

Assignable-cause variation — variation in performance that results from extrinsic causes. Assignable-cause variation is intermittent, unpredictable, and unstable. It is not inherently present in a system; rather, it arises from causes that are not part of the system as designed. Also called exogenous-cause variation and special-cause variation.

Asymmetric encryption — encryption and decryption performed using two different keys, one of which is referred to as the public key and one of which is referred to as the private key. Also known as public-key encryption.

Audit trail — as defined by HIPAA, the data collected and potentially used to facilitate a security audit.

Authorization control — as defined by HIPAA, the mechanism for obtaining consent for the use and disclosure of health information.

Automatic logoff — the termination of an electronic session after a predetermined time of inactivity (for example, 15 minutes).

Autonomation — development of machines with "human intelligence" that stop and alert users when processes do not conform to standards. Point-of-care instruments with "lock-out" features that require quality control testing in order to function are examples of autonomation.

Availability — in the context of HIPAA, the property of a system being accessible and usable upon demand by an authorized user or entity.

Bad outcome — failure to achieve a desired outcome of care.

Batch-and-queue — the mass-production practice of making large lots of a part and then sending the batch to wait in the queue before the next operation in the production process. Contrast with single-piece flow.

Benchmark — as a verb, "benchmark" refers to the process of comparing an individual's or institution's performance to an explicit standard. The standard may be previously demonstrated local performance or an external standard demonstrated by other individuals or facilities. As a noun, "benchmark" refers to higher-than-average performance—a "target"—to which an individual or institution should aspire. A benchmark may be the top quartile of laboratories or individuals, the top decile, or very best performance in the industry.

Bias — the difference between the expected test results and an accepted reference value.

Biological reference interval — the range of test values expected for a designated population of individuals. This is usually the central 95% interval of the distribution of values from individuals who are presumed to be healthy (or normal). For some analytes that reflect high-prevalence conditions (such as cholesterol), significantly fewer than 95% of the population may be "healthy." In this case, the biological reference interval may be something other than the central 95% of values.

Biometric identification — a process for identifying an individual human from a measurement of a physical feature or repeatable actions of the individual (for example, hand geometry, retinal scan, iris scan, fingerprint patterns, facial characteristics, DNA sequence characteristics, voice prints, and handwritten signature).

Business associate — in the context of HIPAA, a person not in the workforce of a covered entity, but who assists the covered entity by performing a function or activity that involves individually identifiable health information received from the covered entity.

Calibration — a process of testing and adjusting an instrument or test system to establish a correlation between the measurement response and the concentration or amount of the substance that is being measured by the test procedure.

Calibration verification — the assaying of materials of known concentration in the same manner as patient specimens to substantiate the instrument or test system's calibration throughout the reportable range for patient test results.

CAP — College of American Pathologists.

Carry-over — the discrete amount of analyte carried by the measuring system from one sample reaction into subsequent sample reactions, thereby erroneously affecting the apparent amounts in subsequent samples.

Cause-and-effect diagram — a diagram that traces the flow of work (generally in a horizontal direction, from left to right) and depicts all of the inputs (causes) that can influence the quality of work. Causes are usually depicted as diagonal lines that intersect with the horizontal path of work flow, giving the overall diagram the appearance of a fish vertebral column with intersecting ribs. Also called a fishbone diagram or Ishikawa diagram.

CDC — Centers for Disease Control and Prevention. The CDC is an agency of the United States Department of Health and Human Services (HHS).

Cells — in the Toyota Production System, the layout of machines of different types, performing different operations in a tight sequence, to permit single-piece flow and flexible deployment of human effort by means of multi-machine working. Contrast with process villages.

Certification — (1) as defined by HIPAA, the technical evaluation performed as part of the validation process that establishes the extent to which a particular computer system or network implementation meets a pre-specified set of security requirements; (2) in the context of CLIA, the written assurance that a laboratory conforms to defined standards.

Challenge — in the context of CLIA-mandated proficiency testing for quantitative tests, an assessment of the amount of substance or analyte present or measured in a sample. For qualitative tests, a challenge means the determination of the presence or the absence of an analyte, specific organism, or attribute in a sample.

Chance-cause variation — see Common-cause variation.

CLIA — Clinical Laboratory Improvement Amendments of 1988.

CLIA certificate for provider-performed microscopy (PPM) procedures — a certificate issued to a laboratory in which a physician, midlevel practitioner, or dentist performs no tests other than PPM procedures and, if desired, waived tests.

CLIA certificate of accreditation — a certificate issued on the basis of the laboratory's accreditation by an accreditation organization approved by the Centers for Medicare and Medicaid Services (CMS) (indicating that the laboratory is approved to meet applicable CLIA requirements).

CLIA certificate of compliance — a certificate issued to a laboratory after an inspection that finds the laboratory to be in compliance with all applicable CLIA condition level requirements.

CLIA certificate of registration — a certificate that enables the entity to conduct moderate or high complexity laboratory testing or both until the entity is determined to be in compliance through a survey by the Centers for Medicare and Medicaid Services (CMS) or its agent or an approved accreditation organization. Also called "CLIA registration certificate."

CLIA certificate of waiver — a certificate issued to a laboratory to perform only waived tests.

CLIA-exempt laboratory — a laboratory that has been licensed or approved by a state where the Centers for Medicare and Medicaid Services (CMS) has determined that the state has enacted laws relating to laboratory requirements that are equal to or more stringent than CLIA requirements.

Clinically reportable range (CRR) — a CAP term that refers to the interval of analyte values that a method can accurately report, allowing for specimen dilution, concentration, or other pretreatment used to extend the direct analytical measurement range (AMR). The CLIA term for the clinically reportable range is the "reportable range."

Close call — see Near miss.

CLSI — Clinical and Laboratory Standards Institute (formerly NCCLS, the National Committee on Clinical Laboratory Standards).

CMS — Centers for Medicare and Medicaid Services. This agency of the federal government is located in Baltimore County, Maryland, and has 10 regional offices. It is responsible for administering the CLIA and HIPAA regulations. CMS is an agency of the United States Department of Health and Human Services (HHS).

CMS agent — an entity with which the Centers for Medicare and Medicaid Services (CMS) arranges to inspect laboratories and assess laboratory activities against CLIA requirements. A CMS agent may be a state survey agency, a private nonprofit organization other than an approved accreditation organization, a component of the Department of Health and Human Services (HHS), or any other governmental component CMS approves for this purpose.

Common-cause variation — variation in a process due to variables inherent within the process itself, rather than an extrinsic disturbance in the process. Common-cause variation can be removed only by making changes in the process itself. Also called endogenous-cause, chance-cause, or systemic-cause variation.

Competence — the demonstrated ability to apply knowledge and skills.

Competency — the ability of an individual to correctly perform assigned tasks, including (as applicable) problem solving and troubleshooting.

Condition level deficiency — in the context of CLIA, noncompliance with one or more condition level requirements.

Condition level requirements — any of the requirements identified as "conditions" in applicable parts of the CLIA regulations.

Confidentiality — the property that information is not made available or disclosed to unauthorized individuals, entities, or processes.

Constraint — see Forcing function.

Context-based access — an access control based on the context of a transaction (as opposed to being based on attributes of the initiator or target). Factors used to grant context-based access might include time of day, location of the user, etc.

Contingency plan — as defined by HIPAA, a plan for responding to a system emergency. The plan includes performing backups, preparing critical facilities that can be used to facilitate continuity of operations in the event of an emergency, and recovering from a disaster.

Continuous quality improvement — depending on context, either a philosophy in which an organization commits to improve quality, or actual demonstrable quality improvement.

Contributing factor — additional reason, beyond the root cause, that an event has occurred.

Control — a process, procedure, policy, or invention designed to provide reasonable assurance that specific objectives are achieved, usually by addressing risks. See Internal control and External control.

Corrective action — action to eliminate the cause of a detected nonconformity or other undesirable situation.

Covered entity — as defined by HIPAA, a health plan, health care clearinghouse, or health care provider who transmits any health information in electronic form.

Credible allegation of compliance — in the context of CLIA, a statement or documentation that (1) is made by a representative of a laboratory that has a history of having maintained a commitment to compliance and of taking corrective action when required, (2) is realistic in terms of its being possible to accomplish the required corrective action between the date of the exit conference and the date of the allegation, and (3) indicates that the problem has been resolved.

Critical value — a range of values of an analyte that signals a correctable life-threatening condition that requires prompt notification and clinical intervention.

Customer — organization or person that receives a product or service.

Cycle time — in the Toyota Production System, the time required to complete one cycle of an operation. If the cycle time for every operation in a complete process can be designed to equal the *takt* time, products can be made in single-piece flow.

Data authentication — the corroboration that data has not been altered or destroyed. Examples of how data corroboration may be assured include the use of a check sum, double keying, a message authentication code, or digital signature.

Data backup — a retrievable exact copy of information.

Data backup plan — a documented and routinely updated plan to create and maintain, for a specific period of time, retrievable exact copies of information.

Data integrity — the property that data has not been altered or destroyed in an unauthorized manner.

Digital signature — an electronic signature based upon cryptographic methods of originator **authentication, computed b**y using a set of rules and a set of parameters such that the identity

Disaster recovery plan — part of an overall contingency plan. The plan for restoring data and access to data in the event of fire, vandalism, natural disaster, or system failure.

Electronic data interchange (EDI) — intercompany computer-to-computer transmission of business information in a standard format. For EDI purists, "computer-to-computer" means direct transmission from the originating application program to the receiving, or processing, application program, and an EDI transmission consists only of business data, not any accompanying verbiage or free-form messages.

Electronic signature — the attribute that is affixed to an electronic document to bind it to a particular person or entity.

Encryption — transforming confidential plaintext into ciphertext to protect it. Also called encipherment. An encryption algorithm combines plaintext with other values called keys, or ciphers, so the data becomes unintelligible. Once encrypted, data can be stored or transmitted over unsecured lines. Decrypting data reverses the encryption algorithm process and makes the plaintext available for further processing.

Equipment control — in the context of HIPAA, documented security procedures for bringing hardware and software into and out of a facility and for maintaining a record of that equipment. This includes, but is not limited to, the marking, handling, and disposal of hardware and storage media.

Equivalency — an accreditation organization's or a state laboratory program's requirements, which when taken as a whole, are equal to or more stringent than the CLIA requirements established by the Centers for Medicare and Medicaid Services (CMS), taken as whole. It is acceptable to CMS for an accreditation organization's or state laboratory program's requirements to be organized differently or otherwise vary from the CLIA requirements, so long as (1) all of the requirements, taken as a whole, would provide at least the same protection as the CLIA requirements, taken as a whole; and (2) a finding of noncompliance with respect to CLIA requirements, taken as a whole, would be matched by a finding of noncompliance with the accreditation or state requirements, taken as a whole.

Error — failure of a planned action to be completed as intended, or use of the wrong plan to achieve an aim. The accumulation of errors results in accidents.

Error of commission — an error that occurs as a result of an action taken. Examples include when a drug is administered at the wrong time, in the wrong dosage, or using the wrong route; surgeries performed on the wrong side of the body; and transfusion errors involving blood cross-matched for another patient.

Error of omission — an error which occurs as a result of an action not taken, for example, when a delay in performing an indicated cesarean section results in a fetal death, when a nurse omits a dose of a medication that should be administered, or when a patient's suicide is associated with a lapse in carrying out frequent patient checks in a psychiatric unit.

Event reporting — as defined by HIPAA, a network message indicating operational irregularities in physical elements of a network, or a response to the occurrence of a significant task, typically the completion of a request for information.

Examination — a set of operations having the object of determining the value or characteristics of a property, such as "sodium concentration" or "Gram stain reactivity."

External control — processes external to the organization that provide reasonable assurance that specific objectives are achieved. Examples include external proficiency testing (helping to assure the objective of analytic proficiency) and external inspections (helping to assure conformance with a set of regulatory or accreditation standards).

External proficiency testing — see Proficiency testing.

Facility security plan — a plan to safeguard premises from unauthorized physical access, and to safeguard the equipment therein from unauthorized physical access, tampering, and theft.

Failure mode — a particular path through which a process or subprocess can fail to provide the anticipated result.

Failure Mode and Effects Analysis (FMEA) — a prospective assessment that identifies and improves steps in a process according to their likelihood of failure and the consequences of failure.

FDA — US Food and Drug Administration. The FDA is an agency of the United States Department of Health and Human Services (HHS).

FDA-cleared or approved test system — a test system cleared or approved by the FDA through the premarket notification (510(k)) or premarket approval (PMA) process for in-vitro diagnostic use. Unless otherwise stated, this also includes test systems exempt from FDA premarket clearance or approval.

Fishbone diagram — see Cause-and-effect diagram.

Five "S" — in the Toyota Production System, five terms beginning with the letter "S" that support visual control. *Seiri* means to separate needed tools, parts, and instructions from unneeded materials, and to remove the latter. *Seiton* means to neatly arrange and identify parts and tools for ease of use. *Seiso* means to conduct a cleanup campaign. *Seiketsu* means to conduct *seiri, seiton,* and *seiso* daily to maintain a workplace in perfect condition. *Shitsuke* means to form the habit of always following *seiketsu, seiri, seiton,* and *seiso.*

Flow — in the Toyota Production System, the progressive completion of tasks along the value stream so that a product proceeds from design to launch, order to delivery, and raw materials into the hands of the customer, with no stoppages, scrap, or backflows.

Flow diagram — see Process map.

Forcing function — the design of an instrument or human interface so that it becomes inoperative unless certain preconditions are met. "Lock-out" devices in glucose meters that require quality control testing as a precondition of patient testing are an example of a forcing function that prevents human error. Forcing functions have also been called constraints, and are the equivalent of *poka yoke* in the Toyota Production System.

Fraud — the intentional material misrepresentation of the truth, or suppression of the truth, to gain an advantage.

Hawthorne effect — an increase in performance produced by the psychological stimulus of being singled out and made to feel important.

Hazard analysis — The process of collecting and evaluating information on hazards associated with the selected process. Part of Failure Mode and Effects Analysis.

Health information — as defined by HIPAA, any information, whether oral or recorded in any form or medium, that (1) is created or received by a health care provider, health plan, public health authority, employer, life insurer, school or university, or health care clearinghouse; and (2) relates to the past, present, or future physical or mental health or condition of an individual, the provision of health care to an individual, or the past, present, or future payment for the provision of health care to an individual.

HHS — United States Department of Health and Human Services. HHS agencies include the Centers for Disease Control and Prevention (CDC), the Centers for Medicare and Medicaid Services (CMS), the US Food and Drug Administration (FDA), and others.

HIPAA — Health Insurance Portability and Accountability Act of 1996.

Human factors — study of the inter-relationships between humans, the tools they use, and the environment in which they live and work.

Human factors design — design of devices or systems to support or enhance human performance. The opposite is a design that forces the user to stretch—to make extra effort—in order to interact successfully with the device or system. Dangerous devices may trip users into unintentional error.

Immediate jeopardy — in the context of CLIA, a situation in which immediate corrective action is necessary because the laboratory's noncompliance with one or more condition level requirements has already caused, is causing, or is likely to cause, at any time, serious injury or harm, or death, to individuals served by the laboratory, or to the health or safety of the general public. This term is synonymous with imminent and serious risk to human health and significant hazard to the public health.

Imprecision — the dispersion of independent results of measurements obtained under specified conditions. Imprecision is expressed numerically as standard deviation or coefficient of variation.

Incident — an individual occurrence or event, in which some process or outcome deviated from the expected.

Individually identifiable health information — health information that identifies the individual, or with respect to which there is a reasonable basis to believe the information can be used to identify the individual.

Information access control — formal documented policies and procedures for granting different levels of access to health care information.

Integrity controls — security mechanism employed to ensure the validity of the information being electronically transmitted or stored.

Intentional unsafe acts — in the context of patient safety, events that threaten patient safety and which result from a criminal act, a purposefully unsafe act, an act related to alcohol or substance abuse or other cause of negligible impairment, or events involving patient abuse.

Intentional violation — in the context of CLIA compliance, knowing and willful noncompliance with any CLIA condition.

Internal audit — as defined by HIPAA, an in-house review of the records of system activity (for example, logins, file accesses, security incidents) maintained by an organization.

Internal control — processes within an organization, effected by owners, managers, and personnel, designed to provide reasonable assurance that specific objectives are achieved. Examples in the laboratory include running quality control specimens along with patient samples (helping to ensure the objective of analytic accuracy) and checking two forms of identification on every patient (helping to ensure the objective of accurate patient identification).

Ishikawa diagram — see Cause-and-effect diagram.

ISO — International Organization for Standardization.

JCAHO — Joint Commission on Accreditation of Healthcare Organizations.

Jidoka — in the Toyota Production System, building quality into the production process. One form of *Jidoka* is stopping the entire production line or process when something goes amiss.

Just-in-time — a system for producing and delivering the right items at the right time in the right amounts so that inventory is minimized. Also referred to as *Kanban*.

Kaizen — in the Toyota Production System, continuous incremental improvement of an activity to create more value with less waste.

Kanban — see Just-in-time.

Key — in cryptography, an input that controls the transformation of data by an encryption algorithm.

Kit — all components of a test that are packaged together.

Laboratory — in the context of CLIA, a facility for the biological, microbiological, serological, chemical, immunohematological, hematological, biophysical, cytological, pathological, or other examination of materials derived from the human body for the purpose of providing information for the diagnosis, prevention, or treatment of any disease or impairment, or the assessment of the health of human beings. Facilities only collecting or preparing specimens (or both), or only serving as a mailing service and not performing testing, are not considered laboratories.

Laboratory director — for laboratories performing nonwaived testing, an individual who meets the qualification requirements of section §493.1405 of CLIA and provides overall management and direction in accordance with section §493.1407 of CLIA. See Exhibit 6 for a list of responsibilities CLIA assigns to the laboratory director.

LAP — Laboratory Accreditation Program of the College of American Pathologists.

Lapse — an error of omission while operating in the schematic control mode.

Latent error — an error in design, organization, training, or maintenance that leads to operator errors and whose effects typically lie dormant in the system for lengthy periods of time. Contrast with active error.

Lean production — see Toyota Production System.

Linear drift — a change in measurement value over time due to factors other than the concentration of the analyte being measured.

Linearity — the ability of a test system to provide results that are directly proportional to the concentration of the analyte in the test sample, over a defined range.

Maintenance records — documentation of repairs and modifications to the physical components of a facility, for example, hardware, instruments, software, walls, doors, locks.

Matrix — all components of a specimen, control, or calibrator, except the analyte.

Matrix effect — the effect (interference) of the matrix on the ability of a procedure to accurately measure an analyte.

Media controls — formal documented policies and procedures that govern the receipt and removal of hardware/software (for example, diskettes, tapes) into and out of a facility.

Medical device — as defined in the Safe Medical Devices Act of 1990, any instrument, apparatus, or other article that is used to prevent, diagnose, mitigate, or treat a disease, or to affect the structure or function of the body, with the exception of drugs. For example, medical devices include, but are not limited to, ventilators, monitors, dialyzers, and any other electronic equipment, implants, thermometers, patient restraints, syringes, catheters, in vitro diagnostic test kits and reagents, disposables, components, parts, accessories, and related software. The Safe Medical Devices Act of 1990 requires that adverse patient events associated with medical devices are to be reported to the US Food and Drug Administration (FDA).

Message authentication — ensuring, typically with a code, that a message received (usually via a network) matches the message sent.

Mistake — an error in judgment or intentional action.

Muda — literally, "waste" in Japanese. In the Toyota Production System, *muda* is any activity that consumes resources but creates no value.

NCCLS — National Committee on Clinical Laboratory Standards. The organization has changed its name to CLSI (Clinical and Laboratory Standards Institute).

Near miss — an error that has the potential to cause patient harm but does not, either by chance or because the error was detected before harm resulted. Some near misses are detected before a test has been reported (eg, a pathologist notices that the tissue on a glass slide does not match the pathology requisition; the labeling error is discovered and corrected before the case is signed out), while others are detected after the result has been reported (eg, a surgeon calls to say that the cancer diagnosis report he or she received does not belong to Mr. Jones, as stated on the pathology report, because Mr. Jones did not have a biopsy). Also referred to as a close call.

Nonwaived test — any test system, assay, or examination that has not been found to meet the statutory criteria specified at section 353(d)(3) of the Public Health Service Act.

Normal range — see Biological reference interval.

Operational definition — a practical method for making determinations, as opposed to some theoretical definition that cannot be applied. An operational definition of acceptable turnaround time for emergency department testing might consist of instructions about how to measure turnaround time of specimens coming from the emergency department, along with an objective standard for what constitutes acceptable turnaround time.

Operator — in the context of CLIA, the individual or group of individuals who oversees all facets of the operation of a laboratory and who bears primary responsibility for the safety and reliability of the results of all specimen testing performed in that laboratory. The term includes (1) a director of the laboratory, if he or she meets the stated criteria; and (2) the members of the board of directors and the officers of a laboratory that is a small corporation under subchapter S of the Internal Revenue Code. In popular use, "operator" refers to testing personnel, as opposed to owners or managers.

Outlier — an observation in a sample so far separated in value from the remainder as to suggest that it may be from a different population or the result of an error in measurement.

Owner — in the context of CLIA, any person who owns any interest in a laboratory except for an interest in a laboratory whose stock and/or securities are publicly traded.

Pareto chart — a histogram that shows the relative importance of different groups of data.

Password — confidential authentication information composed of a string of characters (letters or numbers).

Path of workflow — a unique sequence of processes and procedures necessary to produce a specific service or product.

Patient safety — freedom from accident or injury that results from the delivery of health care.

Patient safety event — an injury, illness, or potential injury that is directly linked to the delivery of health care.

Performance characteristic — a property of a test that is used to describe its quality, eg, accuracy, precision, analytical sensitivity, analytical specificity, reportable range, reference range.

Performance specification — a value or range of values for a performance characteristic, established or verified by the laboratory, that is used to describe the quality of patient test results.

Physical access controls — as defined by HIPAA, the formal documented policies and procedures to be followed to limit physical access to an entity, while ensuring that properly authorized access is allowed.

Physical safeguards — as defined by HIPAA, protection of physical computer systems and related buildings and equipment from fire and other natural and environmental hazards, as well as from intrusion. Also covers the use of locks and keys to control access to computer systems and facilities.

Physician — in the context of CLIA, an individual with a doctor of medicine, doctor of osteopathy, or doctor of podiatric medicine degree who is licensed by the state to practice medicine, osteopathy, or podiatry within the state in which a laboratory is located.

Plan-Do-Study-Act — a rapid, simple method of quality improvement proposed by Shewhart, which involves the design of a change to improve a process ("Plan"), implementation of the change on a test basis ("Do"), evaluation of the impact of the change on process variation and bias ("Study"), and, if the change is successful, implementation on an ongoing basis ("Act"). Plan-Do-Study-Act is sometimes called Plan-Do-Check-Act.

Poka yoke — in the Toyota Production System, mistake-proofing a device or procedure to prevent a defect. This might consist of a computer input application that prevents entry of nonsensical values, or an analyzer that will not test patient samples until quality control testing has been completed satisfactorily. *Poka yoke* is equivalent to the term "forcing function" used by human factors researchers.

Policy — documented statements of an organization's intentions or commitments.

Post-examination procedures — postanalytical phase processes following an examination, including systematic review, formatting and interpretation, authorization for release, reporting and transmission of the results, and storage of samples of the examination.

Potential adverse event — see Near miss.

Precision — the closeness of agreement between independent test results obtained under defined conditions.

Pre-examination procedures — preanalytical phase steps starting with a clinician's request for testing, and including order communication, preparation of the patient, collection of the primary sample, transportation to and within the laboratory, and ending when the analytical examination procedure begins.

Preventive action — action to eliminate the cause of a potential nonconformity or any other undesirable potential situation.

Preventive maintenance — scheduled periodic work on a piece of equipment that is not a result of malfunction or failure and is intended to avert such failure.

Primary sample — specimen.

Principal sanction — the suspension, limitation, or revocation of any type of CLIA certificate, or the cancellation of the laboratory's approval to receive Medicare payment for its services.

Principle — in the context of a procedure, a principle is a tenet upon which the procedure relies. In some cases, the principle is a policy (such as an organizational commitment to comply with a particular regulatory standard or a commitment to honesty); in other cases, the principle may be a scientific or technical fact (such as the fact that the bacterial enzyme catalase catalyzes the conversion of hydrogen peroxide to water and oxygen).

Procedure — documented instructions that an individual follows in order to correctly perform an activity or step in a larger process.

Process — a documented chain of steps that helps an organization carry out its policies or meet an objective. A process specifies the order of steps, the inputs for each step (staff, equipment, materials, information), and the expected outcome of each step. When an individual is responsible for performing a step in the process, instructions for performing the step are described in a procedure.

Process management — the design and implementation of processes to produce a product that consistently meets specifications.

Process map — a visual diagram of a process, indicating each step and decision point. Sometimes called a flow chart or workflow diagram.

Process villages — in the Toyota Production System, process village refers to the undesirable practice of grouping machines or activities by type of operation performed, rather than by its natural place in the workflow. Contrast with cells.

Proficiency testing — a program in which multiple samples or challenges are periodically sent to members of a group of laboratories for analysis and/or identification, in which each laboratory's results are compared with those of other laboratories in the group and/or with an assigned value. Also called external proficiency testing.

Prospective laboratory — in the context of CLIA, a laboratory that is operating under a registration certificate and is seeking any of the three other types of CLIA certificates.

Pull — in the Toyota Production System, a system in which the customer expressing a need creates a progressive cascade of signals down the production chain to stimulate production.

Q-Probes — the brand name of a quality management product produced by the CAP, in which subscribers measure the quality of a particular aspect of laboratory service at one point in time and compare local performance to performance in other institutions.

QSE — see Quality system essentials.

Q-Tracks — the brand name of a quality management product produced by the CAP, in which subscribers periodically measure the quality of a particular aspect of laboratory service, track performance over time, and compare local performance to performance in other institutions.

Quality — all the features of a product that meet the requirements of a customer or the requirements of society (as expressed in applicable laws and regulations).

Quality assurance — a system of quality control activities that promotes the quality of higher-level processes and functions. These higher-level processes are typically composed of multiple steps, each of which may fail and each of which are individually subject to quality control. Quality assurance is best applied to all steps in the laboratory test cycle, including integrity of the test ordering process and collection process, analyses, and the reporting of results, as well as to other important variables that impact quality, such as the training of laboratory personnel.

Quality control — activities that ensure that specific processes and basic functions meet acceptable parameters. Quality control may be applied to an analytic instrument, a centrifuge or water bath, or specimen labeling. Intrinsic to quality control are the development of standards of acceptable performance, a system for measuring performance, and rejection (or remediation) of product that does not meet acceptable standards. Quality control is an integral component of quality assurance.

Quality improvement — an effort to improve the quality of product beyond its current state. Quality may be improved by a properly designed and implemented quality assurance program. Quality may also be improved by redesigning a process—eliminating unnecessary steps or reworking operations that have a high risk of failure.

Quality laboratory practice — any control designed to promote laboratory quality.

Quality management — the application of quality management systems to an operation. Different approaches to managing quality are described in chapter 3 of this manual; all involve the application of one or more quality management systems.

Quality management systems — the processes through which an organization exerts control over the quality of its product and operations, meeting a customer's quality requirements and complying with applicable regulations.

Quality planning — organized research into customers' needs, with development of products that meet those needs, processes that allow the products to be created, and controls that allow the processes to function as intended.

Quality system essentials — in the Clinical and Laboratory Standards Institute (CLSI) formulation, quality system essentials (or QSEs) are necessary elements of a quality management system. An example of a QSE might be adequate policies, processes, and procedures for acquiring and maintaining equipment. QSEs are controls or quality laboratory practices that CLSI considers essential.

Queue time — the time a patient or specimen spends in a line awaiting the next operation.

Referee laboratory — a laboratory currently in compliance with applicable CLIA requirements that has had a record of satisfactory proficiency testing performance for all testing events for at least one year for a specific test, analyte, subspecialty, or specialty, and has been designated by an HHS-approved proficiency testing program for the purpose of determining the correct response for the specimens in a testing event for that specific test, analyte, subspecialty, or specialty.

Reference interval — see Biological reference interval.

Reference range — see Biological reference interval.

Reportable range — a CLIA term for the span of test result values over which the laboratory can establish or verify the accuracy of the instrument or test system measurement response. The CAP term for reportable range is the clinically reportable range (CRR).

Risk analysis — a process through which cost-effective security/control measures are selected, by balancing the costs of various security/control measures against the losses that would be expected if these measures were not in place.

Root cause — the most fundamental reason an event has occurred.

Root cause analysis — a process for identifying the basic or causal factors that underlie variation in performance. A root cause analysis focuses primarily on systems and processes, not individual performance. It progresses from special causes related to a particular incident to common causes embedded within organizational processes, and may identify improvements in processes or systems that decrease the likelihood of such events in the future.

Safety — freedom from accident.

Sample — in proficiency testing, the material contained in a vial, on a slide, or other unit that contains material to be tested by proficiency testing program participants. When possible, samples are of human origin.

Security — as defined by HIPAA, security encompasses all of the safeguards in an information system, including hardware, software, personnel policies, information practice policies, disaster preparedness, and the oversight of all these areas. The purpose of security is to protect both the system and the information it contains from unauthorized access and from misuse.

Security management process — a security management process encompasses the creation, administration and oversight of policies to ensure the prevention, detection, containment, and correction of security breaches. It involves risk analysis and risk management, including the establishment of accountability, management controls (policies and education), electronic controls, physical security, and penalties for the abuse and misuse of assets, both physical and electronic.

Security testing — a process used to determine that the security features of a system are implemented as designed and that they are adequate for a proposed applications environment. This process includes hands-on functional testing, penetration testing, and verification.

Sentinel event — an unexpected occurrence involving death or serious physical or psychological injury, or the risk thereof. Serious injury specifically includes loss of limb or function. The phrase "or the risk thereof" includes any process variation for which a recurrence would carry a significant chance of a serious adverse outcome.

Single-piece flow — a situation in which products or specimens proceed one at a time through the production or testing cycle without interruptions or queues. Contrast with batch-and-queue.

Slip — an error of unconscious action in which an actor does something unintended. A slip is an error of commission while operating in the schematic control mode.

Social facilitation — improved human performance in group settings. The group can be coactors (performing the same task as the subject) or an audience (observing the subject as passive spectators).

Spaghetti chart — a map of the path taken by a specific product or specimen as it travels down the value stream in a mass-production organization, so-called because the product's route typically looks like a plate of spaghetti. In the Toyota Production System, the spaghetti chart is eliminated.

Special-cause variation — see Assignable-cause variation.

Specificity — the ability of a test or procedure to correctly identify or quantify an entity in the presence of interfering phenomena. In quantitative testing, specificity is the ability of a measurement procedure to determine only the component it purports to measure, and not other substances present in the sample. In qualitative or semiquantitative tests, specificity is the method's ability to obtain negative results in concordance with negative results obtained by a reference method.

State licensure — in the context of CLIA, the issuance of a license to, or the approval of, a laboratory by a state laboratory program as meeting standards for licensing or approval established under state law.

State licensure program — in the context of CLIA, a state laboratory licensure or approval program.

State survey agency — the state health agency or other appropriate state or local agency that has an agreement under section 1864 of the Social Security Act and is used by the Centers for Medicare and Medicaid Services (CMS) to perform surveys and inspections.

Statistical control — a state in which all remaining variation is the result of apparently random, unexplainable factors.

Statistical process control — the use of statistical methods to measure (and ultimately control) the quality of a process.

Statistical quality control — see Statistical process control.

Substantial allegation of noncompliance — in the context of CLIA, a complaint from any of a variety of sources (including complaints submitted in person, by telephone, through written correspondence, or in newspaper or magazine articles) that, if substantiated, would have an impact on the health and safety of the general public or of individuals served by a laboratory, and raises doubts as to a laboratory's compliance with any condition level requirement.

Supplier — organization or person that provides a product or a service.

System — a set of interdependent elements interacting to achieve a common aim. Elements of a system may include, but are not limited to, technology, equipment, the environment, policies, procedures, and human operators.

***Takt* time** — in the Toyota Production System, the available production time divided by the rate of customer demand. *Takt* time sets the pace of production to match the rate of customer demand and becomes the heartbeat of any lean production system.

Target value — for proficiency testing of quantitative tests, either the mean of all participant responses after removal of outliers (those responses greater than 3 standard deviations from the original mean), or the mean established by definitive or reference methods acceptable for use in the National Reference System for the Clinical Laboratory (NRSCL) by CLSI. In instances where definitive or reference methods are not available, or a specific method's results demonstrate bias that is not observed with actual patient specimens, as determined by a defensible scientific protocol, a comparative method or a method group ("peer" group) may be used. If the method group is less than 10 participants, "target value" means the overall mean after outlier removal (as defined above), unless acceptable scientific reasons are available to indicate that such an evaluation is not appropriate.

Termination procedures — in the context of HIPAA, formal documented instructions, which include appropriate security measures, for the ending of an employee's employment or an internal/external user's access.

Test system — the instructions and all of the instrumentation, equipment, reagent, and supplies needed to perform an assay or examination and generate test results.

Token — a physical item that is used to prove identity. Typically an electronic device that can be inserted in a door or a computer system to obtain access.

Total quality management (TQM) — a practical philosophy of excellence concerned with how best to organize a business to apply statistical process control to quality and productivity.

Toyota Production System — an example of total quality management applied within an individual company (Toyota). The term "lean production" refers to any production process based on the methods applied at Toyota.

Traceability — a measurement or value that can be related to a stated reference, usually a national or international standard, through an unbroken chain of comparisons, all having stated uncertainties.

Trueness of measurement — closeness of agreement between the average value obtained from a large series of results of measurements and a true value.

Uncertainty of measurement — a parameter associated with the result of a measurement, that characterizes the dispersion of the values that could reasonably be attributed to the measurand/analyte.

Unique user identification — the combination name/number assigned and maintained in security procedures for identifying and tracking individual user identity.

Unsatisfactory proficiency testing performance — failure to attain the minimum satisfactory score for an analyte, test, subspecialty, or specialty for a testing event.

Unsuccessful participation in proficiency testing — in the context of CLIA, any of the following: (1) unsatisfactory performance for the same analyte in two consecutive or two out of three testing events; (2) repeated unsatisfactory overall testing event scores for two consecutive or two out of three testing events for the same specialty or subspecialty; (3) an unsatisfactory testing event score for those subspecialties not graded by analyte (that is, bacteriology, mycobacteriology, virology, parasitology, mycology, blood compatibility, immunohematology, or syphilis serology) for the same subspecialty for two consecutive or two out of three testing events; (4) failure of a laboratory performing gynecologic cytology to meet CLIA standard §493.855.

Unsuccessful proficiency testing performance — failure to attain the minimum satisfactory score for an analyte, test, subspecialty, or specialty for two consecutive or two out of three consecutive testing events.

User-based access — a security mechanism used to grant users of a system access based upon the identity of the user.

Validation — confirmation through a defined process that a method performs as intended.

Value — in the Toyota Production System, a capability provided to a customer at the right time at an appropriate price, as defined in each case by the customer.

Value stream — the activities required to design and provide a specific service, from concept to launch and from order to result. In the laboratory, the value stream includes the activities of suppliers (such as reagent manufacturers) and intermediate customers (such as phlebotomists, technologists, and hands-on caregivers) as well as the ultimate customer (the patient).

Visual control — in the Toyota Production System, the placement in plain view of all tools, parts, production activities, and indicators of production system performance, so the status of the system can be understood at a glance by everyone involved.

Waived test — a test system, assay, or examination that the United States Department of Health and Human Services (HHS) has determined meets the CLIA statutory criteria as specified for waiver under section 353(d)(3) of the Public Health Service Act.

Workflow diagram — see Process map.

Notes and References

1. Nakhleh RE, Fitzgibbons PL. *Quality Management in Anatomic Pathology: Promoting Patient Safety Through Systems Improvement and Error Reduction.* Northfield, Ill: College of American Pathologists; 2005.

2. Contemporary business authors and consultants frequently expand the boundaries of quality management schools, sometimes leaving them unrecognizable. We have endeavored to summarize each approach to quality management in its original form, as described by its original proponents. Even in their original form, many of the major schools of quality management are not easily separated. The Toyota Production System benefited from the work of W. Edwards Deming, who founded the total quality management movement, and also from Henry Ford's innovations. Deming, in turn, developed many of his ideas while working at Western Electric's Hawthorne Works plant, where Shewhart pioneered statistical process control and where, in later years, seminal experiments in industrial psychology and "scientific management" were conducted.

3. A great deal of empiric evidence collected by Shewhart and colleagues supported Shewhart's assertion that processes not in statistical control were more likely to produce defective product than processes that functioned within statistical limits. In addition to numerous studies within Western Electric, Shewhart was able to demonstrate that bakeries that brought their production processes into tight statistical control produced less defective product than bakeries that demonstrated wider variation in product. There is no statistical reason why this should be the case—processes in tight statistical control might converge about a mean that does not meet performance standards. However, in practice, processes in statistical control tend to produce fewer defects.

4. Shewhart recognized that, in some cases, processes in statistical control did not produce product of acceptable quality. In this case, new production processes had to be devised because the old production process, even with all special-cause variation eliminated, was inadequate to produce goods that met required quality standards.

5. Shewhart WA. *Economic Control of Quality of Manufactured Product.* New York: D Van Nostrand Company Inc; 1931. Readers who are looking for a "how-to" manual on statistical quality control will not be satisfied with Shewhart's seminal monograph. Shewhart's writing is dense, and his demanding treatise draws from differential and integral calculus, Alexander Pope on chance, and Aristotle on the manifold nature of quality.

6. Levey S, Jennings ER. The use of control charts in the clinical laboratory. *Am J Clin Pathol.* 1950;20:1059-1066.

7. The steps shown in this figure correspond to recommendations made early in the development of statistical process control methods. A more recent discussion can be found in the NCCLS (now Clinical and Laboratory Standards Institute [CLSI]) document, *Statistical Quality Control for Quantitative Measurements: Principles and Definitions.* Approved Guideline. 2nd ed. Wayne, Pa: NCCLS; 1999.

8. The Pareto chart was originally developed in 1906 by Vilfredo Pareto, a noted Italian economist and sociologist who was also involved with the early stages of the fascist movement. Pareto believed that, for a wide variety of processes, 80% of problems were produced by 20% of causes. The chart was introduced into the total quality management movement by Joseph Juran and is sometimes incorrectly attributed to Juran.

9. Valenstein P. Preanalytic delays as a component of laboratory turnaround time. *Lab Med.* 1990;21:448-451.

10. There are certain circumstances in which it may be permissible to retest a control solution once without rerunning patient specimens. See page 96.

11. Cystatin C has recently been proposed as a marker of renal function that can be measured more reproducibly than creatinine. See Shlipak MG, Sarnak MJ, Katz R, et al. Cystatin C and the risk of death and cardiovascular events among elderly persons. *N Engl J Med.* 2005;352:2049-2060. At the time of this writing, the susceptibility of cystatin C assays to interfering substances has not been adequately studied. Therefore, serum cystatin C is not yet a suitable substitute for creatinine as a marker of renal function.

12. The founders of total quality management have together written dozens of articles and books on the subject. The most readable is Deming WE. *Out of the Crisis.* Cambridge, Mass: MIT Center for Advanced Engineering Study; 1982. A second illuminating source written near the end of Deming's life is Deming WE. *The New Economics for Industry, Government, and Education.* Cambridge, Mass: MIT Center for Advanced Engineering Study; 1994. Joseph Juran was critical of Deming's *Out of Crisis* because he believed it overemphasized statistical process control and did not give sufficient weight to innovative quality thinking from the customer's perspective. For a healthy counterpoint to *Out of Crisis,* read Juran JM. *Planning for Quality.* New York: Free Press; 1988.

13. See Ishikawa K. *Guide to Quality Control.* White Plains, NY: Quality Resources; 1982.

14. See pages 90-92 of Deming. *Out of the Crisis.* op. cit.

15. See pages 322-324 of Deming. *Out of the Crisis.* op. cit.

16. Deming suffered from some glaring misunderstandings of economics, although his deficiencies are not of particular concern to the manger of a clinical laboratory and do not detract from total quality management (TQM) as a quality management tool. Deming misunderstood the role of service industries in international trade and the importance of antitrust safeguards, and too quickly dismissed the importance of formal and transparent financial accounting—a shortcoming that hobbled a number of high-quality Japanese companies during the 1990s.

17. This section was written by Stephen Raab, MD, and Paul Valenstein, MD.

18. Liker J. *The Toyota Way: 14 Management Principles in the World's Greatest Manufacturer.* New York: McGraw-Hill; 2004.

19. The most recent edition of the Womack and Jones book describing the Toyota Production System is Womack JP, Jones DT. *Lean Thinking.* New York: Free Press; 2003. This book was originally published in 1996. Information about the Toyota Production System can also be found at Womack's and Jones' respective web sites (www.lean.org and www.leanuk.org), and in their first book about Toyota's production methods: James P, Womack JP, Jones DT, Roos D. *The Machine That Changed the World: The Story of Lean Production.* New York: Macmillan; 1990.

20. Spear S, Bwen K. Decoding the DNA of the Toyota Production System. *Harvard Business Review.* September-October, 1999.

21. Jennifer LC, Sharbaugh DT, Raab SS. Error-free pathology: applying lean production methods to anatomic pathology. *Clin Lab Med.* 2004;24:865-899.

22. Scholars who have studied the Toyota Production System also credit W. Edwards Deming, who brought statistical process control and total quality management to Japan; Eli Whitney, who introduced the concept of interchangeable parts (as well as the cotton gin); Henry Ford, who pioneered the assembly line—the forerunner of continuous flow in the automobile industry; Frederick Taylor, who emphasized the importance of standardizing work methods; and General Motors' Alfred P. Sloan, who developed business strategies for managing large enterprises.

23. Treadway JC (chairman). *Report of the National Commission on Fraudulent Financial Reporting.* New York: Committee of Sponsoring Organizations of the Treadway Commission; 1987. Available in electronic form free of charge from the COSO web site (www.coso.org).

24. Financial Executives Research Foundation. What is COSO? Issues Alert April 2003. Available at: http://www.fei.org/rf/membersonly/IA_Format.pdf. Accessed November 27, 2004.

25. Committee of Sponsoring Organizations of the Treadway Commission. *Internal Control - Integrated Framework.* New York: American Institute of Certified Public Accountants; 1994. An executive summary is available free of charge from the COSO web site (www.coso.org). The entire report can be ordered from the American Institute of Certified Public Accountants (www.aicpa.org).

26. Because "International Organization for Standardization" would have different abbreviations in different languages ("IOS" in English, "OIN" in French, etc), it was decided at the outset to use a word derived from the Greek *isos* ("equal") to represent the organization. Therefore, whatever the country, whatever the language, the short form of the organization's name is always "ISO."

27. ISO 15189:2003 is also based on ISO 17025:1999 (general requirements for the competence of testing and calibration laboratories) but provides specific requirements for its implementation in medical laboratories. ISO 15189:2003 was developed by ISO technical committee ISO/TC 212, Clinical laboratory testing and in vitro diagnostic test systems, working group WG 1, Quality Management in the Clinical Laboratory, with input from ISO/TC 176, Quality Management and Quality Assurance and ISO's Committee on Conformity Assessment. In 2005, ISO generated a technical reference document (TR 22869:2005) that provides guidance to medical laboratories interested in implementing a quality system to meet the specific technical and management requirements for quality and competence in ISO 15189:2003.

28. The FDA does not always adhere to CLSI antimicrobial susceptibility breakpoints when approving package inserts for antimicrobial drugs. In spite of this, almost all clinical microbiology laboratories in the United States use CLSI interpretive standards for antimicrobial susceptibility testing.

29. Exhibit 5 has been reproduced from the NCCLS (now Clinical and Laboratory Standards Institute [CLSI]) document, *A Quality System Model For Health Care.* Approved Guideline. Wayne, Pa: NCCLS; 2002: HS1-A.

30. This section was written by Deborah Sesok-Pizzini, MD, and Paul Valenstein, MD.

31. The current military standard of FMEA is MIL-STD-1629. The military refers to FMEA as "Failure Mode Effects and Criticality Analysis" (FMECA).

32. Information about the VA patient safety efforts and HFMEA can be found at http://www.va.gov/ncps/index.html.

33. Performance improvement. In: *2002 Comprehensive Accreditation Manual for Hospitals.* Oakbrook Terrace, Ill: Joint Commission on Accreditation of Healthcare Organizations; 2001: 200-201.

34. To address this disparity, it has been recommended that severity-by-probability grids be used for risk mapping. However, these must also be interpreted with caution because the most catastrophic events are not necessarily the most probable.

35. Hofer TP, Hayward RA. Are bad outcomes from questionable clinical decisions preventable medical errors? A case of cascade iatrogenesis. *Ann Intern Med.* 2002;137:327-333.

36. Triplett N. The dynamogenic factors in pacemaking and competition. *Am J Psychol.* 1898;9:507-533.

37. Meumann E. 1904. Haus und Shularbeit: experimente an kindern der volkschule. *Die Deutsche Schule.* 1904;8:278-303, 337-359, 416-431.

38. The Hawthorne Works was the birthplace of many modern innovations, such as the first public address system. The plant also pioneered quality control practices and principles. Two leaders of the quality movement, W. Edwards Deming and Joseph Juran, started their careers at the Hawthorne Works (see section in this chapter on total quality management). Although the Hawthorne Works was closed in 1983 and the site of the main Hawthorne building is now a shopping mall, the old cable plant and water tower remain standing as of this writing.

39. For an in-depth account of the Hawthorne Works experiments, see Gillespie R. *Manufacturing Knowledge: A History of the Hawthorne Experiments.* Cambridge University Press; 1993. Gillespie argues that many of the conclusions drawn by Mayo about the Hawthorne Works experiments were biased by a specific sociopolitical agenda and views about management prevailing at the time.

40. See Novis DA. Detecting and preventing the occurrence of errors in the practices of laboratory medicine and anatomic pathology: 15 years' experience with the College of American Pathologists' Q-Probes and Q-Tracks programs. *Clin Lab Med.* 2004;24:965-978; and Zarbo RJ, Jones BA, Friedberg RV, et al. Q-Tracks: a College of American Pathologists program of continuous laboratory monitoring and longitudinal performance tracking. *Arch Pathol Lab Med.* 2002;126:1036-1044.

41. This section was written by Ron Sirota, MD, and Paul Valenstein, MD.

42. Leape LL. Error in medicine. *JAMA.* 1994;272:1851-1857.

43. Reason J. *Human Error.* Cambridge, England/New York: Cambridge University Press; 1990.

44. Rasmussen J. Skills, rules, knowledge: signals, signs and symbols and other distinctions in human performance models. *IEEE Transactions: Systems, Man & Cybernetics.* 1983;SMV-13:257-266.

45. Bartlett FC. *Remembering: A Study in Experimental and Social Psychology.* Cambridge, England: Cambridge University Press; 1932.

46. Schnitt SJ, Connolly JL, Tavassoli FA, et al. Interobserver reproducibility in the diagnosis of ductal proliferative breast lesions using standardized criteria. *Am J Surg Pathol.* 1992;16:1133-1143.

47. Reason J. *Managing the Risks of Organizational Accidents.* Aldershot, Hampshire, UK: Ashgate Publishing Ltd; 1997.

48. Reason J. Human error: models and management. *BMJ.* 2000;320:768-770.

49. Some of the earliest work in this area was published by Ronan WW. *Training for Emergency Procedures in Multi-Engine Aircraft. AIR-153-53-FR-44.* Pittsburgh, Pa: American Institutes for Research; 1953; and by Grinker RR, Spiegel JP. *Men Under Stress.* New York: McGraw-Hill, 1963.

50. In addition to short-term memory and problem solving, planning is also considered one of the weakest parts of human cognition. Seasoned managers of clinical laboratories recognize that the designers of instruments and test systems cannot anticipate and plan for all possible failures of their products. Therefore, work processes in the laboratory should be developed with the expectation that equipment and test systems will periodically fail, as will the humans who operate these systems.

51. See Sanders CC, Peyret M, Moland ES, et al. Potential impact of the VITEK 2 system and the Advanced Expert System on the clinical laboratory of a university-based hospital. *J Clin Microbiol.* 2001;39:2379-2385. Also see Barry J, Brown A, Ensor V, et al. Comparative evaluation of the VITEK 2 Advanced Expert System (AES) in five UK hospitals. *J Antimicrob Chemother.* 2003;51:1191-1202.

52. Fire alarms in many United States hospitals, which must be regularly tested, are an example of a warning system that lacks specificity and becomes counterproductive; most hospital workers have been trained by frequent tests to ignore fire alarms. Someday tragedy may result.

53. Valenstein P, Howanitz PJ. Ordering accuracy: a College of American Pathologists Q-Probes study of 577 institutions. *Arch Pathol Lab Med.* 1995;119:117-122.

54. Certain forensic and research laboratories that do not issue results for patient management are exempted from CLIA, as is certain drug testing performed by laboratories certified by the Substance Abuse and Mental Health Services Administration (SAMHSA). States that maintain certification programs with standards equal to or more stringent than CLIA may substitute state certification for federal certification. In addition, federal agencies that operate clinical laboratories (including the Veterans Administration) have the right to adopt their own quality standards in lieu of CLIA standards.

55. This definition is found in the Safe Medical Devices Act of 1990.

56. For reporting deviations related to blood products to the FDA, see §606.171 in the November 7, 2000, *Federal Register.* Adverse events associated with medical devices should be reported on FDA Form 3500A. Fatalities associated with transfusion or donation are reported to the FDA's Center for Biologics Evaluation and Research (CBER). Other specific deviations related to biologics must also be reported to the FDA. In general, it is advisable to consult with your institution's risk management department before reporting an adverse event to the FDA.

57. Guidelines related to validation testing of medical software can be found in the FDA publication, *General Principles of Software Validation; Final Guidance for Industry and FDA*

Staff. January 11, 2002. Available at http://www.fda.gov/cdrh/comp/guidance/938.html. Accessed July 25, 2005.

58. Results that rely on certain classes of analyte-specific reagents (Class I ASRs) do not have special reporting requirements. However, results that rely on other classes of ASRs must be reported with certain FDA-specified disclaimers. For more details, consult the CAP LAP checklists and the CAP publication, *Quality Management in Anatomic Pathology: Promoting Patient Safety Through Systems Improvement and Error Reduction* (2005).

59. In order for a hospital to accept Medicare and Medicaid patients, it must meet certain Conditions of Participation (CoPs) established by CMS. In 1965, Congress passed a law awarding the Joint Commission the ability to determine whether hospitals meet CoPs, and most hospitals choose to demonstrate compliance with CoPs by participating in JCAHO's hospital accreditation program. Currently, 49 states allow JCAHO hospital accreditation as a full or partial substitute for meeting health care quality standards and other requirements for state licensure. In 2002, JCAHO accredited 4211 (82%) of Medicare-participating hospitals. The remaining 18% of hospitals chose to be accredited by the American Osteopathic Association (AOA) or were certified by state survey and certification agencies.

60. The JCAHO hospital accreditation program is primarily concerned with assuring compliance with CMS' Conditions of Participation for hospitals. The JCAHO laboratory accreditation program is primarily concerned with assuring laboratory compliance with CLIA standards. JCAHO has done a reasonable job distinguishing between its hospital and laboratory accreditation programs. The JCAHO laboratory accreditation program is optional for laboratories that operate within a JCAHO-accredited hospital, and is discussed in this chapter under the subsection entitled, "Laboratory Accreditation." CAP laboratory accreditation is accepted by JCAHO's hospital accreditation program in lieu of separate JCAHO laboratory accreditation.

61. The specific CLIA requirements for tests to be considered waived are that they "(1) are cleared by FDA for home use; (2) employ methodologies that are so simple and accurate as to render the likelihood of erroneous results negligible; or (3) pose no reasonable risk of harm to the patient if the test is performed incorrectly." The College of American Pathologists takes issue with some of the regulatory language relating to waived tests. The CAP believes that no test is so simple or so inconsequential that it can be exempted from basic quality control and proficiency testing requirements when used by a physician to manage patient care. Even in the case of tests approved for home use, the CAP believes that the consequences of an erroneous result in a physician's hands are greater than the consequences of an erroneous result of a test performed by a lay individual at home. However, this is not the current position of United States regulators. Surveys have shown that approximately 20% of waived laboratories do not perform quality control, and 10% do not follow manufacturers' procedures when performing waived tests, which technically causes the test to become "highly complex" and subject to CLIA quality regulations. However, the majority of waived laboratories do follow manufacturers' recommendations. Regulators have tried to balance the public's interest in test accuracy with the public's interest in ensuring easy access to testing. In recognition of the compliance problems encountered in some waived laboratories, the federal Clinical Laboratory Improvement Advisory Committee has recently developed a set of nonbinding guidelines that waived laboratories will be asked to consider when evaluating or performing waived assays. Because the number of waived tests is expanding rapidly,

the whole area of waived testing will likely receive continued scrutiny by both regulators and the CAP.

62. Waived laboratories must agree to make records available to the United States Department of Health and Human Services (HHS) on request, and to permit announced and unannounced inspections when HHS has reason to believe that the laboratory is being operated in a manner that constitutes an imminent and serious risk to human health, when HHS has received complaints from the public, or when HHS decides to conduct an inspection to determine if the laboratory is performing nonwaived tests or to collect information regarding the appropriateness of waiver of tests. Because of some of the concerns that have been raised about waived laboratories, a number of states have announced plans to increase the inspection of waived laboratories to ensure that only waived testing is being conducted. In addition, some states require inspection of waived laboratories at the time of initial registration.

63. Many laboratorians misunderstand the intent and capabilities of proficiency testing (PT). PT test materials contain nonhuman stabilizers, solvents, and other additives that influence particular test systems in different ways. These influences are called "matrix effects" and are not observed when the same test system is applied to human clinical specimens. An excellent recent series of articles about matrix effects, based on a CAP study of fresh frozen serum specimens, appears in *Archives of Pathology & Laboratory Medicine* (2005;129:292-293, 297-337). Because matrix effects uniquely impact each type of test system, normal PT data cannot be used to determine the accuracy or precision of a particular laboratory's testing or of a particular testing system. PT is designed to measure the proficiency of a laboratory in using its test platform relative to other laboratories using the same platform. PT is not designed to measure accuracy. Some PT materials, such as photomicrographs of microscopic abnormalities, clearly have no matrix effect. These materials look the same to all users. Such PT materials can theoretically be used to measure the accuracy of a laboratory's diagnoses and can potentially be used to measure the accuracy with which individual technologists or pathologists perform visual classification. On a practical level, there are a number of concerns about using PT for this purpose; one major concern is that the number of PT challenges is not sufficient to reliably measure a pathologist's or technologist's accuracy.

64. Laboratories engaged in provider-performed microscopy and no other moderate complexity test or high complexity test receive a certificate of provider-performed microscopy, rather than a certificate of registration.

65. Exceptions to the separate application requirements are provided for (1) laboratories that are not at fixed locations (that is, laboratories that move from testing site to testing site, such as health screening fairs); (2) not-for-profit or federal, state, or local government laboratories that engage in limited public health testing (not more than a combination of 15 moderately complex or waived tests per certificate); and (3) laboratories within a hospital that are located within contiguous buildings on the same campus and under common direction.

66. Laboratories that perform only provider-performed microscopy may receive from CMS a certificate for PPM procedures without undergoing an inspection.

67. Data on file, College of American Pathologists.

68. At the time of this writing, health care accrediting organizations have come under unusual scrutiny. The United States Government Accountability Office (GAO) completed a

study of JCAHO's hospital accreditation program in 2004 and reported that JCAHO's hospital accreditation process did not identify most of the hospital deficiencies in CMS' annual validation survey. Stronger federal oversight of JCAHO was advocated. At the time of this writing, the GAO is known to be investigating laboratory accreditation programs granted deemed status by HHS, including those of the CAP, JCAHO, and COLA, and is expected to issue a report on its findings soon. In Europe, ISO has raised questions about the consistency with which private organizations certify institutions as being ISO compliant.

69. Stahl M, Lund ED, Brandslund I. Reasons for laboratories inability to report results for requested analytic tests. *Clin Chem.* 1998;44:2195-2197.

70. Lapworth R, Teal TK. Laboratory blunders revisited. *Ann Clin Biochem.* 1994;31:78-84.

71. Linden JV, Paul B, Dressler KP. A Report of 104 transfusion errors in New York State. *Transfusion.* 1992;32:601-606.

72. Raab SR, Nakhleh RE, Ruby SG. Patient safety in anatomic pathology: measuring discrepancy frequencies and causes. *Arch Pathol Lab Med.* 2005;129:459-466.

73. We have no evidence to suggest that errors in clinical laboratories are more common than errors in other branches of medicine. In fact, extrapolation from the Institute of Medicine report on medical errors (Kohn LT, Corrigan JM, Donaldson, eds; Committee on Quality of Health Care in America, Institute of Medicine. *To Err Is Human: Building a Safer Health System.* Washington DC: National Academies Press; 2000) suggests that the rate of error in laboratory medicine is significantly less than in other branches of medicine. Nevertheless, the quality of clinical laboratory testing remains a concern to the public and every conscientious laboratory professional.

74. Clearly, laboratory processes of great clinical importance are worth managing even if errors are infrequent. More attention should be applied to properly identifying patients before the administration of blood products than to turnaround time of Pap smear interpretations. This is the case even though patient identification prior to transfusion is much more likely to meet expectations than Pap smear turnaround.

75. Valenstein P, Raab S. *Identification Errors.* Q-Probes (QP51) Data Analysis and Critique. Northfield, Ill: College of American Pathologists; 2005.

76. Ladenson JH. Patients as their own controls: use of the computer to identify "laboratory error." *Clin Chem.* 1975;21:1648-1653.

77. In practice, delta checks are hard to implement as a case-finding method for flagging misidentified specimens. Criteria for rejecting specimens based on delta values must be set very broadly because laboratory values of individual patients often change dramatically in short periods of time. In one study (reference 97), only 0.05% of more than eight million CBC specimens were rejected on the basis of delta checks. This fraction is well below most estimates of the percentage of clinical specimens that are misidentified.

78. Using billable tests as a denominator for identification errors makes sense; in at least one large study, the number of identification errors reported per laboratory over a five-week period was significantly correlated with the number of billable tests the laboratory performed (see reference 75).

79. Data shown in Exhibit 12 are from Dale JC, Renner SW. *Wristband Errors.* Q-Probes (93-10) Data Analysis and Critique. Northfield, Ill: College of American Pathologists; 1993;

see also Dale JC, Renner SW. Wristband errors in small hospitals: a College of American Pathologists' Q-Probes study of quality issues in patient identification. *Lab Med.* 1997;28:203-207; Renner SW, Howanitz PJ, Bachner P. Wristband identification error reporting in 712 hospitals: a College of American Pathologists' Q-Probes study of quality issues in transfusion practice. *Arch Pathol Lab Med.* 1993;117:573-577; and Renner SW, Dale JC. Wristband Identification Reporting Errors: Data Analysis and Critique. Q-Probes Study 95-07. Northfield, Ill: College of American Pathologists; 1995.

80. Howanitz PJ, Renner SW, Walsh MK. Continuous wristband monitoring over 2 years decreases identification errors: a College of American Pathologists Q-Tracks study. *Arch Pathol Lab Med.* 2003;126:809-815.

81. Valenstein P. *Patient Identification Accuracy.* Q-Tracks (QT1) 2004 Annual Summary. Northfield, Ill: College of American Pathologists; 2005.

82. Linden et al. Transfusion errors in New York State. op. cit.

83. Ibojie J, Urbaniak SJ. Comparing near misses with actual mistransfusion events: a more accurate reflection of transfusion errors. *Br J Haematol.* 2000;108:458-460.

84. Murphy MF, Stearn B. Collection of Blood Samples (COBS) data collection carried out on behalf of the International Society of Blood Transfusion (ISBT) Biomedical Excellence for Safer Transfusion (BEST) Committee, part II: rejected and miscollected samples. Available at: http://www.blood.co.uk/hospitals/ services/pages/ClinAud/BEST2.PDF. Accessed July 13, 2003. See also Dzik WH, Murphy MF, Andreu G, et al. Biomedical Excellence for Safer Transfusion (BEST) Working Party of the International Society for Blood Transfusion: an international study of the performance of sample collection from patients. *Vox Sang.* 2003;85:40-47.

85. Lumadue JA, Boyd JS, Ness PM. Adherence to a strict specimen-labeling policy decreases the incidence of erroneous blood grouping of blood bank specimens. *Transfusion.* 1997;37:1169-1172.

86. Khoury M, Burnett L, Mackay MA. Error rates in Australian chemical pathology laboratories. *Med J Aust.* 1996;165:128-130.

87. Nakhleh RE, Zarbo RJ. Surgical pathology specimen identification and accessioning: a College of American Pathologists Q-Probes study of 1,004,115 cases from 417 institutions. *Arch Pathol Lab Med.* 1996;120:227-233.

88. This discussion relies heavily on two recent reviews of identification errors: (1) Valenstein P, Sirota R. Identification errors in pathology and laboratory medicine. *Clin Lab Med.* 2004;24:979-96; (2) Wald H, Shojania K. Prevention of misidentification. In: Wachter RM, ed. *Making Health Care Safer: A Critical Analysis of Patient Safety Practices.* Agency for Healthcare Research and Quality, Contract No. 290-97-0013. Available at: http://www.ahcpr.gov/clinic/ptsafety/pdf/chap43.pdf. Accessed July 10, 2003.

89. Anonymous. The IT revolution: the best thing since the bar-code. *The Economist.* Feb 6, 2003.

90. CLIA 42 CFR 493.1241 Standard: Test request.

91. Data on file, College of American Pathologists Laboratory Accreditation Program.

92. Finn AF, Valenstein PN, Burke MD. Alteration of physician orders by non-physicians. *JAMA.* 1988;259:2549-2552.

93. Valenstein P, Schifman R. *Duplicate Test Orders.* Q-Probes (95-05) Data Analysis and Critique. Northfield, Ill: College of American Pathologists; 1995.

94. Valenstein P, Howanitz PJ. Ordering accuracy: a College of American Pathologists Q-Probes study of 577 institutions. *Arch Pathol Lab Med.* 1995;119:117-122.

95. Valenstein P, Meier F. Outpatient order accuracy: a College of American Pathologists Q-Probes study of requisition order entry accuracy in 660 institutions. *Arch Pathol Lab Med.* 1999;123:1145-1150.

96. Nakhleh RE, Gephardt G, Zarbo RJ. Necessity of clinical information in surgical pathology: a College of American Pathologists Q-Probes study of 771,475 surgical pathology cases from 341 institutions. *Arch Pathol Lab Med.* 1999;123:615-619.

97. Jones BA, Meier FA, Howanitz PJ. Complete blood count specimen acceptability: a College of American Pathologists Q-Probes study of 703 laboratories. *Arch Pathol Lab Med.* 1995:119:203-208.

98. Jones BA, Calam RR, Howanitz PJ. Chemistry specimen acceptability: a College of American Pathologists Q- Probes study of 453 laboratories. *Arch Pathol Lab Med.* 1997;121:19-26.

99. Schifman RB, Strand CL, Meier FA, Howanitz PJ. Blood culture contamination: a College of American Pathologists Q-Probes study involving 640 institutions and 497,134 specimens from adult patients. *Arch Pathol Lab Med.* 1998;122:216-221.

100. Valenstein P, Meier FA. Urine culture contamination. *Arch Pathol Lab Med.* 1998;122:123-129.

101. See *Blood Culture Contamination.* Q-Tracks (QT2) Data Collection Instructions and 2004 Annual Report. Northfield, Ill: College of American Pathologists; 2005.

102. Howanitz PJ, Steindel SJ. Digoxin therapeutic drug monitoring practices: a College of American Pathologists Q-Probes study of 666 institutions and 18,679 toxic levels. *Arch Pathol Lab Med.* 1993;117:684-690.

103. Stankovic AK, Howanitz PJ, Valenstein PN, Meier FA. *Patient Safety with Digoxin Measurements.* Q-Probes (QP044) Data Analysis and Critique. Northfield, Ill: College of American Pathologists; 2005.

104. Dale JC, Novis DA. Outpatient phlebotomy success and reasons for specimen rejection. *Arch Pathol Lab Med.* 2002;126:416-419.

105. See Eyster E, Bernene J. Nosocomial anemia. *JAMA.* 1973;223:73-74; and Hicks JM. Excessive blood drawing for laboratory tests. *N Engl J Med.* 1999;340:1690.

106. Dale JC, Ruby SG. Specimen collection volumes for laboratory tests: a College of American Pathologists study of 140 laboratories. *Arch Pathol Lab Med.* 2003:127:162-168.

107. *Blood Culture Contamination.* Q-Tracks (QT2) 2004 Annual Summary. Northfield, Ill: College of American Pathologists; 2005.

108. *Laboratory Specimen Acceptability.* Q-Tracks (QT3) 2004 Annual Summary. Northfield, Ill: College of American Pathologists; 2005.

109. Valenstein P, Praestgaard A, Lepoff R. Six year trends in expense, productivity, and utilization of seventy three clinical laboratories. *Arch Pathol Lab Med.* 2001;125:1153-1161.

110. See Daniels M, Schroeder SA. Variation among physicians in use of laboratory tests, II: relation to clinical productivity and outcomes of care. *Med Care.* 1977;15:482-487; Hubbell FA, Frye EB, Akin BV, Rucker L. Routine admission laboratory testing for

general medical patients. *Med Care.* 1988;26:619-630; Kaplan EB, Sheiner LB, Boeckmann AJ, et al. The usefulness of preoperative laboratory screening. *JAMA.* 1985;253:3576-3581; and Kroenke K, Hanley JF, Copley JB, et al. Improving house staff ordering of three common laboratory tests: reductions in test ordering need not result in underutilization. *Med Care.* 1987;25:928-935.

111. See Markel SF, Venner AM. A market analysis approach to bidding for capitated clinical laboratory and pathology services contracts. *Arch Pathol Lab Med.* 1995;119:627-634; and Trisolini MG, McNeil BJ, Komaroff AL. The chemistry laboratory: development of average, fixed, and variable costs for incorporation into a management control system. *Med Care.* 1987;25:286-299.

112. See College of American Pathologists. Laboratory Management Index Program 1995 - 2005. Northfield, Ill: College of American Pathologists; Peredy TR; Powers RD. Bedside diagnostic testing of body fluids. *Am J Emerg Med.* 1997;15:400-407; Portugal B. *Benchmarking Hospital Laboratory Financial Performance.* AHA. 012882. Chicago, Ill: American Hospital Association; 1993; and Zimmerman JE, Seneff MG, Sun X, Wagner DP, Knaus WA. Evaluating laboratory usage in the intensive care unit: patient and institutional characteristics that influence frequency of blood sampling. *Crit Care Med.* 1997;25:737-748.

113. Third Report of the National Cholesterol Education Program (NCEP) Expert Panel on Detection, Evaluation, and Treatment of High Blood Cholesterol in Adults (Adult Treatment Panel III). National Institute of Health Publication No. 02-5215. September 2002.

114. Valenstein PJ, Walsh MK, Meier F. Heparin monitoring and patient safety: a College of American Pathologists Q-Probes study of 3,431 patients at 140 institutions. *Arch Pathol Lab Med.* 2004;128:397-402.

115. See *Blood Product Wastage.* Q-Tracks (QT4) Annual Summary. Northfield, Ill: College of American Pathologists. (Different years have different authors; data shown in Exhibit 31 are from the 2004 annual report, issued in 2005.)

116. See Novis DA, Renner SW, Friedberg, RC, Saladino, AJ, Walsh, MK. Quality indicators of fresh frozen plasma and platelet utilization: three College of American Pathologists Q-Probes studies of 8,981,796 units of fresh frozen plasma and platelets in 1639 hospitals. *Arch Pathol Lab Med.* 2002;126:527-532; and Novis DA, Renner S, Friedberg R, Walsh M, Saladino A. Quality indicators of blood utilization: three College of American Pathologists Q-Probes studies of 12,288,404 red blood cell units in 1,639 hospitals. *Arch Pathol Lab Med.* 2002;126:150-156.

117. Friedberg RC, Jones BA, Walsh MK. Type and screen completion for scheduled surgical procedures: a College of American Pathologists Q-Probes study of 8941 type and screen tests in 108 institutions. *Arch Pathol Lab Med.* 2003;127:533-540.

118. Schifman RB, Bachner P, Howanitz PJ. Blood culture quality improvement: a College of American Pathologists Q-Probes study involving 909 institutions and 289,572 blood culture sets. *Arch Pathol Lab Med.* 1996;120:999-1002.

119. Novis DA, Dale JC, Schifman RB, Ruby SG, Walsh MK. Solitary blood cultures: a College of American Pathologists Q-Probes study of 132,778 blood culture sets in 333 small hospitals. *Arch Pathol Lab Med.* 2001;125:1285-1289.

120. The ADA recommendation for monitoring glycohemoglobin has been criticized for being too aggressive. Some health service researchers believe that a large number of diabetics can be adequately managed with less intensive glycohemoglobin monitoring and more attention applied to blood pressure control.

121. Valenstein PN, Pappas, AA, Howanitz, PJ. Interinstitutional variation in glycohemoglobin monitoring and glycemic control of diabetic patients. *Arch Pathol Lab Med.* 2001;125;191-197.

122. Valenstein P, Pfaller M, Yungbluth M. The use and abuse of stool microbiology: a College American Pathologists Q-Probes study of 601 institutions. *Arch Pathol Lab Med.* 1996;120:206-211.

123. Valenstein P, Schifman RB. Duplicate laboratory orders: a College of American Pathologists Q-Probes study of thyrotropin requests in 502 institutions. *Arch Pathol Lab Med.* 1996;120:917-921.

124. Everett GD, Chang PF, de Blois CS, Holets TD. A comparative study of laboratory utilization behavior of "on- service" and "off-service" housestaff physicians. *Med Care.* 1983;21:1187-1191.

125. Valenstein P, Leiken A, Lehmann C. Test-ordering by multiple physicians increases unnecessary laboratory examinations. *Arch Pathol Lab Med.* 1988;112:238-241.

126. Epstein AM, Begg CB, McNeil BJ. The effects of group size on test ordering for hypertensive patients. *N Engl J Med.* 1983;309:464-468.

127. Hartley RM, Epstein AM, Harris CM, McNeil BJ. Differences in ambulatory test ordering in England and America: role of doctors' beliefs and attitudes. *Am J Med.* 1987;82:513-517.

128. See Zaat JO, van Eijk JT. General practitioners' uncertainty, risk preference, and use of laboratory tests. *Med Care.* 1992;30:846-854; and Ornstein SM, Markert GP, Johnson AH, Rust PF, Afrin LB. The effect of physician personality on laboratory test ordering for hypertensive patients. *Med Care.* 1988;26:536-543.

129. Yarnold PR, Martin GJ, Feinglass J, et al. First-year residents' caring, medical knowledge, and clinical judgment in relation to laboratory utilization. *Acad Med.* 1994;69:996-998.

130. See Epstein AM, McNeil BJ. Relationship of beliefs and behavior in test ordering. *Am J Med.* 1986;80:865-870; and Schectman JM, Elinsky EG, Pawlson LG. Self-reported versus actual test ordering behavior among primary care clinicians. *QRB Qual Rev Bull.* 1992;18:60-62.

131. See Sherman H. Surveillance effects on community physician test ordering. *Med Care.* 1984;22:80-83; and McGillivray DL, Roberts-Brauer R, Kramer MS. Diagnostic test ordering in the evaluation of febrile children: physician and environmental factors. *Am J Dis Child.* 1993;147:870-874.

132. See Grossman RM. A review of physician cost-containment strategies for laboratory testing. *Med Care.* 1983;21:783-802; Axt-Adam P, van der Wouden JC, van der Does E. Influencing behavior of physicians ordering laboratory tests: a literature study. *Med Care.* 1993;31:784-794; Valenstein P. Managing physician use of laboratory testing. *Clin Lab Med.* 1996;16:749-771; and Greco PJ, Eisenberg JM. Changing physicians' practices. *New Engl J Med.* 1993;329:1271-1274.

133. See Schroeder SA, Myers LP, McPhee SJ, et al. The failure of physician education as a cost containment strategy. *JAMA*. 1984;252:225-230; Malcolm L, Wright L, Seers M, Davies L, Guthrie J. Laboratory expenditure in Pegasus Medical Group: a comparison of high and low users of laboratory tests with academics. *N Z Med J*. 2000;113:79-81; Davis MA, Thomson MA, Oxman AD, Haynes RB. Evidence for the effectiveness of CME: a review of 50 randomized controlled trials. *JAMA*. 1992;268:1111-1117; and Tunis SR, Hayward RS, Wilson MC, et al. Internists' attitudes about clinical practice guidelines. *Ann Intern Med*. 1994;120:956-963.

134. Laposata ME, Laposata M, Van Cott ME, Buchnet ES, Kashalo MS, Dighe AS. Physician survey of a laboratory medicine interpretive service and evaluation of the influence of interpretations on laboratory test ordering. *Arch Pathol Lab Med*. 2004;128:1424-1427.

135. See Wones RG. Failure of low-cost audits with feedback to reduce laboratory test utilization. *Med Care*. 1987;25:78-82; and Beck JR. Does feedback reduce inappropriate test ordering? *Arch Pathol Lab Med*. 1993;117:33-34.

136. See Grivell AR, Forgie HJ, Fraser CG, Berry MN. Effect of feedback to clinical staff of information in clinical biochemistry requesting patterns. *Clin Chem*. 1981;27:1717-1720; Berwick DM, Coltin K. Feedback reduces test use in a health maintenance organization. *JAMA*. 1986;255:1450-1454; Eisenberg JM, Williams SV, Garner L, Viale R, Smits H. Computer-based audit to detect and correct overutilization of laboratory tests. *Med Care*. 1977;15:915-921; Spiegel JS, Shapiro, MF, Berman B, Greenfield S. Changing physician test ordering in a university hospital: an intervention of physician participation, explicit criteria, and feedback. *Arch Intern Med*. 1989;149:549-553; and Winkens RA, Pop P, Grol RP, Kester AD, Knottnerus JA. Effect of feedback on test ordering behavior of general practitioners. *Br Med J*. 1992;304:1093-1096.

137. Lomas J, Enkin M, Anderson GM, Hannah WJ, Vayda E, Singer J. Opinion leaders vs audit and feedback to implement practice guidelines: delivery after previous cesarian section. *JAMA*. 1991;265:2202-2207.

138. Cohen DI, Jones P, Littenberg M, Neuhauser D. Does cost information reduce physician test usage? *Med Care*. 1982;20:286-292.

139. Cummings KM, Frisof KB, Long MJ, Hrynkiewich G. The effects of price information on physicians' test-ordering behavior: ordering of diagnostic tests. *Med Care*. 1982;20:293-301.

140. Tierney WM, Miller ME, McDonald CJ. The effect on test ordering of informing physicians of the charges for outpatient diagnostic tests. *N Engl J Med*. 1990;322:1499-1504.

141. Marton KI, Tul V, Sox HC Jr. Modifying test-ordering behavior in the outpatient medical clinic: a controlled trial of two educational interventions. *Arch Intern Med*. 1985;145:816-821.

142. Novich M, Gillis L, Tauber AI. The laboratory test justified: an effective means to reduce routine laboratory testing. *Am J Clin Pathol*. 1985;84:756-759.

143. See Wong ET, McCarron MM, Shaw ST Jr. Ordering of laboratory tests in a teaching hospital: can it be improved? *JAMA*. 1983;249:3076-3080; Hardwick SF, Morrison JI, Tydeman J, Cassidy PA, Chase WH. Structuring complexity of testing: a process oriented approach to limiting unnecessary laboratory use. *Am J Med Technol*.

1982;48:605-608; and van Gend JM, van Pelt J, Cleef TH, Mangnus TM. Quality improvement project in laboratory diagnosis by family physicians' leads to decrease in number of laboratory tests. *Ned Tijdschr Geneeskd.* 1996;140:495-500.

144. Zaat JO, van Eijk JT, Bonte HA. Laboratory test form design influences test ordering by general practitioners in the Netherlands. *Med Care.* 1992;30:189-198.

145. See Wilson GA, McDonald CJ, McCabe GP Jr. The effect of immediate access to a computerized medical record on physician test ordering: a controlled clinical trial in the emergency room. *Am J Public Health.* 1982;72:698-702; and Tierney WM, Miller ME, Overhange JM, McDonald CJ. Physician inpatient order writing on microcomputer workstations: effects on resource utilization. *JAMA.* 1993;269:379-383.

146. Marx WH, DeMaintenon NL, Mooney KF, et al. Cost reduction and outcome improvement in the intensive care unit. *J Trauma.* 1999;46:625-629.

147. Mehari SM, Havill JH, Montgomery C. A written guideline implementation can lead to reductions in laboratory testing in an intensive care unit. *Anaesth Intensive Care.* 1997;25:33-37.

148. Barie PS, Hydo LJ. Lessons learned: durability and progress of a program for ancillary cost reduction in surgical critical care. *J Trauma.* 1997;43:590-594.

149. Exhibit 38 consists of tasks that managers of laboratories in the United States should complete before placing new tests into production. Additional tasks not directly related to quality (eg, setting up billing, medical necessity checking, ABN) are not included in the Exhibit. In developing Exhibit 38, we have adopted the CAP position that all tests should be subject to basic quality practices, including so-called waived tests; CLIA does not require validation of waived test systems. For technical reasons, CLIA does not require validation of test systems placed in service before April 24, 2003, but we have adopted the view that all tests currently used clinically should be validated. We have not advocated several of the tasks included in evolving ISO standards that are not binding upon US laboratories, such as including statements in reports that quantify analytic uncertainty of each laboratory result.

150. CLIA 42 CFR 493.1253 (page 1036 of the October 1, 2003, *Federal Register*) requires that laboratories verify the "accuracy" of a test system. However, the term "accuracy" is not formally defined in CLIA regulations. For quantitative tests, "accuracy" can be established by testing reference materials (the most common method), comparing results of tests performed by the laboratory against the results of a reference method, or comparing split sample results with results obtained from another method that is shown to provide clinically valid results. The technical term for what we are calling accuracy is "trueness of measurement." Trueness refers to how closely the average value obtained from a large series of measurements comes to the true value. Technically, "accuracy" refers only to how closely one particular value comes to the true value.

151. Howanitz PJ. *Physician Satisfaction with Clinical Laboratory Services.* Q-Probes (02-QP17) Data Analysis and Critique. Northfield, Ill: College of American Pathologists; 2002.

152. CLIA 42 CFR 493.1253 (page 1036 of the October 1, 2003, Federal Register) requires that laboratories verify the "precision" of a test system. Precision can be assessed by measuring the day-to-day, run-to-run, and within-run variation by repeat testing of known patient samples over time; testing the same QC material repeatedly over time; or repeat testing of calibration materials over time. When a test has a subjective interpretation or is subject to other influence by operators, reproducibility testing should

include repeat testing performed by different operators. Operator variance does not need to be evaluated for fully automated systems that are not user dependent.

153. A formal discussion of how to estimate precision can be found in the NCCLS (now Clinical and Laboratory Standards Institute [CLSI]) document, *Evaluation of Precision Performance of Quantitative Measurement Methods.* Approved Guideline. 2nd ed. Wayne, Pa: NCCLS; 2004.

154. A theoretical argument can be advanced that it is important to test the same sample multiple times with a qualitative system, to see if the system produces the same identification. However, for FDA-approved qualitative test systems, this sort of validation normally is not conducted.

155. 2005 CAP Proficiency Testing survey CF1/CG2. Data on file, College of American Pathologists.

156. MDRD is an abbreviation for the "Modification of Diet in Renal Disease Study Group."

157. During 2004, CAP inspectors cited 1.6% of hematology sections for failing to perform checks to ensure that INR and other values were calculated properly; 13 laboratories were cited for calculating the INR incorrectly (failing to use the appropriate PT mean or the correct ISI). Data on file, College of American Pathologists.

158. CLIA 42 CFR 493.1251(b)(14); page 3706 of the January 24, 2003, *Federal Register.*

159. CLIA 42 CFR 493.1253(3); page 3707 of the January 24, 2003, *Federal Register.* The quality management program for each assay should provide reasonable assurance that the test system is functioning properly; however, no quality management program can provide absolute assurance that every result is accurate. Intermittent and short-lived instrument malfunction or unusual patient interferences will adversely influence rare results.

160. Exactly what constitutes a "significant change" to a test system that requires recalibration is not well defined, and is the subject of some debate. An entire change of reagents or a complete replacement of the physical test instrument should initiate recalibration. But what about a change of a single reagent, the replacement of a defective part of an analyzer, or a decision to move an analyzer across the room or to another building? In these situations, the decision to recalibrate an instrument lies with the professional judgment of the laboratory director, although exactly how the laboratory director is supposed to make this professional judgment is not at all clear.

161. Data cited are from Jones BA, Howanitz PJ. Bedside glucose monitoring quality control practices: a College of American Pathologists Q-Probes study of program quality control documentation, program characteristics, and accuracy performance in 544 institutions. *Arch Pathol Lab Med.* 1996;120:339-345. Similar results were obtained in a later study of smaller hospitals by Novis DA, Jones BA. Interinstitutional comparison of bedside blood glucose monitoring program characteristics, accuracy performance, and quality control documentation: a College of American Pathologists Q-Probes study of bedside blood glucose monitoring performed in 226 small hospitals. *Arch Pathol Lab Med.* 1998;122:495-502.

162. If a laboratory can convincingly demonstrate that a test system is so stable that daily controls are not required, testing of physical control specimens at a lesser frequency is permitted by CLIA. However, demonstrating system stability is not always an easy undertaking; depending on the specifics of a test system, it may take 60 days of daily testing to establish that a system is so stable that daily quality control is not required.

Consult the "Equivalent Quality Control" section of CLIA 1988 for details (January 23, 2003, revision in the *Federal Register* and State Operations Manual, Appendix C-Interpretive Guidelines, §493.1256). Laboratory directors should keep in mind their obligation to retest clinical specimens when physical control testing fails to yield expected reactions or levels. If physical controls are run less often than daily, this retesting may pose a considerable burden. Regulations related to "equivalent quality control" are evolving, and there is controversy about when nontraditional quality control activities can be safely substituted for traditional "wet" testing of external quality control reagents.

163. This rule was originally described by Shewhart and is abbreviated as 1_{3S}. The "1" signifies that 1 result outside the control limit is sufficient to "trip" the control rule, and the "3S" signifies that the control limit consists of 3 standard deviations from the mean. A control rule abbreviated "2_{2S}" indicates that 2 successive results that are both 2 standard deviations from the mean will violate the control rule.

164. Westgard JO, Barry PL, Hunt MR. A multi-rule Shewhart chart for quality control in clinical chemistry. *Clin Chem.* 1981;27:493-501. For quantitative analyses that are performed manually, the multi-rule described by Westgard et al is an improvement over the simple 1_{3S} rule described by Shewhart (1 point, 3 or more standard deviations from the mean).

165. Occasionally, variation during the manufacturing of a single lot will cause failure of only some product within the same lot. Also, improper storage of reagents, kits, or media may cause the failure of only some product within the same lot. More commonly, however, laboratories experience failures when new lots of consumables are introduced into test systems.

166. Limitations of PT include: (1) External PT is required only for the primary test system a laboratory uses to measure an analyte. Backup test systems are not subject to PT. (2) For any given PT challenge, only a single instrument, set of reagents, and operator will be tested. On another day, with another operator, instrument, or reagent lot, performance may differ. (3) When PT is applied to certain qualitative tests, such as HIV or hepatitis testing, moderate linear "drift" may be present without causing deficient PT performance. This drift may impact patient results that fall close to decision points (positive vs negative), even though PT results are not be impacted, because the target value of the PT specimen is further from the decision point than some patient results. (4) Matrix effects prevent PT from measuring the analytic accuracy of a laboratory's result. PT measures the proficiency of a laboratory in using its test system, compared with peers, but does not measure the accuracy of the laboratory's result. (5) Similarly, PT does not measure the quality of an analytic test system, and aggregate PT results cannot normally be used to compare test platforms. (6) PT testing is insensitive to interfering substances that may be present in specimen collection tubes, but not present in the containers used to distribute PT materials. For example, increased surfactant concentrations in certain lots of a widely used specimen collection tube recently interfered with several FDA-approved thyroid function assays. PT specimens, which were shipped in their own containers, were unaffected. (7) Finally, when PT testing indicates a problem within a laboratory, the information usually arrives too late to correct many hundreds of patient results that may have already been released to caregivers.

167. CLIA 42 CFR 493.801; page 1002 of the October 1, 2003, *Federal Register.*

168. Parham S. Test tube interference shows "chink in armor." *CAP Today.* January 2005.

169. Stankovic et al. *Patient Safety with Digoxin Measurements.* Q-Probes. op. cit.

170. Cembrowski GS, Howanitz PJH. *Postanalytical QA: Hypercalcemia.* Q-Probes (QP91-08A) Data Analysis and Critique. Northfield, Ill: College of American Pathologists; 2002.

171. Survey conducted by the College of American Pathologists in 2001. Data on file, College of American Pathologists.

172. For a more in-depth discussion of this topic, see the NCCLS (now Clinical and Laboratory Standards Institute [CLSI]) document, *How to Define and Determine Reference Intervals in the Clinical Laboratory.* Approved Standard. Wayne, Pa: NCCLS; 2000: C28-A2. This publication describes considerations that should enter into the conduct of a reference interval study, based largely on the seminal work of HE Solberg that was published in the late 1980s and early 1990s.

173. Of course, there are small differences in the potassium values determined by different test platforms. But for the purposes of setting reference ranges, these differences are not clinically important.

174. See Exhibit 42 for a discussion about the regulatory issues surrounding local validation of reference ranges. Laboratory directors who choose not to perform local validation studies should be mindful of the fact that some manufacturer-supplied reference ranges are wrong or not applicable to the local population of patients served by the laboratory. Laboratory directors should consider the source and quality of manufacturer-supplied normal ranges when using these ranges in lieu of a local validation study.

175. As a general rule, unless very large samples of patients are tested, it is preferable to calculate the "normal" range using the mean value of the population's results plus or minus 2 standard deviations, rather than the actual central 95% of the values from the population that was tested. However, manufacturer's recommendations should also be considered when performing reference range validation studies.

176. The reference range for international normalized ratio (INR) is in the same class as the reference range for cholesterol; both are decision based and method independent. The INR (when properly calculated!) does not vary significantly with the test platform or reagent used, although the ISI attached to lots of thromboplastin reagents does not completely correct lot-to-lot reagent variability. INR decision breakpoints have been established to help clinicians adjust anticoagulants for common clinical conditions (eg, deep venous thrombosis, prosthetic cardiac valve). The studies validating these breakpoints do not need to be replicated locally.

177. CLIA 42 CFR 493.1291; page 1047 of the October 1, 2003, *Federal Register.*

178. Laboratories having a single CLIA certificate for multiple sites/locations must have a system in place to identify which tests were performed at each site. A code to identify the name and address of the laboratory performing testing is acceptable as long as the code is clearly annotated on the patient test report. Regulations specify that all sites should be listed when different parts of a single test are performed at multiple sites (such as a tissue slide that is prepared in one CLIA site and interpreted by a pathologist at a different CLIA site).

179. The authors recognize that the question of what constitutes a laboratory "report" is a murky area, and our recommendations about how required information should be

exchanged will evolve as technology and regulations change. The College of American Pathologists does not have a formal position on this issue, apart from the more general reporting requirements listed in the CAP Laboratory Accreditation standards and inspection checklist questions.

180. See, for example, Zarbo RJ. Inter-institutional assessment of colorectal carcinoma surgical pathology report adequacy: a College of American Pathologists Q-Probes study of practice patterns from 532 laboratories and 15,940 reports. *Arch Pathol Lab Med.* 1992;116:1113-1119; Gephardt GN, Baker PB. Lung carcinoma surgical pathology report adequacy: a College of American Pathologists Q-Probes study of over 8300 cases from 464 institutions. *Arch Pathol Lab Med.* 1996;120:922-927; and Nakhleh RE, Jones B, Zarbo R. Mammographically directed breast biopsies: a College of American Pathologists Q-Probes study of clinical physician expectations and of specimen handling and reporting characteristics in 434 institutions. *Arch Pathol Lab Med.* 1997;121:11-18.

181. See Association of Directors of Anatomic and Surgical Pathology. Standardization of the surgical pathology report. *Am J Surg Pathol.* 1992;16:84-86; and Rosai J. Standardized reporting of surgical pathology diagnosis for the major tumor types: a proposal. *Am J Clin Pathol.* 1993;100:240-255.

182. See 2005 Laboratory Services National Patient Safety Goals of the Joint Commission on Accreditation of Healthcare Organizations (JCAHO). Available at: www.jcaho.org.

183. Modern commercial airplane cockpits contain video display terminals that present flight information in a form that could not be duplicated with physical gauges.

184. See Ruby SG. Clinician interpretation of pathology reports: confusion or comprehension? *Arch Pathol Lab Med.* 2000;124:947-948.

185. There are numerous examples of collection dates and times being confused with report dates and times. We have also seen clinicians confuse poorly formatted times (such as "134" for 1:34 p.m.) with a numeric test result.

186. We recognize that the date and time of specimen receipt and result verification may occasionally be useful to caregivers. In microbiology, these dates and times can alert physicians to prolonged transport or prolonged incubation before detection, which suggests low inoculum. Our point is that this information is usually not used in clinical decision making and is apt to be confused with the date and time of specimen collection. For this reason, the date of receipt, verification, and reporting should be displayed separately from test results.

187. Powsner SM, Costa J, Homer RJ. Clinicians are from Mars and pathologists are from Venus: clinician interpretation of pathology reports. *Arch Pathol Lab Med.* 2000;124:1040-1046.

188. Markel SF, Hirsch SD. Synoptic surgical pathology reporting. *Hum Pathol.* 1991;22: 807-810.

189. Improving the accuracy of communication among caregivers is one of the 2005 Laboratory Services National Patient Safety Goals of the Joint Commission on Accreditation of Healthcare Organizations (JCAHO). For telephone results, laboratories are required to verify the complete result by having the person receiving the result "read back" the complete test result.

190. See 2005 Laboratory Services National Patient Safety Goals of the Joint Commission on Accreditation of Healthcare Organizations (JCAHO). Available at: www.jcaho.org.

Exceptions are provided for computer-generated abbreviations and values because the potential for transcription error or misinterpretation is small. JCAHO permits a free text anatomic pathology report to use trailing zeroes to describe the size of a thyroid nodule (1.0 cm) or the Breslow depth of an invasive melanoma (0.30 mm), if the trailing zero indicates the precision of measurement.

191. Kost GJ. Critical limits for urgent clinician notification at US medical centers. *JAMA.* 1990;263:704-707.

192. Lundberg GD. When to panic over abnormal values. *MLO Med Lab Obs.* 1972;4:47-54.

193. Lundberg GD. *Managing the Patient-Focused Laboratory.* Oradell, NJ: Medical Economics Books; 1975.

194. Howanitz PJ, Steindel SJ, Heard NV. Laboratory critical values policies and procedures: a College of American Pathologists Q-Probes study in 623 institutions. *Arch Pathol Lab Med.* 2002;126:663-669.

195. Linden et al. Transfusion errors in New York State. op. cit.

196. Williamson LM, Lowe S, Love EM, Cohen H, Soldan K, McClelland DBL, Skacel P, Barbara JAJ. Serious hazards of transfusion (SHOT) initiative: analysis of the first two annual reports. *BMJ.* 1999;319:16-19.

197. Data posted on the Joint Commission on Accreditation of Healthcare Organizations web site, www.jcaho.org, accessed April 15, 2005. Because reporting of sentinel events to JCAHO is voluntary, these data may be influenced by selection bias.

198. Shulman IA, Saxena S, Ramer L. Assessing blood administering practices. *Arch Pathol Lab Med.* 1999;123:595-598.

199. Novis DA, Miller KA, Howanitz PJ, Renner SW, Walsh MK. Audit of transfusion procedures in 660 hospitals: a College of American Pathologists Q-Probes study of patient identification and vital sign monitoring frequencies in 16,494 transfusions. *Arch Pathol Lab Med.* 2003;127:541-548.

200. See Stainsby D, Williamson L, Jones H, Cohen H. 6 Years of SHOT reporting—its influence on UK blood safety. *Transfus Apheresis Sci.* 2004;31:123-131; and Wagner SJ. Transfusion-transmitted bacterial infection: risks, sources and interventions. *Vox Sang.* 2004;86:157-163.

201. Burk MD. Clinical laboratory consultation: appropriateness to laboratory medicine. *Clin Chem Acta.* 2003;333:125-129.

202. Howanitz PJ, Cembrowski GS. Postanalytical quality improvement: a College of American Pathologists Q-Probes study of elevated calcium results in 525 institutions. *Arch Pathol Lab Med.* 2000; 124:504-510.

203. Jones BA, Novis DA. Follow-up of abnormal gynecologic cytology: a College of American Pathologists Q-Probes study of 16,132 cases from 306 laboratories. *Arch Pathol Lab Med.* 2000;124:665-671.

204. Laposata M. Patient-specific narrative interpretations of complex clinical laboratory evaluations: who is competent to provide them? *Clin Chem.* 2004;50:471-472.

205. Kratz A, Laposata M. Enhanced clinical consulting—moving toward the core competencies of laboratory professionals. *Clin Chim Acta.* 2002;21:117-125.

206. Lim EM, Sikaris KA, Gill J, et al. Quality assessment of interpretative commenting in clinical chemistry. *Clin Chem.* 2004;50:632-637.

207. Chenhsu RY, Chiang SC, Chou MH, et al. Long-term treatment with warfarin in Chinese population. *Ann Pharmacother.* 2000;34:1395-1401.

208. Balas EA, Krishna S, Kretschmer RA, Cheek TR, Lobach DF, Boren SA. Computerized knowledge management in diabetes care. *Med Care.* 2004;42:610-621.

209. Readers should not conclude that a reporting error has occurred whenever a second pathologist's review of a surgical pathology case results in a diagnosis that does not agree with the original diagnosis. When a discrepancy is discovered through re-examination, the first or the second interpretation may be in error.

210. Yuan S, Astion ML, Schapiro J, Limaye AP. Clinical impact associated with corrected results in clinical microbiology testing. *J Clin Microbiol.* 2005;43:2188-2193.

211. Howanitz PJ, Walker K, Bachner P. Quantification of errors in laboratory reports: a quality improvement study of the College of American Pathologists' Q Probes program. *Arch Pathol Lab Med.* 1992;116:694-700.

212. CLIA 42 CFR 493.1291.

213. The CAP recognizes that clinical decisions or actions may have been based on a previously reported incorrect result. For this reason, the CAP currently requires as a condition of laboratory accreditation that all initially reported numerical values be reproduced on subsequent reports. This includes incorrect test results, reference intervals, and even short interpretive comments that were later corrected, so that clinicians can compare the incorrect results with the revised information. However, the CAP emphasizes that the previous information in the revised report must be identified as such, and while the original data must be present in revised paper reports, it may be linked electronically or logically to the revised information in electronic reports so as to minimize confusion.

214. We are aware of some health care information systems that display incorrect results first on computer screens, and require that caregivers scroll down to visualize corrected values. It would be difficult to design a less safe system. Some computer systems are configured in a way that requires clinicians to view preliminary reports before final reports can be seen. This procedure is almost as troubling.

215. CLIA 42 CFR 493.1291 states: "When errors in the reported patient test results are detected, the laboratory must do the following: (1) Promptly notify the authorized person ordering the test and, if applicable, the individual using the test results of reporting errors. (2) Issue corrected reports promptly to the authorized person ordering the test and, if applicable, the individual using the test results. (3) Maintain duplicates of the original report, as well as the corrected report."

216. CAP standards for laboratory accreditation specify that for "extensive interpretive or textual data (eg, surgical pathology reports), replicating the entire original and corrected pathology reports may be cumbersome and render the revised report format difficult to interpret. In such cases, a comment in the corrected report summarizing the previous information and the reason for the correction may be more appropriate than repeating the entire original report." Published studies suggest errors are less common in institutions committed to removing errant surgical pathology reports entirely from the clinical record. (See Nakhleh RE, Zarbo RJ. Amended reports in surgical pathology and implications for diagnostic error detection and avoidance: a College of American Pathologists Q-Probes study of 1,667,547 accessioned cases in 359 laboratories. *Arch Pathol Lab Med.* 1998;122:303-309.)

217. Howanitz PJ, Valenstein, P. *Competency of Point-of-Care (POC) Glucose Testing Personnel.* Q-Probes Data Analysis and Critique. Northfield, Ill: College of American Pathologists; 2005.

218. Haun DE, Leach A. Performing poorly but testing perfectly. *Clin Leadersh Manag Rev.* 2003;17:85-87.

219. CLIA 42 CFR 493.1413; page 1053 of the October 1, 2003, *Federal Register.*

220. Howanitz PJ, Valenstein P, Fine G. Employee competence and performance-based assessment. *Arch Pathol Lab Med.* 2000;124:195-202.

221. Federal Air Regulations, Part 125-Certification and Operations: Airplanes Having a Seating Capacity of 20 or More Passengers or a Maximum Payload Capacity of 6,000 Pounds or More. Washington, DC: US Government Printing Office; 1997.

222. Valenstein P, Sours R, Wilkinson DF. Staffing benchmarks for clinical laboratories: a College of American Pathologists Q-Probes study of staffing at 151 institutions. *Arch Pathol Lab Med.* 2005;129:467-473.

223. For a readable and not too technical discussion of the major issues in computer security, see Schneier B. *Secrets and Lies.* New York: John Wiley & Sons; 2000.

224. Valenstein P, Aller R, Treling C. Laboratory computer availability. *Arch Pathol Lab Med.* 1996;120:626-632.

225. Valenstein P, Walsh M. Six-year trends in laboratory computer availability: a College of American Pathologists Q-Probes study. *Arch Pathol Lab Med.* 2003;127:157-161.

226. American Society for Testing and Materials. Standard practice for reporting reliability of clinical laboratory computer systems. Standard E 1246 88. *Annual Book of ASTM Standards.* Vol 14.01. Philadelphia, Pa: American Society for Testing and Materials; 1988.

227. Kilbridge P. Computer crash: lessons from a system failure. *N Engl J Med.* 2003;348:881-882.

228. Lo B, Dornbrand L, Dubler NN. HIPAA and patient care: the role for professional judgment. *JAMA.* 2005;293:1766-1771.

229. This "business associate agreement" is required because the enabling HIPAA legislation applied only to health care providers, health care plans, and health care clearinghouses. If Congress had passed legislation requiring all citizens and entities to comply with the terms of HIPAA, business associate agreements would probably be unnecessary.

230. *Laboratory Instruments and Data Management Systems: Design of Software User Interfaces and End-User Software Systems Validation, Operation, and Monitoring.* Approved Guideline. 2nd ed. Wayne, Pa: NCCLS; 2003.

231. *General Principles of Software Validation.* op. cit.

232. Both HS1-A and GP26-A3 are available from the Clinical and Laboratory Standards Institute (CLSI, formerly NCCLS), 940 W. Valley Rd, Suite 1400, Wayne, Pa; or at www.clsi.org.

233. Hallam K. Turnaround time: speeding up, but is it fast enough? *MLO Med Lab Obs.* 1988;20:28-34.

234. Barnett RN. Medical significance of laboratory results. *Am J Clin Pathol.* 1968;50:671-676.

235. Barnett RN, Bimmell M, Peracca M, Rosemann K. Time intervals between ordering and obtaining laboratory test results. *Pathologist*. 1975;29:3-8.

236. Selker HP, Beshansky JR, Pauker SG, Kassirer JP. The epidemiology of delays in a teaching hospital. *Med Care*. 1989;27:112-129.

237. Valenstein P. Laboratory turnaround time. *Am J Clin Pathol*. 1996;105:676-688.

238. Valenstein PN, Emancipator KA. Sensitivity, specificity, and reproducibility of four measures of laboratory turnaround time. *Am J Clin Pathol*. 1989;91:452-457.

239. Barnett RN, McIver DD, Gorton WL. The medical usefulness of stat tests. *Am J Clin Pathol*. 1978;69:520-524.

240. Howanitz PJ, Cembrowski GS, Steindel SJ, Long TA. Physician goals and laboratory test turnaround times: a College of American Pathologists Q-Probes study of 2763 clinicians and 722 institutions. *Arch Pathol Lab Med*. 1993;117:22-28.

241. Howanitz PJ, Steindel SJ. Interlaboratory performance and laboratorians' expectations for stat turnaround times: a College of American Pathologists Q-Probes study of four cerebrospinal fluid determinations. *Arch Pathol Lab Med*. 1991;115:977-983.

242. Hilborne LH, Oye RK, McArdle JE, Repinski JA, Rodgerson DO. Use of specimen turnaround time as a component of laboratory quality: a comparison of clinician expectations with laboratory performance. *Am J Clin Pathol*. 1989;92:613-618.

243. Valenstein PN. Meeting clinicians' demands for faster turnaround time. *Am J Clin Pathol*. 1990;93:842.

244. Steindel SJ, Howanitz PJ. *Emergency Department Turnaround Time*. Q-Probes (93-03) Data Analysis and Critique. Northfield, Ill: College of American Pathologists; 1993.

245. Novis DA, Jones BA, Dale JC, Walsh MK. Biochemical markers of myocardial injury test turnaround time: a College of American Pathologists Q-Probes study of 7020 troponin and 4368 creatine kinase-MB determinations in 159 institutions. *Arch Pathol Lab Med*. 2004;128:158-164.

246. Valenstein P, Walsh M. Five-year follow-up of routine outpatient test turnaround time: a College of American Pathologists Q-Probes study. *Arch Pathol Lab Med*. 2003;127:1421-1423.

247. Zarbo RJ, Gephart GN. *Surgical Pathology Routine Biopsy Turnaround Time*. Q-Probes (92-09) Data Analysis and Critique. Northfield, Ill: College of American Pathologists; 1992.

248. Saladino AJ, Zarbo RJ. *Surgical Pathology Diagnosis Turnaround Time*. Q-Probes (93-11) Data Analysis and Critique. Northfield, Ill: College of American Pathologists; 1993.

249. Jones BA, Valenstein P, Steindel S. Gynecologic cytology turnaround time: a College of American Pathologists Q-Probes study of 371 laboratories. *Arch Pathol Lab Med*. 1999;123:682-686.

250. Jones BA, Novis DA. Nongynecologic cytology turnaround time: a College of American Pathologists Q-Probes study of 180 laboratories. *Arch Pathol Lab Med*. 2001;125:1279-1284.

251. Baker PB, Zarbo RJ. *Autopsy Timeliness and Permit Adequacy*. Q-Probes (92-03) Data Analysis and Critique. Northfield, Ill: College of American Pathologists; 1992.

252. Baker PJ, Zarbo RJ. *Autopsy Report Adequacy*. Q-Probes (90-09A) Data Analysis and Critique. Northfield, Ill: College of American Pathologists;1990.

253. Schifman RB, Valenstein PN. *Laboratory Diagnosis of Tuberculosis.* Q-Probes (94-05) Data Analysis and Critique. Northfield, Ill: College of American Pathologists; 1994.

254. Novis DA, Friedberg RC, Renner SW, Meier FA, Walsh MK. Operating room blood delivery turnaround time: a College of American Pathologists Q-Probes study of 12,647 units of blood components in 466 institutions. *Arch Pathol Lab Med.* 2002;126:909-914.

255. Novis DA, Walsh MK, Dale JC, Howanitz PJ. Continuous monitoring of stat and routine outlier turnaround times: two College of American Pathologists Q-Tracks monitors in 291 hospitals. *Arch Pathol Lab Med.* 2004;128:621-626.

256. Bluth EI, Lambert DJ, Lohmann TP, et al. Improvement in 'stat' laboratory turnaround time: a model continuous quality improvement project. *Arch Intern Med.* 1992;152:837-840.

257. Models of pathologist relationships with clinical laboratories are discussed extensively in the CAP publication, *Professional Relations Manual.* 12th ed. Northfield, Ill: College of American Pathologists; 2003.

258. CLIA additionally defines the roles of a "technical supervisor" for high complexity laboratories, "testing personnel," "cytology manager," and "cytology testing personnel."

259. Sirota RL. The Institute of Medicine's report on medical error: implications for pathology. *Arch Pathol Lab Med.* 2000;124:1674-1678.

260. Much of this discussion is adapted from the works of James Reason (references 43, 47, and 48).

261. Berwick DM. Continuous improvement as an ideal in health care. *N Engl J Med.* 1989;320:53-56.

262. This section was written by Bruce Jones, MD, and Paul Valenstein, MD.

263. See CAP December 2004 LAP checklist question GEN.20367: "Have the referring physicians' or patients' satisfaction with the laboratory service been measured within the past 2 years?"; and 1998 JCAHO Hospital Manual PI 3.2.6.

264. Valenstein PN, personal experience contracting for laboratory services with more than ten health maintenance organizations.

265. Fowler FJ. *Survey Research Methods.* 2nd ed. London: SAGE Publications; 1993.

266. Steindel SJ, Howanitz PJ. Physician satisfaction and emergency department laboratory test turnaround time. *Arch Pathol Lab Med.* 2001;125:863-871.

267. Dale JC, Howanitz PJ. *Physician Satisfaction with Phlebotomy Service.* Q-Probes Study Data Analysis and Critique. Northfield, Ill: College of American Pathologists; 1995.

268. Valenstein PN. *Patient Satisfaction with Outpatient Specimen Collection.* Q-Tracks (QT7) Annual Summary. Northfield, Ill: College of American Pathologists; 2004.

269. Jones BA, Ruby SG. *Hospital Nursing Satisfaction with Clinical Laboratory Services.* Q-Probes (QP041) Data Analysis and Critique. Northfield, Ill: College of American Pathologists; 2004.

270. For example, turnaround time expectations of providers are more tightly correlated with current service levels than with the severity of patient illness. Patients in smaller hospitals tend to have lower Medicare case mix indexes (less resource-intensive disease). Yet test turnaround time in smaller hospitals tends to be faster than turnaround time in larger institutions, and physicians who practice in smaller hospitals have the most stringent turnaround time expectations.

271. Wachter RM, Shojania KG. *Internal Bleeding.* New York: Rugged Land LLC; 2004.

272. See Kaplan H, Barach P. Incident reporting: science or protoscience? Ten years later. *Qual Saf Health Care.* 2002;11:144-145; Kaplan H, Fastman B. Organization of event reporting data for sense making and system improvement. *Qual Saf Health Care.* 2003;12:68-72; and Barach P, Smal S. Reporting and preventing medical mishaps: lessons from non-medical near miss reporting systems. *BMJ.* 2000;320:759-763.

273. CAP LAP checklist item GEN.13806.

274. The accounting profession has thoughtfully considered the strengths and limitations of internal control systems. Some of the limitations of a quality management plan we describe are drawn from COSO's publication, *Internal Control - Integrated Framework* (reference 25).

275. CLIA assigns the laboratory director in the United States has statutory responsibility for overseeing the quality of laboratory operations. The CAP Laboratory Accreditation Program also requires that the laboratory director approve the quality plan (CAP LAP checklist item GEN.13806).

276. The contents of the quality management plan recommended in this manual conform generally to the requirements of ISO standard 15189. However, the plans in this manual are designed primarily to meet United States regulatory requirements and not ISO requirements.

277. CAP LAP checklist item GEN.19602.

278. See Womack JP, Jones DT. *Lean Thinking.* New York: Free Press; 2003 (lean production terminology); JCAHO web site, www.jcaho.org (sentinel event and some patient safety terminology); Nakhleh RE, Fitzgibbons PL, eds. *Quality Management in Anatomic Pathology: Promoting Patient Safety Through Systems Improvement and Error Reduction.* Northfield, Ill: College of American Pathologists; 2005 (quality assurance terminology); the Institute of Medicine web site, www.iom.edu (patient safety terminology); Centers for Medicare and Medicaid Services. *Survey Procedures and Interpretive Guidelines for Laboratories and Laboratory Services.* US Government Printing Office; 2004 (CLIA and related regulatory terminology); Centers for Medicare and Medicaid Services (HIPAA and related regulatory terminology); NCCLS documents HIS-A (vol. 22, no. 13), GP26-A3 (vol. 24, no. 3), and GP22-A2 (vol. 24, no. 35) (Clinical and Laboratory Standards Institute [CLSI, formerly NCCLS] quality standards and terminology); ISO 9001: 2001 (quality and quality management terminology). Some of the definitions in the glossary have been taken verbatim from the aforementioned sources, while others have been modified based on the authors' personal experience or to reconcile conflicting definitions provided by different sources.

Index

*Page numbers with *e* indicate exhibits; page numbers with *f* indicate figures.

Clinical Laboratory Improvement Amendments
(CLIA) (1988), 49, 202
    on accurate order communication, 70
    certificate for provider-performed
        microscopy (PPM) procedures, 202
    certificate of accreditation, 202
    certificate of compliance, 56, 57, 202
    certificate of registration, 56, 203
    certificate of waiver, 56, 203
    external proficiency testing and, 97
    on incident management systems, 162
    on laboratory types, 52
    on personnel competency, 126-128
    on procedures for correcting reporting errors,
        120, 121
    quality control and, 94-95
    quality standards and, 51
    required report elements, 105-106, 105*e*
    requirements for establishing reference
        ranges, 100
    responsibilities of clinical consultant under,
        151*e*
    responsibilities of laboratory director under,
        53*e*
    responsibilities of technical consultant under,
        151*e*
    risk assessment and, 169
    on specimen collection and handling, 73
CLIA-exempt laboratory, 203
Clinically reportable range (CRR), 90-91, 203
Clinical materials, retention of, 132-133
Clinical pathology
    identification errors in, 66-67
    retention of records and clinical materials in,
        133
    turnaround time of selected procedures in,
        148*e*, 149*e*, 150*e*
Close call, 203
Clostridium difficile toxin testing, 84
COLA, 57
Collection devices, interactions of test systems
    with, 99
College of American Pathologists (CAP), 1, 34
    anonymous reporting system, 129, 163
    awareness of compliance problem, 58
    customer surveys and, 155
    development of incident reporting system by,
        163
    Laboratory Accreditation Program (LAP),
        55, 59-60, 202
        checklists, 169
        external inspection process, 129
        inspection checklists, 106

Laboratory General Checklist, 134
    patient safety goals of, 63*e*
    on quality management plans, 167
    requirements for reports, 105
    risk assessment and, 169
National Laboratory Patient Safety Goals,
    63, 63*e*, 106, 110
proficiency testing (PT) program, 55-56,
    59-60
regulatory context of programs, 59-60
Committee of Sponsoring Organizations of the
Treadway Commission (COSO), 32
    appraisal of framework, 33-34
    history of, 32
    key points, 32
Common-cause variation, 18, 146, 203
Communication. *See also* Order communication
    case history of failure in, 12-14
    clear formatting of information in reports,
        107
    in COSO, 33
    follow-up, in incident reporting, 164
    in quality management plans, 170, 186
    quality of, 114
Competence, 203
Competency, 203
    assessing, in laboratory personnel, 126-128,
        126*e*, 127*e*
Complaints
    management system for, 162
    monitoring, 170
Complete blood count specimens, reasons for
    rejected, 74*e*
Complexity
    of laboratories, 52
    of tests, 51-52
Compliance, CLIA certificate of, 56, 57, 202
Compliance officer, designation of, 140
Computerized physician order entry (CPOE)
    systems, 73
    turnaround time and, 150
Computers
    availability of systems, in laboratories, 136*e*
    in customization of laboratory reports, 110
    data integrity and, 138
    impact of downtime, on laboratory
        operations, 136*e*, 137-138, 137*e*
Computer software, user validation of new, 141-
142
Condition level deficiency, 203
Condition level requirements, 203
Conditions of Participation, 57
Confidentiality of information, 134-137, 203

Dell Computer Corporation, lean production methods in, 29
Delta checks in clinical chemistry and hematology, 64
Deming, W. Edwards, 18, 26-27, 28
    14 points for management of quality, 28*e*
Detectability, in FMEA, 39
Diabetics, glycohemoglobin monitoring in, 83, 84*e*
Digital signature, 204
Digoxin specimen collection, timing, 76, 77*e*, 79
Direct one-on-one conversations in assessing customer opinions, 156
Disaster recovery plan, 205
Documentation of calls on critical results, 114
Document control, principles of, 143, 143*e*
Dodge, H.F., 18
Double-checking computer orders, 72
Duplicate testing, 85, 85*e*

E

Educational interventions in changing physician behavior, 86
Electronic data interchange (EDI), 205
Electronic quality control, 95
Electronic signature, 205
Emergency department
    physicians, satisfaction with laboratory services, 158
    turnaround time of selected general laboratory tests, 148*e*
Encryption, 205
Equipment control, 205
Equivalency, 205
Error reduction, system approach to, 46-48
Errors, 205. *See also* Human error research; Identification errors
    active, 45
    of automatic action, 43-44
    of commission, 205
    correcting reporting, 119-122
    factors known to promote, 46-48
    human, 39, 43-48, 123-124
    of judgment, 44-45
    knowledge-based, 45
    laboratory, 61, 121
    latent, 45, 92, 141, 209
    of omission, 205
Established tests, ongoing quality management of, 93-99, 94*e*
Event reporting, 206
Events, 162
Examination, 206

External accuracy testing, 98
External control, 185, 206
External inspections, 55
Externally developed surveys of customers, 156
External proficiency testing, 55-56, 97-98, 206

F

Facility security plan, 206
Failure mode, 39, 206
Failure mode and effects analysis (FMEA), 38-40, 206
    appraisal of, 40
    classic, 38-39
    history of, 38
    key points, 38-39
    modern, 39
Federal regulations, 49-50
Feedback, 47
    clinical, in improving ordering of laboratory services, 86
    financial, in promoting appropriate ordering of laboratory services, 86
    on incidents, 163
    of monitoring results, 42
    risk assessment of, from laboratory customers, 169
Field testing of surveys, 157
Financial Executives International, 32
Financial feedback in promoting appropriate ordering of laboratory services, 86
Fishbone diagram, 19, 206
Five "S," 206
Flow, 206
Flow chart, 19, 20*f*
Flow diagram, 206
Focus group in assessing customers opinions, 156
Follow-up communication in addressing incidents, 164
Food and Drug Administration (FDA), 49, 206
    classification of test systems by, 51
    510(k) premarket approval process, 50
    Good Manufacturing Practices (GMP) / Quality System (QS) Regulation, 7, 49, 96
    medical device and biologics regulation by, 49-50
Food and Drug Administration (FDA), cleared or approved test system, 206
Forcing functions, 47, 206
Ford, Henry, 30
Ford Motor Company, 30
Fraud, 128-129, 207
    case history, 14-16
    controls for preventing, 128*e*

communication in, 42

concurrent, 42

extinction in, 42

history of, 40-41

ongoing, 67, 68*e*, 72, 79, 86, 86*e*

passive, 43

in promoting appropriate ordering of laboratory services, 86

in quality management plan, 170

in reducing identification errors, 67-68

Motivation of laboratory personnel, 130-131

Muda, 209

Multi-rule procedures, quality control and, 95

Multi-site operations, quality plan of, 168

N

Narrative interpretations, of test results, 118*e*

National Adverse Event Reporting Systems, 164-165

National Association of Accountants, 32

National Bureau of Standards, 35

National Cholesterol Education Project (NCEP), 81

National Committee on Clinical Laboratory Standards (NCCLS), 35, 209. *See also* Clinical and Laboratory Standards Institute (CLSI)

National Institute of Standards and Technology (NIST), 35

National Laboratory Patient Safety Goals, 63, 63*e*, 92, 106, 110

National proficiency testing (PT) program in gynecological cytology, 128

National Reference System for the Clinical Laboratory, 35-36

National Standardizing Association, 34

NCCLS. *See* Clinical and Laboratory Standards Institute (CLSI)

Near miss, 209-210

New employees, introduction of, into laboratory, 124-126, 125*e*

New tests, 88-93, 88*e*

analytic accuracy of, 89

analytic precision of, 89-90

analytic sensitivity and specificity, 91

backup plan for, 92

calculations, 91-92

reportable range, 90-91, 91*e*

Nonwaived tests, 51-52, 210

Normal ranges, 99, 210

Nurses

satisfaction with laboratory services, 160, 161*e*

turnaround time expectations of, 148

O

Occurrence, 39, 162

Occurrence management, 162-165

Ohno, Taiichi, 30

Ongoing monitoring of error rates, 67, 68*e*, 72, 79, 86, 86*e*

Ongoing quality management

of established tests, 93-99, 94*e*

of information systems, 142-143

for laboratory directors, 93

of personnel, 126-131, 126*e*, 127*e*, 128*e*, 131*e*

Open-ended surveys in assessing customers opinions, 156

Operational definition, 210

Operators, 210

Order communication, 70-73

accuracy of

during hospitalization, 71*e*

for outpatients, 72*e*

CLIA regulations on, 70

control measures to improve, 72-73

magnitude of risks, 71-72, 71*e*, 72*e*

Order mnemonics in improving order communication, 73

Organizational culture, 48

impact on error and patient safety, 48, 153-154

and quality management plan implementation, 172

Outliers, 210

Outpatients

accuracy of order communication for, 72*e*

phlebotomy in, 76-77, 77*e*

urine culture contamination in, 76*e*

Owners, of laboratory, 210

P

Panic values, 110. *See also* Critical values

Pap smears

competency testing and, 128

procedural follow-up of abnormal results, 118*e*

retention of records and clinical materials in, 132*e*

turnaround time of, 149*e*

Pareto chart. *See* Pareto diagram

Pareto diagram, 19, 20*f,* 27, 210

in managing turnaround time, 150

Password, 210

Path of workflow, 210

Toyota Production System (lean production), 29-32, 34, 216
    appraisal of, 31-32
    history of, 30
    key points, 30-31
Traceability, 216
Tracer methodology, 55
Trailing indicator, 162
Transfusion medicine
    identification errors in, 64, 66
    interinstitutional variation in staffing for, 131*e*
    monitoring vital signs in patients, 115-116, 116*e*
    retention of records and clinical materials in, 133
    turnaround time in, 150*e*
Treadway, James C., Jr., 32
Treadway Commission, 32
Treatment, confidentiality and, 139
Troponin-I assays
    case study, 6-8
    establishing reference range of, 103-104
Trueness of measurement, 216
Turnaround time, 145-150
    controls for, 150, 169
    goals of, 147-150
    measuring, 145-147, 146*f*
    median, desired by caregivers, 147*e*
    nurses' interest in, 155, 160
    of selected anatomic pathology procedures, 149*e*
    of selected general laboratory tests, 148*e*
    of selected microbiology procedures, 149*e*
    in transfusion medicine, 150*e*

U

Uncertainty of measurement, 216
Unfractionated heparin, monitoring patients receiving, 81*e*
Unique user identification, 216
Unsatisfactory proficiency testing performance, 216
Unsuccessful proficiency testing performance, 217
Urine culture contamination
    in outpatients, 76*e*
    rates of, 75-76
Usability testing, 45-46
User-based access, 217

V

Validation, 217
    of computer systems, 141-142, 142*e*
    of new tests, 88-93
Values, 217
    critical, 111, 112*e*, 114, 204
    mean, 95
    target, 215-216
Value stream, 217
Variation
    assignable-cause, 18, 19, 21, 24, 95
    causes of, 19, 21
    chance-cause, 18, 146
    common-cause, 18, 146
    special-cause, 18, 19, 21, 24, 95
    types of, 18
Visual controls, 30, 217
Vital signs, monitoring, in transfused patients, 115-116, 116*e*
Vulnerabilities, cumulative effect of, 39

W

Waived laboratories, 52, 55, 56
Waived tests, 51, 52, 217
Web-based procedure manuals, 145
Western Electric Company, 17-18
Workflow, path of, and patient safety, 37
Workflow diagram, 217
Written competency plans, institutional adherence to, 127
Wrong-site surgeries, 51, 165
Wrong-site/wrong-patient procedures, resulting from laboratory operations, 165

X

X-bar control chart, 21
    for continuous variables, 22*e*
    in monitoring turnaround time, 147

From the CAP Press ...

An Essential Resource for the Clinical Laboratory

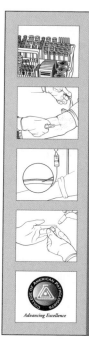

**So You're Going
to Collect a
Blood Specimen**

An Introduction
to Phlebotomy

Eleventh Edition

FOR 30 YEARS, *So You're Going to Collect a Blood Specimen: An Introduction to Phlebotomy* has served as a basic text and functional reference guide for phlebotomy. In this latest edition, emphasis is placed on safety considerations for phlebotomists, other health care professionals, and patients. The text is well illustrated, providing step-by-step instruction for obtaining blood. Following the procedures outlined in this manual will minimize patient discomfort, assure specimen integrity, and, insofar as is currently possible, provide protection against potential hazards of infectious disease. Incorporated in the text are the latest standards and regulations from CLSI, OSHA, HIPAA, the CDC, and the CAP. Also included is a comprehensive, up-to-date, recommended order of draw for multiple specimen collection.

Contents Include:

- How Blood Is Collected
- Identification and Labeling of the Blood Specimen Tube
- Common Blood Collection Tubes
- Order of Draw for Multiple Specimens
- Timed Specimens
- The Venipuncture from an Arm Vein
- Difficult Venipunctures
- Skin Punctures
- Blood Cultures
- Obtaining Blood from Babies
- Collecting Blood Specimens in Special Patient Care Areas
- Drawing Blood from Existing Intravascular Devices
- Standard Precautions and Disposal of Used Materials

EDITOR *Frederick L. Kiechle, MD, PhD, FCAP,* is the Chairman of the Department of Clinical Pathology at William Beaumont Hospital and the Medical Director for the Beaumont Reference Laboratory in Royal Oak, Michigan. Dr. Kiechle formerly was the chair of the College of American Pathologists Patient Preparation and Specimen Handling Editorial Board. He has been the editor of *So You're Going to Collect a Blood Specimen* since 1994.

So You're Going to Collect a Blood Specimen: An Introduction to Phlebotomy, 11th edition
Softcover; 72 Pages; 30 Illustrations and Tables; 2005
ISBN: 0930304845
Price: $25.00; CAP Members: $15.00
Quantity Discounts Available
Item Number: PUB212

To Purchase CAP Publications ...
Call the College of American Pathologists at 1-800-323-4040, option 1#.

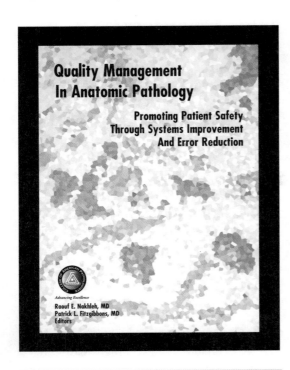